Nursing Management and Leadership in Action

Nursing Management and Leadership in Action

LAURA MAE DOUGLASS, R.N., B.A., M.S., Ph.D.

Director, R.N. Refresher Program, The Good Samaritan Hospital
of Santa Clara Valley, San Jose, California; formerly Chairman,
Division of Nursing, Point Loma College, San Diego, California;
Professor and Curriculum Coordinator, San Jose State University,
San Jose, California, and President of California Board of
Registered Nursing

EM OLIVIA BEVIS, R.N., B.S., M.A., F.A.A.N.

Professor and Head, Department of Nursing,
Georgia Southern College, Statesboro, Georgia

FOURTH EDITION

with **46** illustrations

The C. V. Mosby Company

ST. LOUIS · TORONTO · LONDON   1983

MOSBY

A TRADITION OF PUBLISHING EXCELLENCE

Senior editor: Chester L. Dow
Assistant editor: Sally Gaines
Manuscript editor: Nelle Garrecht
Book design: Jeanne Bush
Cover design: Diane Beasley
Production: Mary Stueck

FOURTH EDITION

The C.V. Mosby Company
11830 Westline Industrial Drive, St. Louis, Missouri 63141

Library of Congress Cataloging in Publication Data

Douglass, Laura Mae.
  Nursing management and leadership in action.

  Includes bibliographies and index.
    1. Nursing service administration. 2. Leader-
ship. I. Bevis, Em Olivia. II. Title. [DNLM:
1. Leadership. 2. Nursing. WY 105 D737t]
RT89.D67 1983   362.1'73068   82-8024
ISBN 0-8016-1450-3   AACR2

VT/VH/VH 9 8 7 6 5 4 3 2 1   03/D/326

To
My colleagues and nursing staff
at The Good Samaritan Hospital of Santa Clara Valley
whose contribution to my professional development
can never be fully recognized.
LMD

To
Ada Fort and Lois Wilder
for their continuing affection and encouragement.
EOB

Preface

Many things have happened to nursing in the years since this book was first published in 1970 under the title *Team Leadership in Action*. Rapid changes are sweeping all the health-related disciplines. Nursing is attempting to devise care delivery systems that will better meet the needs of health consumers and provide continuity, comprehension, and quality. New practice modes are marked by autonomy, authority, and accountability. Nurses practice some form of collaborative care in most areas of the country, and more and more agencies and individuals are structuring delivery systems that will provide the client with better services and the nurse with greater challenge and satisfaction. Consequently, this book has enlarged its focus from leadership to the broader spectrum of leadership and management in nursing. Principles of leadership and management apply regardless of the specific nursing care delivery system in use at a given agency.

Education of nurses has traditionally emphasized the study of knowledge and skills of patient care and assumed that the graduate could function in management and leadership roles with minimal preparation. This preparation was expected to be provided by the employer, who in turn anticipated that the graduate would be able to function in a leadership capacity from the first day of employment with only brief orientation to agency routine and policy. Lack of sufficient leadership preparation has resulted in the nurse's frustration and disenchantment with leadership activities and in disillusionment for the employer whose expectations have not been met. Most nurses are promoted through the bureaucratic hierarchy to lower, middle, and higher management positions on the basis of nursing care skills rather than administrative and managerial knowledge and ability. Efforts to remedy this situation are being exerted by individuals, schools of nursing, professional organizations, and employing institutions. This book is designed to assist in this effort.

One goal of nursing education is to teach the use of foresight. Anticipating the result of behaviors and the effective use of self requires the ability to predict outcomes and therefore to behave in a way that will produce the desired results. This text attempts to meet this educational goal by offering administra-

tive principles that will enable the nurse-leader to mobilize appropriate resources for the benefit of those who need health care.

Several new dimensions have been added to this book. In addition to
updating predictive principles in accordance with current theory and practice,
we have provided many illustrations that apply principles to nursing practice.
Figures and tables have been added to each chapter, along with guidelines for
functioning in the varied managerial roles. New content has been added to some
chapters and two new chapters have been created.

In Chapter 1, a conceptual framework for the book presents the basic
hypothesis on which the remaining content is based: *Formulation and use of
predictive principles promote a cognitive habit that enables the nurse who uses
them to become an effective leader and manager, able to cope with the complexities of day-to-day nursing activities.* A predictive principle is defined as a set
of cause-and-effect relationships that can be used to predict consequences of
nurse decision making.

Chapter 2 defines management, organizational structure, and strategies
necessary for effective management. An additional focus for this edition is the
role preparation of nurse-managers for high-level positions. A practical tool is
offered in the section on budget. This tool shows how to keep budgets current
through the use of logs. A section containing the topics of contractual agreements for jobs, resolution of conflict, and striking nurses has been added to aid
the nursing leader to cope with these increasingly common work-stressors.

Chapter 3 is new and contains material devoted to the staffing process,
its philosophy, standards, job satisfactions, dissatisfactions, and guidance in developing staffing patterns. Examples are given of how various staffing methods
are used by hospitals throughout the country to attract and retain qualified personnel. The nurse is also guided through the process of scheduling hours for a
nursing work force.

Chapter 4 focuses on the teaching-learning process. Emphasis is given to
formulation and use of objectives and to motivation and reinforcement of nursing staff. Legal aspects of client teaching have been added, along with new material on conducting orientation and preceptor training programs which are useful
in retention of personnel and in promotion of job satisfaction.

Chapter 5 addresses individual and group communication strategies
useful to leaders and managers. Several communication models are presented to
give the nurse an eclectic approach. New material concerning the informal
communications system and its use has been added.

Chapter 6 is designed to help the nurse delegate responsibility compe-
tently and with assurance, and to measure results of delegated activities. The
nurse is introduced to the process of delegation, given a description of educational preparation of nurses in the work force, led through a discussion of
various systems used to provide nursing care, including their advantages and

disadvantages, and provided with examples and explanations of how to assign workloads and tasks to nursing members using the various care-giving systems.

Chapter 7 has a change of focus in that the content is confined to evaluation of nursing personnel. Legal responsibilities of evaluation are discussed, examples of job descriptions of head nurses and team leaders are given to illustrate how they relate to the evaluation process, sample criteria for evaluation of nursing personnel are included, and tools and samples used for collecting and processing data are provided. A detailed section on the performance review session between nurse and supervisor is presented. Specific guidelines for preparing, conducting, and following up performance review sessions are added. An example of a coaching program is included.

Chapter 8 presents the basic ground rules for change, conditions necessary to changing, basic organizational patterns for changing, and planning strategies to effect the process of change.

Chapter 9, as rewritten, now explains more fully the meaning of authority, power, and influence; and personality, behavioral, and situational factors that influence leadership are explored. The nurse is provided with predictive principles, theory, and tools for selection of a leadership style that best suits her, the follower, and the work situation. The section on self-awareness has been retained, along with the inclusion of a means for translating individual needs into an objective approach to leadership.

Chapter 10 attacks the all-too-common problem of nurse attrition and its prevention and cure. Burnout, dropout, and runaway, common consequences of workplace problems, are examined.

No attempt has been made to cover the entire field of the subjects implied by the chapter headings. We have carefully selected materials that we consider to be most useful to nurses. The book continues to be designed for use by students, staff nurses, supervisory staff, independent nurse practitioners, and teachers.

For convenience the feminine pronoun has been used throughout this book to refer to nursing personnel. We are aware of the many men who are also active and successful in this field and intend to include them notwithstanding the traditional choice of pronoun.

We are especially grateful to Julian for the many evenings and weekends he devoted to editorial work for this book. As a result of his contribution, we believe the content to be more succinct and easily read. We are grateful as well to family, friends, and colleagues who gave their understanding, support, and time so this book could be written. We take this opportunity to thank our students, whose need inspired the book and whose studies helped us grow, and to thank the nursing staff of the hospitals in which supervision and nursing are practiced.

Laura Mae Douglass
Em Olivia Bevis

Contents

4 Predictive principles of teaching and learning, 117

5 Predictive principles of effective communication: interpersonal and group, 169

6 Predictive principles for delegation of assignments and authority, 234

7 Predictive principles for evaluation of nursing personnel, 273

8 Predictive principles for changing, 312

chapter one

Conceptual framework
for the nurse-manager
and leader

All nurses today function as leaders and managers. Health agencies in every setting and of every type expect nurses to be leaders of patients, nursing teams, and health teams, as well as being involved in community groups. Nurses are also managers of environments, budgets, time, and equipment.

Leadership and management are learned behavior patterns. To function effectively the nurse must acquire fundamental principles that make management and leadership learned processes rather than a series of duties described and listed in a policy manual. Principles of effective management and leadership and their use can be learned by both the student and the experienced nurse. Every nurse's knowledge, skill, and experience can be organized so that the quality of management and leadership ability is improved. The development of management and leadership ability may be achieved through the following:

1. Formulating principles of management and leadership based on a sound body of knowledge (input)
2. Utilizing these principles systematically to solve problems (operation)
3. Obtaining evaluative information (feedback)

Learning principles of management and leadership through the traditional cognitive methods is insufficient. The terms "management" and "leadership" imply behaviors; they imply interaction with people. The term "manager" implies systematic operations. Therefore the knowledge and skills of management and leadership must be acquired where people work together, where behaviors and operations can be practiced.

This chapter establishes a conceptual framework from which the remainder of the book derives its form and structure. Basically the authors and readers must be able to meet on conceptual and theoretical common ground. John Stuart Mills' admonition, "... above all, to insist upon having the meaning of a word clearly understood before using it, and the meaning of a proposition before assenting to it,"* clearly bespeaks the obvious need to set about a simple but scholarly task. That task is one of coming to grips with key concepts and hypotheses (meanings and propositions) prior to elaborating ideas that are both consequences of and subsequent to theoretical or conceptual constructs. Meanings and propositions will be provided for management and leadership; for the nature of roles and role assumptions; for theories generally, with particular emphasis on predictive theories or predictive principles; and for problem solving and decision making.

Defining leadership and management

June Bailey and her associates at the University of California, San Francisco, define leadership as follows:

Within the conceptual framework of the Power/Authority/Influence Model, we define leadership as a set of *actions* that influence members of a group to move toward goal setting and goal attainment. Inherent in the *actions* are situational variables; personal, organizational, and social power bases; formal and functional bases of authority; and accountability. Other elements in the spectrum of leadership actions are sound managerial and human relations and the use of influence strategies that will promote a willingness to follow so that individual and organizational goals can be achieved. Thus, leadership is viewed as multidimensional, encompassing the wise use of power, managerial functions, and human relations processes.†

Leadership can be defined by the behaviors manifested by leaders, by characteristics, or by role enactment. Leadership that is defined only by leadership behavior becomes nonfunctional; in other words, behavior alone cannot be operationalized. If leadership is a learned behavior and therefore can be taught, then it follows that leadership must be defined in some way that makes it feasible to operationalize the definition. For this reason, Dr. Bailey's definition is a highly valuable one. Fig. 1-1 is a model of the interactive flow of the components of leadership as defined. Note that the set of actions (processes), the organizational structure (human relationships), and the task (goal setting-goal attainment functions) are all placed within the context of the characteristics and values of the leader and the led, and all the foregoing are placed within the larger context of the external environment.

Management is the manipulation of people, environments, equipment, budgets, and time. It involves many of the same skills as leadership but has a wider range of function, a wider variety of roles, and a more legitimate source of

---

*From Mills' inaugural address as Rector, University of St. Andrews, February 1, 1867.
†From Claus, K.E., and Bailey, J.T.: Power and influence in health care: a new approach to leadership, St. Louis, 1977, The C.V. Mosby Co.

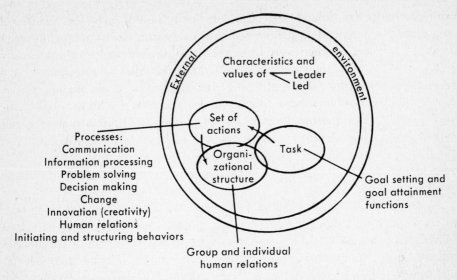

Fig. 1-1. Model of the interactive flow of the components of leadership.

power and authority. In any organization or agency management involves the following:

1. Planning and providing professional services within the mission and goals of the agency
2. Providing the continuity of those services
3. Providing for the quality control of those services
4. Managing the budgets and business and financial arrangements that make the services possible
5. Safeguarding the legality of the services
6. Coordinating the environmental services such as equipment, housekeeping, maintenance, and parking
7. Ensuring that support materials, supplies, and services are available
8. Providing for the improvement of the quality of services through educational programs, library, and dissemination of information

In addition, management is directly involved in the logistics of nursing care. This means (1) purchasing supplies and materials; (2) transporting these supplies and materials to the areas where they are needed; (3) maintaining storerooms (central supply rooms—CSRs) and supply depots where adequate materials and equipment are on hand; and (4) coordinating dietary, housekeeping, laboratory, and medical services so that nursing services dovetail with them.

Good managers are better if they are also good leaders; however, good leaders may or may not have the knowledge and skills to be managers. Many of the processes that leaders and managers use are the same. However, most of the functions that managers carry out are not ordinarily functions of the nurse-leader. Traditionally, nursing leadership has been the term used for lower level management—team leaders, primary caregivers, assistant head nurses, and staff nurses. Middle management—head nurses and supervisors—have generally been referred to as supervisory personnel, and their roles and functions have been differentiated from those of lower management or nurse-leaders. Upper level management—directors of nursing service and their assistants—have usually been referred to as administrators, and their roles and functions are covered in books on nursing administration. In essence, all managers, regardless of their level or functioning, utilize similar processes. This book concentrates on the common elements of all managerial levels and focuses on middle and lower level management.

Leadership can be assumed. In some groups, it tends to shift from person to person, depending on such relative factors as the area of expertise needed, the energy level of the participants, and the charisma of the people involved. Leadership can be an opportunity of the moment, a dynamic thing that shifts from one person to another as the situation and circumstances demand. Management, on the other hand, is a legitimately designated position. Managers obtain their authority from two sources: supervisors and subordinates. Managers are sometimes elected by the people they lead; they are always confirmed in their position by those who employ them and pay their salaries. Sometimes managers are not elected but are imposed from above. This does not relieve the managers of the constant necessity to validate their power base with those they manage. Managers not cognizant of the two sources from which their power is derived will fail to meet the objectives of one group and will therefore jeopardize the whole enterprise or their own positions in the organization.

For convenience, the components of leadership and management behaviors have been grouped and dealt with in this book in a variety of ways in appropriate places. Roles, theory levels, predictive principle formulation, conceptual framework, problem solving, and decision making are covered in this chapter.

Management principles are covered in Chapter 2; Chapter 3 deals with the various ways to cope with staffing patterns; Chapter 4 discusses the teaching of individuals and groups; communications and group dynamics are covered in Chapter 5; delegating authority and evaluating personnel are discussed in Chapters 6 and 7; organizing for and facilitating change and principles of leadership behaviors are examined in Chapters 8 and 9; Chapter 10 deals with the difficult problem of nurse attrition. These ten topics examine the principles and processes necessary to the middle and lower management nurse. The topics, though separated in the book, in reality are interrelated and mutually supportive for they are, in fact, normal, practical life processes people use in everyday life. *Management and leadership involve the ability to use the processes of life to facilitate the movement of a person, a group, a family, or a community toward the establishment and attainment of a goal. Nursing management and leadership in-*

volve the ability to use the processes of life to facilitate the movement of a person, a group, a family, or a community toward the establishment and attainment of goals pertaining to health. This includes the manipulation of all factors related to goal attainment.

Process—a theory about the nature of things

Inevitably, words must be used to define other words, and in the definitions of both management and leadership the words "process" and "processing" are used. The word "process" has become popular in education and in nursing during the last twenty years. People refer to *process* teaching, *processing* information, the *process* of problem solving, nursing *process*, and so on. One has but to connect the various ways the word is used and examine the context of its use to observe that the common denominator of meaning is flow or, as Alfred North Whitehead labels it, flux.* Process is change toward an objective using feedback. Change—flow, flux, dynamics—is in the nature of all things. Some things flow more rapidly than others; the flow of time, measured by the rising and setting of the sun, is more rapid than the flow or change of granite. But even granite, that symbol of permanence, decomposes and crumbles; thus it becomes part of the flux of nature.

Each change, each product of flux, is new and unique from its antecedents; therefore flux is the creative thrust of life. This creativity—uniqueness—comes about from the interaction and mutually inclusive nature of processes. The result of interaction is that each process does indeed affect the "new" product. Take, for instance, the processes included in the definitions of leadership and management. The process of relating to other humans includes elements of the process of communicating (see Fig. 1-2). One cannot communicate without processing information; for example, "to relate to" means (1) to perceive; (2) to validate, classify, sort, and interpret the perceptions (which is one way to process data); (3) to solve problems by thinking of alternative responses to the perceived messages; (4) to weigh the consequences of each possible response; and (5) to choose a response and respond to the other human being. Thus in a single encounter in reacting to another human being, the processes of communication, information processing, problem solving, and decision making have all been used to initiate and structure one unique, new, transient act or behavior. Fig. 1-2 depicts how single processes interact, intertwine, and combine to produce a single new episode—a unique act or behavior. *A process has purpose, organization, and outcome. The purpose is the goal; the organization is the way in which many components or other processes unite to produce the unique outcome. The whole of the three components flows inexorably into the next life episode.*

---

*Whitehead, A.N.: Process and reality, New York, 1929, Macmillan Publishing Co., Inc.

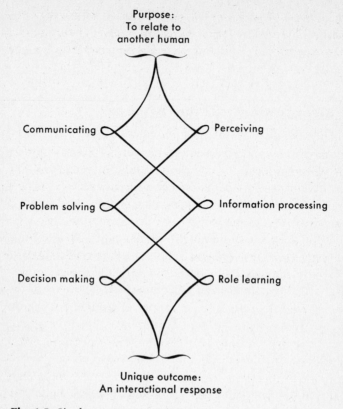

Fig. 1-2. Single processes combining to make a new process.

One of the most common examples used to illustrate the nature of processes is the phenomenon of human reproduction. The purpose of reproduction is to continue the species. Each reproductive episode or successful birth produces a new, unique human being; yet siblings are created from the same antecedents or ancestors. The antecedents or ancestors combine in uniquely organized ways and provide endless genetic combinations to produce an infinite number of possible products, or children—each child different from his or her sibling.

This concept of flux and flow and the unstoppable nature of this flow are beautifully expressed in the *Rubaiyat* of Omar Khayyám. The entire work is an expression of the flux of life. Captured in these few lines is part of that expression:

> The Moving Finger writes; and, having writ,
> Moves on: nor all your Piety nor Wit
>   Shall lure it back to cancel half a Line,
> Nor all your Tears wash out a Word of it.

To summarize, a process is a phenomenon of life that has purpose, organization, and innovative outcome and each innovative outcome is a result of many unique factors combining in an organized and preestablished pattern. All managers use process. They combine many factors in ways that produce desired results.

Learning leadership and management roles

Leadership and management roles, like other roles, comprise an organized set of behaviors assigned to or assumed by a person. The role of leader can be assumed, but the role of manager is always assigned. The management position can be attained by job description, but the role of leader is often attained by the power that knowledge and skill generate, by assumption of the role, or by investment of power by others. The leadership role is interactional in nature and cannot be learned or enacted out of the social context of complementary roles. In other words every leader, to be a leader, must have someone, some group, to lead. The role of being led is the role that complements the role of leader. A leader must learn not only the leadership behaviors that enable the assumption of the leadership role, but also the role of the led. Only through learning the complementary role can a leader know and enact the leadership role appropriately.

A role is learned using an entire role set, which includes the role of *leader or manager,* the *complementary* role, and the *audience* (interested others). The complementary role of the led creates the expectation of leadership behavior. Every patient who is led by a nurse has certain behavioral expectations for the nurse, which are communicated in overt and covert ways. The patient may communicate the expectation that the nurse will act as information giver, disciplinarian, nurturer or mother figure, authority person, teacher, decision maker, or advocate or will display any number of other behaviors or functions. Understanding the complementary role of those led increases the nurse's ability to perform that role.

The audience, or interested others, performs vital functions, even though this group is neither the leader nor the led. The audience may be families, supervisors, administrators, patients, or colleagues, depending on who plays the complementary role of the led. For instance, if the patient is in the complementary role of the led, then families, supervisors, administrators, and colleagues will be the audience. The audience performs the following functions: (1) creates the social reality of the role; (2) gives cues for leadership behaviors, expectations, and role enactment; (3) provides social reinforcement through praise, approval, participation, and rewards; and (4) contributes to the maintenance of the leadership in behavior.

Roles can be either ascribed or achieved. *Ascribed* roles are the roles people are born to or are granted through socialization. The roles of son, daughter, or child are examples of ascribed roles attained through the process of socialization. *Achieved* roles, on the other hand, are roles one aspires to or earns. The role of nurse, for example, is an achieved role. One sets out to learn the nurse role; similarly, one sets out to learn the leader role. Achieved roles are more complex than ascribed roles in that they are superimposed on the ascribed. Women nurses bring to the role of nurse-leader the characteristics and behaviors of the ascribed roles of women in this society—mother, daughter, sister. For men nurses there is a similar superimposition of achieved role of nurse-leader on the ascribed roles of men—father, brother, son.

One of the obvious problems of learning a professional role such as nursing is that role preconceptions of anticipatory socialization are simpler and more stereotyped than the role's reality. The person aspiring to the nurse's role may envision a Sue Barton or a Cherry Ames, both highly stereotyped misconceptions of reality. Therefore a conflict arises because preconceived role expectations do not conform to the complex reality of the role as it must be enacted. Further complications arise when previous learning of ascribed roles conflicts with the learning needs of the achieved roles.

This pyramiding of roles (see Fig. 1-3) produces highly complex identity and behavioral learning situations. A clear picture of the various roles being played in one life episode enables the player to establish role priorities or role combinations compatible with role expectations of the audience and complementary role players.

According to theorists, roles must be learned as a whole, total, organized pattern—including both the cognitive and behavioral components. Learning bits and pieces of a role can occur as separate learning episodes, but the success of role enactment depends on the learner's ability to integrate the total set. In other words, learning bits and pieces must be followed by learning the interrelationship of these bits and pieces and insights and behaviors with the total field, or

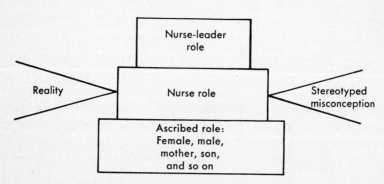

Fig. 1-3. Nurse roles in relation to reality and stereotyped misconception.

pattern. The implication for learning leadership and management roles is that this learning must occur in a manner that facilitates interaction, either real or simulated, with all characters: leader, led, and audience. Learning each of these roles independently of the others will not result in the ability to enact the leadership role successfully. Practice, with coaching, in situations in which occur all elements of the leadership set of behaviors is necessary for the leadership role to be achieved.

Defining roles*

The concept of roles in nursing has been defined in a variety of ways but has usually focused on describing the actions nurses perform. As the nurse's responsibilities have changed and expanded, so have the activities, so that descriptive definitions no longer serve the purpose of facilitating role enactment or of making role change. A brief discussion of definitions of role will demonstrate the differences and will highlight the implications the definition has for the nurse's ability to function in a role or to make role change.

Normative definitions. Defining roles using normative criteria means roles are viewed as fixed and standardized. Rules or expectations for behavior associated with a given position or office govern the individual's way of functioning. Cultural norms, the result of values and attitudes ascribed by society, act as a guide for the conduct of the occupant of the role. These same values and attitudes assign roles a status; the rights and privileges that constitute the status of the role must be assumed by the occupant of the role if an overt expression of the rule is to fit the expected norm.

Defining the nurse's role using normative criteria means the nurse's performance is determined by prescribed societal expectations and attitudes. The nurse who deviates from this view may find it difficult to enact the role. For example, men are readily accepted in the role of physician but are sometimes labeled "gay" or "queer" in the nurse's role. Assertive women nurses are often labeled "castrating"; nurses with organizational skills are seen as cold and impersonal; and nurses who cry are viewed as "out of control." In each of the examples, the behaviors labeled were not part of the cultural norm for the nurse role. Labeling is used in an attempt to explain deviant behavior. In time and with change in societal attitude and expectations, these behaviors may be accepted as the norm.

Role congruency, the compatibility of one role with another, is more likely to occur when role definitions are normative. The "role taker" simply follows the prescribed and predetermined set of expectations. He accepts the

*This section is from Bower, F.L.: Nursing process roles and functions of the nurse. In Bower, F.L., and Bevis, E.O.: Fundamentals of nursing: concepts, roles and functions, St. Louis, 1979, The C.V. Mosby Co., pp. 178-181.

expected role behaviors and the rights and privileges that accompany the role and performs accordingly. The role taker knows what to do, and the reciprocal role enactors get what they expect. There are no role conflicts, discrepancies, or role strains. Of course, role change is difficult. In fact, role change depends on the redefinition of the role by *others*.

Perhaps one of the reasons role change for the nurse has been so difficult is that most people have viewed the nurse role from a normative stance.

Situational definitions. Another way to define role is to use situational criteria. A situational definition of role refers to the pattern or type of social behavior that is appropriate in terms of the demands and expectations of the situation in which the role is enacted. Like normative definitions, situational definitions are based on norms, but in this case the norms are set in relationship to the particular set of circumstances of the situation. Defining the nurse's role using situational criteria means the nurse's performance is prescribed and performed in light of its fit with the situation. The nurse in the hospital setting may act quite differently with the client and his family than when in the client's home. In the hospital the nurse is "at home" and has many resources, whereas in the home the nurse is the "visitor" with a very different set of resources.

Acute situations demand role behavior different from that of nonacute ones. In acute situations the nurse's performance may be very different from that when there is time to seek the help of others. For instance, in situations where childbirth is imminent the nurse delivers the baby. If time allowed, that same mother-to-be would be referred to a physician.

Role congruency with situational definitions is variable. Since all those involved in the situation take their cues from "what is happening," conflict could occur if two people responded to the same "cue." Conversely, the situation could define exactly who is to do what. For example, a cardiac arrest in a coronary care unit precipitates actions by nurses and physicians in very definite ways.

Role change with situational definitions is easy. Since the situation defines the performance, the players act in a variety of ways. There are no set norms or prescribed performance expectations—no limits on what the players are sanctioned to do. Unfortunately, this means many persons can decide to perform the same act. The nurse practitioner's role can be defined situationally, since the nurse practitioner and the physician may perform the same act, depending on the situation.

Functional definition. Using a functional perspective to define roles means roles are defined by what players do. Roles are not defined by norms or situations but by how an individual performs when given a particular function to accomplish. Role is the manner in which a person actually functions. Role is influenced by factors other than the stipulation of the office. Role performance has important consequences for the functioning of the group in which the role is performed and important personal consequences for the individual who performs it. Unlike the other definitions, which define role in terms of demands and expectations, functional definitions of role are concerned only with what functions the role player performs. For instance, a coordinator coordinates, teachers teach, and planners plan.

Nurses' roles are often defined in functional terms. Such labels as facilitator, leader, change agent, listener, validator, assessor, data gatherer, and evaluator are used to describe the many nursing roles nurses play. Most recently, nurses have assumed the role of consumer advocate. If nurses' roles were to be defined functionally, the list would be long and encompassing.

In a traditional sense, congruency is difficult with functional definitions, since distinct differences in roles are lacking. Roles overlap as people acting in different positions play the same role. Congruency does occur if there is agreement among the role players that there are no distinct standardized rules to follow or limits on what they can do. A role diffusion results, with functions being enacted by the one who accepts the responsibility, regardless of position or status.

This molding of roles across positions has implications for role learning. Individuals do not have rules of behavior for performance or specified expectations as models for role enactment. Role-specific behaviors are nonexistent. The role aspirant must learn the new role by learning the appropriate role behavior. Appropriate role behaviors are learned in the context of acting out what is *thought* to be appropriate rather than what *should* be done. There are trial and error attempts in role taking. Some individuals find this freedom to determine roles to be stimulating and challenging. For others, it is anxiety provoking.

Functional definitions of role tend to facilitate role change. Since there are no prescribed expectations, the individual is free to try new behaviors. The usual constraints of culturally accepted norms are not present, so the individual defines role by the behavior displayed. This means roles are shared by persons of different status groups and positions. For example, the nurse, physician, psychologist, and psychiatrist diagnose; the administrator, dietician, physical therapist, and nurse are planners; the teacher, student, lawyer, and nurse evaluate. It is possible that people in all these positions are fulfilling many of the same roles. Their differences are not delineated by what they do (functional roles) but by what position they occupy (teacher, physician, nurse, etc.).

Interactional definition. From the standpoint of an interactional definition, roles become more than a prescription for the behavior expected of a person occupying a given position. Role is conceptualized as a constellation of behaviors that emerge out of an interaction between self and others. Role identification becomes the function of how others act and not merely the behavior of self. The individual acts out the role based on the purpose or meaning assigned to the behavior as it relates to the relevant others. For example, the role of nurse may be meaningless or misinterpreted unless it is reciprocated by the role of client. Therefore the interactional concept of role permits the perception and enactment of role as reflective of the other role in the situation.

The interactional concept of role does not deny that certain patterns of behavior are perceived as appropriate for a person occupying a particular position, nor does it imply an expectation-conformity model is incorrect. It does suggest, however, that these approaches are incomplete, since they describe only one of the several bases on which interaction can proceed.

Similarly, role learning and role conflict are viewed in a somewhat different light by the interactionist. Roles are not learned as rules of behavior for performance in isolation. Roles are learned in pairs. In the process of learning a role the role taker learns the role of the relevant other. Thus the recruit in the process of learning the nurse's role is also developing some sense of the behaviors, expectations, attitudes, and desires of the client role.

Role conflict in an interactional framework consists of making compromises so that viable relationships with relevant others can be maintained. Unlike the other definitions of role, the role enacter in an interactional sense does not have to abandon one role in favor of another. The individual is able to shift, alter, and utilize different behaviors within and between role enactment so that conflict is avoided or resolved without too much difficulty.

•   •   •

Although the four definitions presented here offer different views of the concept of role, there are three basic similarities in all the definitions. Individuals assume roles (1) in social locations, (2) with reference to expectations, and (3) with behavior related to the nature of the expectations.

These four definitions of role enactment (normative, situational, functional, and interactional) are presented with the realization that the nurse performs many roles and that role enactment, role change, and role conflict depend on the frame of reference of those who work with or influence the nurse's scope of practice.

Theories—the basis of leadership and management activity*

A theory is an invention of humans. Human beings theorize to explain or speculate about what something is; what it is like or what its characteristics and attributes are; how something exists in relation to other things; what circumstances or conditions will make things behave in certain ways and what will prevent them from behaving in certain other ways; and, finally, how they can be used in life situations. In other words, a theory enables the nurse to work with

*This discussion on theory is adapted from Bevis, E.O.: Curriculum building in nursing: a process, ed. 3, St. Louis, 1982, The C.V. Mosby Co.; and derived and synthesized from the works of Dickoff, James, and Wiedenbach; Gagne; and Abdulla and Levine (see bibliography).

others in speculating about problems, to devise hypotheses about alternative solutions to those problems, and to develop ways to test those hypotheses in nursing actions.

The word "theory" can be used in many different ways. People use "theory" to separate the cognitive components from the practical or activity components of a discipline. Sometimes "theory" is used to indicate the speculative as opposed to the proved; sometimes it is used to refer to guesses or hypotheses about how simpler concepts or laws relate to one another; sometimes it is used to mean predictions about how things are going to behave; and sometimes it is used to prescribe ways to make certain behaviors occur. "Theory" has many definitions because it is a complex phenomenon, and all the definitions or meanings just listed do refer to one or more of its aspects (sometimes referred to as levels). Theories evolve through a hierarchy of serial levels. They are still theories, regardless of their level of development. An analogy to this phenomenon of theory levels can be found in Erik Erikson's theory of human development. Human development theory maintains that success in life or human maturity is attained when each central task of development is accomplished, at least in part, in its proper order. Further, full maturity is not attained until these tasks of development are minimally accomplished. In the same manner the attainment of the highest level of theories depends on the successful completion of each prior level of that theory. *Skilled leadership and management exploit a given theory or hypothesis by testing out in practice the validity of the prediction.*

The four levels or phases of theories in practice disciplines

Four stages of development are necessary for a theory to reach its full maturity and thus be optimally useful in management practice. These theory levels are (1) factor isolating, (2) factor relating, (3) situation relating, and (4) situation producing. Basically, nurse management practice relies on the third and fourth levels. The third level is *predictive* theory, and the fourth level is *prescriptive* theory. These two levels enable the nurse to formulate action hypotheses and to construct or prescribe ways in which one can create the environment or series of events that will allow the prediction (action hypothesis) to come true. However, since a theory to be workable—to have reached its full maturity and have some chance at validity—must have evolved through the prior levels of development, the nurse needs to have a working knowledge of all four levels of theories. In this way, hypotheses (or predictive principles) have a much higher validity and reliability than those formulated in the limbo of the third and fourth levels without reference to or cognizance of the prior two levels.

James Dickoff, Patricia James, and Ernestine Wiedenbach's classic article in *Nursing Research** provides the best source for a clear explanation of theory

---
*Dickoff, J., James, P., and Wiedenbach, E.: Theory in a practice discipline. Part I. Practice oriented theory, Nurs. Res. **17**(5):415-435, 1968.

levels. Presented here is a highly simplified summary of the levels of theory in practice disciplines, as presented in their article.

Level I—Factor-isolating theories. Level I has two activities: (1) naming, or labeling, and (2) classifying, or categorizing.

Naming. The function of the naming stage is to allow an idea or object to be perceived and talked about or referred to. Once something is named, it is mentionable. One must isolate identifying aspects or factors to recognize that a thing is what it is and not something else—thus the title of this level: factor-isolating theories. Names may be assigned for a variety of reasons: (1) the order of discovery (such as microbes and organisms); (2) the discoverer or inventor (such as Cushing's disease or Bowman's capsule); (3) function (such as heart-lung machine or computer); (4) similarity to other things that have previously been identified and named (such as kidney basin or kidney bean); and (5) description (such as spider-web angioma).

Classifying. The second activity in level I is classifying. Classifying is sorting, categorizing, or grouping things according to some commonality. Classifying by commonality requires that the factors or attributes of an object, idea, or thing be *isolated.* The second activity is not possible without the first, that of perceiving and naming, having occurred. Categorizing requires one to identify what something is and what it is not. Categories can be grouped just as single items can be grouped. Grouping or categorizing is possible because of some common denominator or unifying factor. Thus a hierarchy of categories is formed. (*Acute inflammatory response* is a large category that contains subcategories such as *fever* or *local edema;* cancer is classified in stages.)

Level II—Factor-relating theories. Level II also contains two activities: (1) depicting, or describing, and (2) relating factors. This level of theory building depicts or describes how one, single, named and classified thing (factor) relates to another single, named and classified thing (factor); thus the title of this level: factor-relating theories. For example, a description of the face requires communication of how the eyes sit in relation to the nose, mouth, ears, and forehead. This level of theory describes relationships to other factors. In other words, it is a "natural history" of any given subject. Any descriptive science, such as anatomy, is an example of factor-relating theory.

Level III—Situation-relating theories. Level III is concerned with causal relationships. It relates one situation to another in a way that allows for prediction. One of the essential ingredients of this level is causal-connecting statements that give a basis for prediction. Prediction is a statement of causal or consequential connections between two states of affairs or two concepts. This level of theory reveals what conditions, circumstances, or behaviors (for example, the cost in time, energy, effort, pain) will promote or inhibit the occurrence of an event or consequence. Dickoff, James, and Wiedenbach consider this level of theory building to be of "incredible importance" to practice. Predictive principles, the format for this book, are in reality third level theories. They are guides for developing realistic alternatives for nursing actions and are essential to the judgments and decisions of leadership and management. Simply stated, third level theories tell you that if "A" occurs, "B" will occur. Third level theories explain what promotes, speeds up, has a catalytic effect, slows down, inhibits, highly correlates with, or prevents something from happening. Promoting or inhibiting theories indicate under what circumstances things will occur and with what speed and effort. Examples are: "Increasing pressure over the blood vessels in the arm allows blood pressure to be determined with the aid of a sphygmomanometer"; "Use of a calm voice and manner with an anxious patient helps reduce anxiety."

Level IV—Situation-producing theories. Level IV, the final level of theory building, comprises prescriptive theories; it is the level at which theories come to maturity. This level of theory indicates how one arranges the environment and circumstances so that the desired goal is achieved. Situation-producing theories have three aspects—goal, prescription, and survey list.

Goal. The goal aspect is the simple establishment of a goal. It is the primary act of any problem-solving organism. The nurse-manager and leader is a goal-oriented person whose behavior is geared toward helping those he or she leads in goal identification and attainment.

Prescription. The prescription aspect is a diagram or road map of the specific activities and directions that, when completed, will produce the results predicted in level III (predictive theories) and achieve the desired goal. Prescriptions can be the actual directions for carrying out a plan necessary to achieve a goal. Both leaders and managers provide prescriptions. The prescriptions of leaders involve lower level work—usually at the direct client level. The prescriptions of managers involve manipulations of all factors enabling successful direct client care. For example, prescriptions for administering lipids, log-rolling a patient, or administering a medication by bolus are the culminating steps of theory building.

Survey list. The survey list contains the dimensions, knowledge, and other resources that might be helpful in structuring or completing the activity and provides the basis for judgments about alternatives in achieving the established goal. Managerial level survey lists are more extensive and far-reaching, involve many other people and departments, and include financial as well as environmental and staff considerations. Leadership level survey lists involve resources and factors directly related to client care.

Summary on theorizing

This book uses predictive theories as its format. Instructions in the construction and use of predictive theories are provided for the nurse learning leadership and management. These instructions will show how second level theories are used in constructing third level theories. Problem solving is also one of the primary conceptual constructs of this book. Subsequent discussions will show how problem solving and decision making are, in essence, fourth level theories. Problem solving produces the judgments and decisions necessary to select the series of actions that will achieve the desired result. In other words, the final act of problem solving is the selection of the series of actions or behaviors (prescriptions) that will produce the desired situation as predicted in the third level of theory building.

Predictive principles

Utilization of predictive principles in problem solving is based on a knowledge and understanding of theory levels and problem solving. Understanding the composition of a predictive principle and the actions involved in using it is to acquire a *working definition*, or a definition that can be made operational. Real understanding of a definition comes when one has acquired the ability to use the definition in suitable activities. Some activities requiring the use of the definition of a predictive principle are identifying principles either in the literature or in use, constructing specific principles using the component parts (lower level theories) appropriately, and using principles in solving problems.

The following section begins with a working definition of a predictive principle and proceeds through the use of principles in solving a problem. This is designed to guide the nurse to an increased understanding of principles and enables the practitioner to use principles in activities that require leadership.

Definition

For use in this book, *a predictive principle is defined as a set of circumstances, conditions, or behaviors that produces a given, definable outcome.* A principle expresses relationships of conditions, circumstances, or behaviors to predictable consequences. A predictive theory is a nursing action hypothesis. Predictive principles differ from facts or concepts in that a fact or concept need only be valid, whereas a predictive principle, in addition to being valid, must predict outcomes. Principles are derived from authoritative sources or through scientific observation, experimentation, or compilation of data. Predictive principles are third level theories.

The predictive relationships that exist between the circumstances, conditions, or behaviors and the predicted outcome or consequence of those circumstances, conditions, or behaviors can best be articulated by the use of an active verb or verb clause that is causal connecting in a predictive way.

Predictive relationships may also be shown in two other ways:
1. "If-then"—if this happens, then that will happen. (*If* breathing stops, *then* the O_2 supply to the brain is absent. *If* very explicit directions are given, *then* the recipient has the necessary guidelines for following.)

2. Proportions—the greater or less (fewer) this, the greater or less (fewer) that. (*The greater the* swelling of leg tissues within a cast, *the greater the* pressure of the leg on the cast. *A lesser than* justified pay scale results in a shortage of *(fewer)* nurses to meet the demand.)

Developing principles

In the development of principles three separate stages of cognitive activity are required. These three stages are also the first three levels of theory building.

1. Identifying or accumulating facts and experiences or isolating and classifying factors (level I theory)
2. Depicting and describing factors or experience commonalities and relationships (a high-order conceptualization and level II theory)
3. Relating circumstances, conditions, and behaviors (situations) to consequences (level III theory)

Facts and theories can be fairly easily and rapidly identified and acquired through processes that enable and promote recall. Experiences (mental, emotional, and physical) allow for the further acquisition or retention of facts by using learned material. Acquisition of facts could include such information as anatomy, physiology, or hospital or agency structure.

When facts begin to form a pattern and are applicable to several experiences, they become the second stage of cognitive activity, the formation of concepts. For use in this book, *a concept is a classification of experiences that have similar properties:* the recognition of common elements for the purpose of useful classification. Concepts can be communicated to others. They can be converted into words or phrases that represent the ideas, objects, characteristics, or behaviors held together in groupings by the common elements. Concepts are the way people categorize experiences so that mental filing systems have organization. Concepts grow and enlarge as the number and variety of an individual's experiences increase. As an example, a compilation of facts, experiences, and observations concerning anatomy and physiology and the individual's perception form the basis for the concept of pain. Facts related to hospital or agency structure serve as a basis for the formation of the concept of hierarchy. This activity is level II theory.

The third stage in the development of principles is relating concepts to predict outcomes. This is a complex but useful thinking process because predictive principles show the relationship between concepts. *A predictive principle shows the relationship between the concept(s) drawn from some conditions, circumstances, or behaviors and the concept(s) of the predicted outcome.* The concepts of *motivation* and *learning* will be used for illustrative purposes.

Motivation is a condition and learning is an outcome. Many discussions of the relationship motivation has to learning can be found in the literature. An observer of the learning process quickly recognizes that there is an inherent relationship between motivation and learning. The effect these two concepts have on each other can be expressed in a principle; the components are separated in example 1.

EXAMPLE 1

Conditions, circumstances, and behaviors triad	*Active verb phase*	*Predicted outcome*
Being motivated	influences	learning

This principle is simple and direct but lacks specificity and direction. The use of *qualifiers* gives principles increased usefulness. This is illustrated in the following:

EXAMPLE 2

Qualifiers	*Conditions, circumstances, and behaviors triad*	*Active verb phase*	*Qualifiers*	*Predicted outcome*
Being highly	motivated	influences	the rate of	learning

In the examples used thus far the condition has always been on the left and the predicted outcome on the right. This is not necessary to the construction of a principle. To change the order of the concepts one need only change the orientation of the active verb phase. The order of the concepts used in example 1 can be reversed as follows:

EXAMPLE 3

Predicted outcome	*Active verb phase*	*Conditions, circumstances, and behaviors triad*
The rate of learning	is influenced by	being highly motivated

The definition of a principle and the examples of principles used imply that the conditions, circumstances, and behaviors (CCB) triad with its qualifiers describes the environment, activities, knowledge, skills, or state of being necessary to make the predicted outcomes occur. The CCB triad is the concept subject matter and contains the necessary qualifying descriptions for the formation of principles. The CCB triad and its qualifiers can be positive or negative. Some words that indicate positive action are *facilitate, precipitate, aid, result in, determine, assist, influence, promote, ensure, contribute to, enhance,* and *enable.* Note that most of the action words suggested have limitations by definition. For instance, *facilitate* means to "make easy or less difficult," whereas *ensure* means to "make certain." The difference is important because the choice of the connecting action words helps to determine the validity of the principle. Some action words that indicate negative action are *inhibit, prevent, discourage, negate, invalidate, obviate, preclude, deter,* and *damage.* Active verbs, in addition to indicating the positive or negative direction of the activity, can, with qualifying phrases, indicate person. *Person* is the one who perpetrates the activity, for example, the nurse, the learner, the patient, the ancillary worker, the student, or the group. It is not essential that person be indicated but to do so promotes clarity and specificity. The following illustrates how different active verbs and persons alter the principle:

EXAMPLE 4

Conditions, circumstances, and behaviors triad	*Active verb phase and person(s)*	*Predicted outcome*
Having knowledge pertinent to to the current situation	(a) ensures that the leader makes (b) aids the group in making (c) promotes the making of (d) facilitates the making of (e) results in the group's making (f) helps the nurse-leader to make (g) enables the group to make	valid judgments and decisions

Example 4 indicates the variety of ways cause-and-effect relationships of a principle may be linked together. Choices depend on the situation under consideration.

Clarity is achieved through accurate, concise statements of principles that are positive instead of negative, are logical in their sequence, and contain connecting words and phrases that produce valid principles.

Using principles in nursing process

Nursing process, in essence, is dealing appropriately with nursing problems to bring about effective solutions. Organizing ideas and facts into predictive principles enables the nurse to have a clear, categorized fund of knowledge for immediate use in solving nursing problems. However, the acquisition of a body of knowledge in the form of practical and usable predictions is only part of the problem facing the nurse who wishes to be a proficient leader and manager. Predictive principles will have relevance only if the nurse judiciously applies them to identified problems. Predictive principles are guides for developing realistic alternatives of action. The use of predictive principles is a process that requires (1) identification of the real problem; (2) selection of the appropriate, valid, and relevant principle(s); (3) identification of alternatives for action sequential to the selected principle(s); (4) the ability to select one or more of the alternatives; and (5) the ability to prescribe the ways and means to actualize the alternative selected.

Initially this is a slow, laborious process, but through repeated application to various types of problems the process becomes a behavior habit. Habits of thinking beget habits of behavior. Habits are developed after thoughts or activities are repeated in the same pattern or way until the behaviors become customary. Habits are characterized by automatism (without deliberation). Any skill, whether intellectual or manual, involves habits. (Even bed making or preparing a medication for injection was a slow process for the nurse at first.)

The mechanics of problem solving (nursing process) using predictive principles is a habit, not a reflex. While reflexes are inborn and inherent in the nervous system, habits are learned. The answers to problems or possible alternatives of action do not materialize automatically; it is the *process* of arriving at the best possible alternatives that becomes the habit. When this process becomes habitual, the nurse faced with nursing problems will automatically use the predictive principles approach to nursing process. This means that each step in the process may lose its identity, become blurred, and not be conscious; nevertheless, the process takes place. Arriving at this degree of skill requires consistent, repeated, conscious practice.

Acquiring skill in problem solving must be reconciled with the needs of patients and the demands of agencies for ongoing nursing services. Nurses cannot cease activities or leave patients or co-workers in suspended animation and adjourn to the library to read about a topic and formulate principles. Real nursing problems usually require some immediate action. Formulating and acquiring a list of principles, learning an organized methodology for problem solving, and enlarging the problem-solving tool chest and the critical thinking necessary to select the most effective nursing interventions are skills that must be learned initially in situations that permit time and freedom to err. One effective method is to allot a specified interval when the involved personnel are relieved of nursing responsibilities and can work through the nursing process. Reality can be preserved by using problem situations observed in practice by the involved nurses.

Learning nursing process by using real problems in the class or conference room is a simulated problem-solving situation. Simulation, for the purpose of learning the role of problem solver, allows for the practice of skills in a safe, nonthreatening environment. Neither the nurse nor the patient or client can be severely damaged in a simulated environment. Mistakes in judgment, errors of commission or omission, are without deadly consequences. Yet actual practice, an essential ingredient for learning any role, can be available. In the simulated learning situation, coaching can take place, complementary roles can be learned, the audience (classmates) can participate, and competence in decision making and other leadership skills can be acquired. However, although competence can be gained in simulated situations, only in reality can confidence for that role be attained.

After learning principles and the use of principles in solving nursing problems, nurses can use their skill to solve simple problems within the real situation with success and without disruption of necessary activities. Solving of complex problems frequently takes time and involves groups of people. The results of this group effort are (1) an increased awareness by the group of nursing problems, (2) increased quality of nursing services for patients, (3) broadening and deepening of the individual caregiver's nursing skill, and (4) utilization of each caregiver's potential contribution to patient care. Management problems are handled by individual managers or committees, depending on the circumstances, the urgency, and the complexity of the problem.

Problem solving is a process. A process is an organization of many components, parts, other processes, and tasks to achieve an explicit purpose. The outcome of this combination of many factors is one unique episode, act, task, factor, thing, person, or process. The discussion of the processes of problem solving will be clearer if problems are divided into two categories—obvious and obscure. *Obvious* problems are problems open to view. In nursing, they usually originate from procedures, schedules, timing, machinery, and work loads. *Obscure* problems are most frequently problems of behavior, communication, or interpersonal relations. Obscure problems are usually complicated by emotional overtones and loss of objectivity. In general, the more human interaction in an event or situation, the more difficult the identification and solution of the problem. Even overt problems may be difficult for the nurse to identify because of strong distracting stimuli or inattention to or breakdown in the processes preliminary to identifying the problem.

The processes that produce clear and accurate problem identification are the same for both obvious and obscure problems; however, the steps may be much more protracted when identifying obscure problems.

Problems are continually being solved by every individual. It is impossible to go through life without some kind of successful problem solving, either conscious or unconscious, formal or informal. Problem solving is one of the most important elements of leadership and management. It becomes increasingly important that nurses enter the practice of nursing prepared to engage in an organized problem-solving process. One of the basic tenets of any group practice of nursing is that groups collectively are more productive, more efficient, and more effective than the sum of their individual members. The inclusion of other nursing caregivers in problem solving whenever possible or appropriate ensures group commitment to the solution. This activity also improves esprit de corps, taps the abilities of each individual member, and gives the group the benefit of diverse thinking. The group process is slow at first but functions more rapidly as the group gains skill in problem solving together.

Problem solving has two aspects that nursing leaders and managers must utilize: (1) the tools, or heuristics, of problem solving and (2) the facets, or phases, of problem solving.

Problem-solving heuristics

Problem-solving heuristics are tools, techniques, or devices people use to solve problems. Whereas problem-solving facets or stages are aspects of problem solving (such as assessment, problem identification, and data gathering), problem-solving heuristics are the activities one uses to complete the tasks appropriate to each facet. For instance, some tools one might choose to use for assessment are looking, observing, questioning, or assuming. For problem identification, one might use the activities of guessing, supposing, analyzing, categorizing, synthesizing, or generalizing. Characteristically, every leader and every person being led has favorite problem-solving tools. Some people are impulsive and just leap in; some think the problem through from the beginning to the conclusion; and some work backward from a possible solution to the necessary supporting data. Some people tend to meditate or cogitate over problems; others let an idea incubate and come to a decision without conscious thought ("sleep on it"). The wider the range of problem-solving heuristics available to the leader, the more likely she or he will be to have the tools to arrive at adequate decisions. No one heuristic or device is better than another; each has its use, depending on the group, the leader, the problem, and the situation. Every leader must take inventory of problem-solving tools, especially those used most frequently. The leader needs to watch and talk with others to find out what tools others use. By adding to one's own tool chest and helping others add to theirs, the nurse will expand problem-solving skills and be more effective in facilitating the problem solving of others.

Facets or phases of nursing process

Nursing process has four phases, facets, or stages. The term "facets" is used here because the terms "phases" and "stages" communicate an order to the sequence of activities. Although listed here from problem identification to the judgment or decision, actual nursing process is seldom followed in that set sequence. The human mind tends to work backward and forward between aspects of problem solving until completion or decision is reached. The development of data, alternatives, and other considerations throws light on aspects of the problem previously developed, so that the whole changes; this flux is the process nature of problem solving. Each facet of nursing process contains the tasks necessary for successful completion of that facet. No facet is static; each is dynamic, for information uncovered in one facet may alter the significance of information uncovered in previous facets.

The following four facets of nursing process are in sequential form, and the tasks necessary to each are given. The following nursing problem is considered throughout to illustrate the use of this process.

Problem: An aide on a nursing team failed to give oral care to the patients assigned to her.

Problem-solving facet I: Problem identification (assessment)

Following are the tasks involved in problem identification:
1. Observe an event or situation.
2. Obtain relevant, valid, accurate, detailed descriptions from appropriate people or sources.

3. Write a description of the situation.
4. Discard irrelevant or questionable data.
5. Isolate the tentative problem and state it concisely.

Task 1—*Observe an event or situation.* The first task of the problem identification facet is the recognition that a problem needs to be identified. It seems unnecessary to say that one must have a problem before the problem can be solved, but it is an important maxim. Problems, by definition, are a question or a perplexity. This means a process, activity, or normal progression of events has been interrupted, altered, or disturbed in some way. It means someone believes that the situation is not optimal or that expectations have not been met.

Nursing students are often given case histories of patients with directions to identify the nursing problems. In reality, these students are being asked to identify areas of nursing care necessary to the health of the patient. Specific problems cannot be identified without an event or situation in which a team leader's normal expectations have not been met:

> While functioning as a leader of a team of nursing personnel on an acute medical care unit, the nurse notes that an aide on the team is not giving oral care to the patients assigned to her.

The team leader having observed this event or situation proceeds to task 2.

Task 2—*Obtain relevant, valid, accurate, detailed descriptions from appropriate people or sources.* Accurate descriptions and observations are the forte of nursing; however, continued practice and study in this realm are necessary for maintaining and improving skill. Teaching observational skills to all nursing caregivers will result in increasingly better nursing care. After one nurse had repeatedly sensitized the ancillary personnel to accurate descriptions, an aide was asked in casual conversation if she had seen the director of nurses' new car. The aide answered that she had. The nurse then inquired about the color and the aide responded that it was "blue on the side toward me." Although the aide's answer was facetious, this kind of cautious accuracy will increase the speed and validity of solving nursing problems through accurate and objective observations and reports.

Good results can be obtained if effective interviewing skills are exercised. Descriptions of situations collected from all individuals concerned can become confused and subjective if inappropriate questions are posed. Desired information can be obtained if the leader asks such questions as "What happened?" "What preceded the event?" "What followed then?" "What else was going on while this was occurring?" "How did you feel about the incident?" Further data can be obtained by focusing statements such as "Tell me more about that," "Help me to understand the events." Sometimes simple listening postures and sounds are enough. Oh? Yes? And then . . . ?

Open-ended questions and statements such as these will assist the nurse and those involved to separate feelings from facts, achieve objectivity, and formulate a more vivid description of the problem.

For example, the nurse gathers the following descriptive information from appropriate sources:

1. There are twenty patients assigned to the nursing team on the given day; all but five are seriously ill.
2. Basic technical care to be administered to the twenty patients includes ten complete bed baths, five partial bed baths, five showers, and twenty beds to be changed; seven patients must be fed their meals.
3. One nurses' aide scheduled to work on the team failed to report to work because of illness. A replacement was not available.
4. Some team members had complained of overwork and expressed feelings of injustice.
5. The aide not giving oral care has been employed in this health agency for one month.

Task 3—Write a description of the situation. The nurse will find it helpful to take notes on the descriptions of the event as reported by all those concerned with the problem situation. Summarizing the descriptions in a short, concise, clear paragraph that contains all relevant material will aid in clarifying the event. When events are in written form, it is much easier to identify material that does not contribute to the description of the problem situation. Writing helps to crystalize thinking and is a valuable step in problem identification. A paragraph description of the problem situation is written here:

An aide who has been employed one month is not giving oral care to patients assigned to her. Team members feel overworked with one unreplaced absent member. There are twenty patients, ten who need complete care and seven who need feeding.

Task 4—Discard irrelevant or questionable data. Data that are irrelevant or of questionable use in identifying the problem may be of considerable use when gathering data for the solution of the problem. Superfluous material in the descriptive situation increases the confusion and difficulty of isolating the problem. These same data may be helpful at a different stage of problem solving. Here is the described situation with noncontributory material deleted:

An aide who has been employed one month is not giving oral care to patients assigned to her.

Task 5—Isolate the tentative problem and state it concisely. Problem identification is a dynamic, not static, process. As information is gathered subsequent to the implementation of principles, it may become necessary to alter the original identified problem so that reality and accuracy are preserved. Identified problems should always be considered tentative or subject to change by the group or leader. When identified problems are labeled "tentative," there is greater willingness on the part of those participating in problem solving to change the identification of the problem. Groups and individuals can change the identified "tentative" problem with less embarrassment and fewer feelings of inadequacy than they can a "definite" problem.

The temptation for the beginning problem solver is to put conclusions about why the aide is not giving oral care into the statement of the problem. Following are two possible erroneous statements of the problem:

1. Aide not giving oral care because she resents her work load.
2. Aide inadequately oriented to ward routines and does not know she should give oral care.

Such guessing wastes time in idle speculation and leads to a search for substantiation of the hypothesis rather than selection of the appropriate principles and consequent activities necessary to the efficient and objective solution of the problem. Problems are easier to solve if stated as questions. Following is a concise statement of the problem:

How to ensure that oral care is given to patients.

Problem-solving facet II: Selection of appropriate principles (theorizing)

Following are the tasks involved in selecting the appropriate principles:
1. Determine topics or area of principles relevant to the subject.
2. Formulate the principles of the determined area or topic from authoritative sources appropriate to the tentative problem, or select appropriate list of principles from a cumulative file.
3. Select the specific principles applicable to the problem based on validity, relevance, and practicality.
4. List principles in the order they may be used most effectively.

Selection of appropriate principles depends totally on the proper identification of the problem. Principles useful to the solution of the problem will be selected only if the correct problem has been identified.

Task 1—Determine topics or area of principles relevant to the subject. Selection of the topic or subject of the principles is made by determining the subject area to which the problem relates. For example, if the nurse concerned in this situation had identified the problem as "inadequate orientation," the principle area would have been "teaching-learning." Had the problem been identified as "resentment of work load," the principle area would have been "team spirit." However, failure to properly carry out a job assignment clearly identifies the area of necessary principles as "delegation of authority."

Task 2—Formulate the principles of the determined area or topic from authoritative sources appropriate to the tentative problem, or select appropriate list of principles from a cumulative file. Leaders who utilize the principles method of problem solving accumulate many principles from which to draw. If a list has been compiled, it should be examined for inclusiveness. Additional principles needed must be formulated from authoritative sources and added to the list.

Nursing problems frequently require utilization of principles from several subject areas. In the interest of simplicity a problem has been chosen that can be satisfactorily solved using principles from one subject area. The following is a partial list of principles of delegation of assignments and authority from Chapter 6.

1. Performance of assigned tasks effectively depends on sufficient influence, power, and authority.
2. The nurse's belief that ultimate accountability lies with her determines the scope and limitations she sets for her leadership.
3. Decentralization of power allows for a greater amount of delegation.
4. Understanding the categories and roles of nursing personnel enables the delegator to select the type and number of personnel appropriate to the job.
5. Written descriptions of policies, procedures, and guidelines by which an employee may handle situations promote ease of operation for the caregiver and control of the authority delegated by the nurse.
6. Staff member participation in the formulation of policies, job descriptions, and procedures increases use of policies and improves job satisfaction.
7. The philosophy and policies of a health agency determine the pattern of nursing care delivery system to be provided.
8. Guidelines such as established channels, methods, and provision for communication within an agency enable the nurse-manager to delegate tasks and authority appropriately.
9. The number of workers and span of control depend upon consideration of factors that most affect the work group.
10. Formulation of objectives for care that are realistic for the health agency, patients, and nursing personnel assures successful goal accomplishment.
11. Utilization of nursing care plans provides the mechanism for making nurse assignments according to patient needs and the order of priorities.
12. A systematic planning process enables effective delegation for work implementation.
13. Assignment of patient care and support services to increasing personnel depends upon the pattern or system of nursing care in force.
14. Consideration of safety factors and instructions regarding emergency situations prepare nursing staff to employ preventive measures and to cope with emergency situations.
15. The delegator's availability to staff members results in assistance, teaching, counsel, and evaluation where necessary.
16. Centralized control of incidental task requests prevents maldistribution of workloads.
17. A balance between variety and continuity of assignment increases motivation and productivity.

18. Consideration for each caregiver's preferences and areas of expertise influences morale.
19. Centralization of information storage and retrieval systems allows for efficient assessment, delegation, and implementation of tasks.
20. Clear and concise directions enhance task delegation.
21. Frequent evaluation of performance using criteria influences the quality of care and the level of actual performance of care activities.

Task 3—Select the specific principles applicable to the problem based on validity, relevance, and practicality. It is apparent that only selected principles within an area apply to a given problem. Some problems may require the use of only one or two principles for a solution to be reached; others may require many principles. The number of principles selected depends on the nature of the problem.

After careful consideration the nurse decides that the problem can be solved using principles 4, 5, 8, 9, 11, 12, 15, and 21. The others are not relevant.

The nurse will evaluate each principle selected using the criteria of validity, relevance, and practicality. Principle 11 will be used as a model.

PRINCIPLE: A systematic planning process enables effective delegation for work implementation.

This principle is valid because if planning is not systematic and plans are not followed, mistrust develops rapidly in a group and morale decreases. For example, if the delegator had been unaware of the activities of each nurses' aide, all team members may have been confronted for an explanation of the lack of good hygienic care. The use of this haphazard approach not only may offend the workers who are doing their jobs correctly but also may cause the team member involved to feel justified in offering retaliatory remarks such as "You should have known that these patients were mine; you assigned them to me, so why didn't you come to me for an explanation?" The new employee may also feel insecure in her position and therefore take other means of self-defense; these usually involve "grapevine" activity that undermines the nurse as an effective leader and manager.

The principle is relevant, for if the team leader knows to whom the responsibility for the patients involved is delegated, immediate personal contact can be established with that particular team member. The nurse can then obtain immediate feedback about what is going on and why it is occurring.

The principle is practical because systematic planning will work at the time and place needed within the natural limits of the situation.

Task 4—List principles in the order they may be used most effectively. Principles show outcomes, and outcomes usually have a logical, necessary, desirable sequence. For example, the nurse has channels-of-communication guidelines established by the agency; using those guidelines ensures that actions are within designated authority. Using established, designated lines of authority the nurse must take steps to ensure that the job descriptions, policies, and procedures include the assigned tasks and are available to each aide. The process of arranging principles in their logical order of use continues until all selected principles are arranged in an ordered sequence. The order in which the principles selected for the example problem can be most effectively used is as follows:

1. Understanding the categories and roles of nursing personnel enables the delegator to select the type and number of personnel appropriate to the job. (4)
2. Written descriptions of policies, procedures, and guidelines by which an employee may handle situations promote ease of operation for the caregiver and control of the authority delegated by the nurse. (5)
3. Guidelines such as established channels, methods, and provision for communication within an agency enable the nurse-manager to delegate tasks and authority appropriately. (8)
4. The number of workers and span of control depend upon consideration of factors that most affect the work group. (9)
5. Utilization of nursing care plans provides the mechanism for making nurse assignments according to patient needs and the order of priorities. (11)
6. A systematic planning process enables effective delegation for work implementation. (12)
7. The delegator's availability to staff members results in assistance, teaching, counsel, and evaluation where necessary. (15)
8. Frequent evaluation of performance using criteria influences the quality of care and the level of actual performance of care activities. (21)

Flexibility in both selection and order of application of principles is important. The result of an action dictated by a principle may necessitate substitution of one or more subsequent principles. The nurse familiar with all the important principles of a given area or topic finds flexibility easy to maintain.

Problem-solving facet III: Determining alternatives for action (planning)

Following are the tasks involved in determining alternatives for action:
1. Determine all alternative courses of action that are a natural consequence of each principle.
2. Determine who will select the course of action.
3. Select the courses of action to be instigated and establish a serial order for implementation.
4. Evaluate selected alternatives for practicality. This requires determining if the proposed courses of action are:
   a. within the philosophy of the agency
   b. supported by the administration

   c. reasonable investment of time, energy, equipment, and money
   d. technologically current, yet within the abilities of the group
   e. assessed for safety and predictability of risk
   f. legally and morally acceptable to the nurse, group, and patient
   g. planned in conjunction with those who are most concerned with
      the problem (physician, patient's family, social services, occupational therapy, physical therapy, or rehabilitation personnel)

Facet III is a planning facet. Determining alternatives for action is a selective process in which one deliberates about the principles and the possible courses of action that arise from the principles, decides who must select the course of action, and attempts to establish the best *order* for implementing actions. Facet III is not the facet in which intervention behaviors occur; it is the facet in which plans, preparations, and decisions about intervention are made. Rapid judgments and decisions can be made by the nurse, or discussions may be held with appropriate people.

Task 1—Determine all alternative courses of action that are a natural consequence of each principle. Since a "principle" is by definition a circumstance, condition, or behavior that produces a given definable outcome, activities are the natural extension of a principle. The activity consequence of a principle can take any number of forms, depending on the specific problem and ramifications of that problem. Consideration of a variety of alternative courses of action increases the probability of choosing a workable course of action. However, any activity that is considered must comply with the dictates of its antecedent principle.

In the example used here the following principle has been selected as the model: The delegator's availability to staff members results in assistance, teaching, counsel, and evaluation where necessary. This principle indicates that the delegator's availability is a condition necessary to teaching, counsel, and evaluation. Availability can be achieved in a variety of ways, depending on the people and circumstances involved. Behaviors that lead to availability are tailored to each problem or situation.

Following are some suggested alternatives for establishing availability in the example situation:

1. Go immediately to the aide and ask for a conference.
2. Wait until there is a natural pause in her work and ask her to come for a conference.
3. Wait until her work is over for the morning and request a conference.
4. Go to the aide and tell her you wish to speak to her as soon as she is free.
5. Give her a note asking her to come and see you as soon as possible.

The best way to demonstrate availability depends on the people involved and the circumstances. The nurse must consider all alternatives and select the best for each situation.

Task 2—*Determine who will select the course of action.* Selecting the course of action to be taken may not always be the responsibility of the nurse. If the situation involves policy, procedure, patient safety or treatment, or cultural, religious, emotional, or interpersonal matters, the nurse may be compelled by policy, law, safety of the patient, or good judgment to involve other people in the selection of the appropriate course of action. In this example the *nurse* will be the one to choose the alternatives to be used.

Task 3—*Select the courses of action to be instigated and establish a serial order for implementation.* As shown in task 1, each principle has one or more courses of action. In task 3 the nurse must select the most effective actions from the list suggested in task 1. When the decision is made concerning the available alternative to be used, the order in which the courses of action are to be actualized must be determined. These activities are nursing action prescriptions and are, in part, level IV of theory building. The selected courses of action derived from the selected principles and arranged in the appropriate order for this situation would be as follows:

1. Seek out the aide in question.
2. Arrange a meeting in private with the aide.
3. Gather data that would determine the aide's:
   a. level of understanding of role
   b. ability to fulfill expectations
   c. reaction to the incident
   d. rationale for omission
4. Request the aide to give oral care to patients assigned to her (providing necessary assistance, teaching, and supervision).
5. Evaluate overall patient assignment to ensure continuing orientation and practice commensurate with experience and ability of all personnel.
6. Establish time for future conference.

Task 4—*Evaluate selected alternatives for practicality.* Practicality is an important consideration. Prescribed action must be possible within a given framework at a specific time and place. "Common sense" or intuition is not sufficient. Social, physical, and biologic science factors must be considered when testing principles for practicality. The practicality of any plan of action can be assessed through the use of the following criteria:

a. *Within the philosophy of the agency.* If the selected alternative is not within the philosophy of the agency, it is inappropriate for the nurse to pursue that particular action. Policy is not the same as philosophy, but it reflects philosophy. For example, the agency philosophy may state that basic nursing care is to be provided or administered to every patient. Policy would then dictate that the one assigned to give care would follow through with the commitment.

b. *Supported by the administration.* Administration and high level management backing usually implies that policies and procedures have been formulated and orientation has been provided. In the situation under question the nurse's aide, although a new employee, would have been exposed to appropriate procedure through in-service programs and supervision and would have had an opportunity to review the procedure manual any time a need was felt.

c. *Reasonable investment of time, energy, equipment, and money.* Nurses have responsibilities for providing care to patients. Regardless of the agency involved, each patient is entitled to receive services according to his or her needs and the commitment of the agency to meet those needs.

The nurse need not expend time and energy to determine whether the service of oral hygiene should have been administered. All data support the need for this service. The next logical step is to investigate equipment. Were supplies available for the administration of oral hygiene? If not, why not? If so, why were they not used? The economic factor could play a part in this situation, depending on the philosophy of the institution. The health agency might expect patients to provide their own equipment. If so, do the patients have supplies? When the institution provides equipment, supplies cannot be considered always available or unlimited in number. These are areas in which energy need be expended. The nurse should have someone available to check nonnursing details, but in every case the responsibility for determining facts lies with the delegator of authority.

When emergencies arise, such as a reduction in the number of personnel, some goals are sacrificed and priorities among patients' needs are established. The authority figure will have the knowledge necessary to make judgments about the importance of oral hygiene in providing for the needs of an ill patient.

The leader of the nursing team will seek out the nurse's aide to find answers about why oral hygiene was not administered to the assigned patients.

d. *Technologically current, yet within the abilities of the group.* The field of technology includes scientific knowledge and mechanical and procedural skills. The investigator must know if the nurse's aide failed to administer oral hygienic care because of a lack of knowledge or skill. If lack of knowledge or skill is the reason, remedial steps are in order. The leader knows there has been a breakdown in initial or continuing orientation.

There is a lag between current technology and workers' knowledge and abilities to implement technology. The field of oral hygiene has moved away from a simple gargle or a few strokes of a brush into a procedure that depends on knowledge of anatomy and physiology, bacteriology, and dental hygiene. Patients have a right to the most technologically advanced care available, and nurses and employers need to keep abreast of advancements in order to provide the best care possible.

e. *Assessed for safety and predictability of risk.* Safety is always a primary consideration in selecting nursing interventions. Safety cannot be assumed for any act that has inherent risk. When selecting a realistic, usable alternative of action, one must consider what the gains and losses will be for patient, family, nurse, and hospital. Weighing risks and ascertaining the alternative that gives greatest benefit to the recipient of the action, with the least possibility of damage, can become quite complicated. The process can be compared to item pricing. In purchasing a pair of shoes, one wishes to know how much quality and service can be obtained for how much money. All shoes cost something. The question becomes "Is the expected purchase worth the price?" There are times when the contemplated actions are simply not worth the risks involved, whether a health and safety risk or a social-interpersonal risk.

In the situation under consideration the team leader, in telling the aide about the omission of mouth care and asking for clarification, risks several things, among which are the following:

1. Offending or embarrassing the aide
2. Damaging rapport or relationships
3. Being placed in the vulnerable position of being asked why oral hygiene is important

If the omission is allowed to continue and nothing is done, the nurse risks the following:

1. Reinforcing unacceptable behavior by silent consent
2. Allowing patient health, hygiene, and comfort to suffer
3. Criticism from team members who do give mouth care

Implementation of alternatives for each principle carries with it risks that must be evaluated. Actions and interventions will then be actualized in full knowledge of the risks, and preparation can be made in anticipation of consequences.

f. *Legally and morally acceptable to the nurse, group, and patient.* Since nursing practice is governed by local, state, and federal regulations, most personnel are aware of basic laws concerning the practice of nursing. There are ample sources of reference if legal or moral issues become a question.

In the nursing situation posed the nurse must be convinced that the nurse's aide did not omit oral hygienic care because of laziness. Serious moral and legal implications are presented if negligence is established. The supervisor of care realizes the possibilities of infection, malnutrition, and other problems that can occur as a result of omission of this important part of care.

g. *Planned in conjunction with those who are most concerned with the problem.* Many alternative solutions to problems involve members of other disciplines, whether the problem be patient centered or organization oriented.

In the nursing situation under discussion the nurse's aide may need additional classes with the in-service education department, more supervision from the nurse, or participation in group discussion with members of the nursing team. All three alternatives may be desirable.

Problem-solving facet IV: Implementing plans (intervention)

Following are the tasks involved in implementing intervention:
1. Assume the responsibility for coordinating or implementing activities.
2. Determine what must be done to establish authority to implement the plan.
3. Establish time and place for follow-up, reassessment, and evaluation of activities.
4. Implement plans.
5. Reassess, evaluate, follow up, and revise plans according to data.

Facet IV is the action facet. All work prior to this phase has been in preparation. Facet IV is that phase in which the nurse and the nursing group have responsibility for actualizing the philosophies, objectives, principles, and plans that have been previously determined. Facet IV is equivalent to the situation-producing theories (level IV) of theory building. They are prescriptive theories, which include prescription, implementation, and evaluation of a nursing intervention.

Action requires not only implementing behaviors but also concurrent evaluation of the effectiveness of the action. Formalized reassessment depends in part on data gathered during action. The following tasks of facet IV are the crux of the problem-solving process and the proof of the validity of all foregoing facets.

Task 1—Assume responsibility for coordinating or implementing activities. A responsible leader and manager is essential to smooth implementation of alternatives. Often intervention activities occur over a period of several weeks. Patient problems are seldom solved quickly, and interdepartmental problems within an agency require continued effort; these activities require a manager who will be responsible for seeing that efforts are ongoing. This does not imply that the nurse who assumes this responsibility will do all the work. It implies only that the manager will see that the planned activities are carried out.

The nurse in the problem example is the organizational person most familiar with the situation and nearest to the level of operation. The responsibility for implementation and follow-through belongs at this level. Frequently managers "pass the buck" for any number of reasons to those who might assume the responsibility for implementation. The head nurse or in-service education instructor is the most likely recipient of "buck passing" from lower level management. The nurse must fully assume leadership responsibilities and act with the authority of the role. Any activities relevant to patient care must be instigated and coordinated by the team leader or primary nurse.

Task 2—Determine what must be done to establish authority to implement the plan. To carry out a selected alternative the authority to implement an activity must be clearly established through the proper channels and lines of authority. Written memos are the best means of clearing channels or informing appropriate people, regardless of the friendliness of relationships with line or staff people, other departments, or physicians. Conversations, both in person and on the telephone, that establish the authority to implement should be followed by a memo referring to the phone call or conversation and summarizing the content. These memos should be kept for future reference. Trust and good relationships are maintained through the use of good business practices. Good records reinforce memory and provide a reference source. Reliance on memory alone is a shaky foundation for any relationship because it permits misunderstanding to occur without revealing to the participants that a misunderstanding exists and, therefore, clarification is not possible. Memos reveal misunderstandings and allow the participants to clarify positions immediately. The memo also serves as a reminder of commitments or activities in progress. In this example, authority to act is invested with the position of team leader, and no other channels need be cleared.

Task 3—Establish time and place for follow-up, reassessment, and evaluation of activities. Establishing a time and place for follow-up and reassessment is important to ensure continuing awareness of and continuity in handling the problem. Crisis situations invariably draw the strongest and most immediate response, and situations that have ceased to be crises are often delegated to places of less importance and are not followed through to completion. This practice increases the possibility that the same situation will again become a crisis. Planned follow-up establishes a system whereby further complications can be avoided and continued growth can be promoted.

Plans for follow-up and reassessment are most important when groups are involved in problem solving. Planning times for this important activity gives the group a sense of continuity. It provides target dates and motivates individuals to think in realistic terms about what they can contribute to such a conference. This activity not only underlines the importance of the planned intervention but also allows the group to evaluate effectiveness and further plan other activities or even reassess the problem (see principle 8, facet II, task 4, pp. 27-28).

Task 4—Implement plans. The problem is identified, the principles selected, the alternatives established and chosen, authority clearly defined, and implementation is under way. Nurses who are implementing plans and are wary of forgetting a part of the planned implementation may wish to make a list. This list, if made, should be kept small and brief.

When groups are involved, roles need to be clearly defined in the perpetration of a plan of action so that each person knows what every other person is doing. If all are to participate, *how* each will participate needs to be discussed so that guidelines for action are established and each person can fit within the framework.

In the situation under discussion the nurse would find the appropriate aide, take her aside, and privately find out the information necessary. Basing actions on the findings of the interview, the leader would provide the necessary equipment, assistance, teaching, or supervision and arrange for the aide to give the oral care to the patients assigned to her. The team leader would arrange for further evaluation, assessment, and follow-up and evaluate the overall patient assignment.

       Task 5—Reassess, evaluate, follow up, and revise plans according to data (evaluation). Task 5 occurs after the initial actions that deal with the immediate situation and is designed to determine if the problem has been adequately solved or if alterations in plans need to be made. Participation by all concerned is important to the success of this task. Retrospective as well as concurrent evaluation is necessary to the solution of any problem. The nurse's evaluation, together with the aide's evaluation, will serve as a guide to determine the relevancy and effectiveness of all the problem-solving steps. Revision of plans may be necessary because of further developments, such as more trust and better communications, additional data, or the rapidity with which the aide learns. Procedure manuals or orientation programs may need review, or patient assignments may need more planning. This information may not become apparent until follow-up conferences are conducted in which all people concerned honestly attempt to evaluate the entire situation. From such conferences may come continuity and progress for the entire unit or a redefinition of the problem and subsequent problem-solving actvities.

Conceptual frameworks—a guide to nursing care decisions

       Conceptual frameworks were once the exclusive domain of nursing education. Graduate students were required to construct conceptual frameworks for papers, theses, and dissertations. Schools of nursing are required to have conceptual frameworks from which curriculum is derived in order to have a unifying mechanism and decision-making strategy for their plans for learning. With increasing frequency, health care institutions are formulating philosophies and conceptual frameworks to enable management to make decisions that are consistent with the philosophy, mission, and goals of the agency, responsive to the needs of the setting and clients, and consistent in the type and quality of health care desired.

       The conceptual framework is an interrelated system of premises that provides guidelines or ground rules for making all nursing care and organizational decisions. It is derived from a philosophy and is the conceptualization and articulation of concepts, facts, propositions, postulates, theories, phenomena, and variables relevant to a specific nursing care system. It describes the relationships these concepts and theories have to one another and to the nursing care given in each agency. It is the structure that provides the map for all managerial

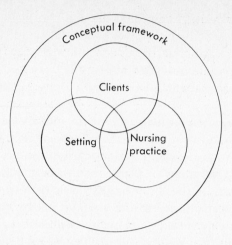

Fig. 1-4. The Chater model for conceptual frameworks.

and staff nurse level decisions. It is like the framing of a house that outlines the specifications and the decision-making guidelines for the walls, rooms, forms, and functions of the house. The conceptual framework provides the perimeters (limits and constraints) and parameters (values) for nursing care, giving consistency and integrity to the entire nursing department. The conceptual framework of each department of nursing or health care agency differs, at least slightly, from that of every other agency, even though large areas of similarity may exist because of the nature of nursing.

Just as each person has a frame of reference that is influenced by his or her culture—life experiences, ethnicity, philosophy, and personality—so each nursing service agency is influenced by its "culture"—its philosophical set, the clients it serves, the community it serves, and the type of nursing care it offers. These elements, when brought together, comprise an implied and expressed value system and provide explicit decision-making rules for nursing care. According to Chater* there are three areas that provide concepts, theories, and decision-making guidelines (a conceptual framework) for curriculum building. These same three areas are useful for devising a conceptual framework for nursing practice. Progressive nursing care agencies such as the University of California Hospital at San Francisco, Nursing Service Department, have successfully used the Chater model for devising a conceptual framework for nursing service. The three areas that Chater recommends for inclusion in a conceptual framework are as follows:

---

*Chater, S.: A conceptual framework for curriculum development, Nurs. Outlook **23:**428-433, July 1975.

1. Setting or context
2. Clients
3. Conceptualization of nursing practice, or the knowledge base

Fig. 1-4 is a diagram of the Chater model.

Much nursing literature, when referring to a conceptual framework for nursing, seems to refer only to the knowledge base, or conceptualization, of nursing practice. Most authors communicate concepts and theories relevant to this area to the exclusion of the other two factors represented in the Chater model, which are equally influential in nursing service decision making. Nursing service departments successful in the delivery of care are responsive to all three areas identified by Chater.

All nursing service departments operate under conceptual frameworks; however, some are clearly articulated, and some simply exist and are understood. The three areas of the Chater model may be applied in nursing process in specific ways, as shown here.

Setting

The setting of nursing practice refers to various things. One is the agency or institution that houses the nursing service department. The type of agency, the kinds of services offered, the composition of the sponsoring group, the budget constraints, and the philosophy, mission, and goals are the major elements for consideration about the sponsoring agency. A large teaching general hospital would have a mission, a philosophy, and goals different from those of a small specialty hospital such as an eye, ear, nose, and throat hospital. Parochial institutions such as Mount Sinai Hospital or Holy Cross Hospital would have philosophies and missions different from those of large, state-supported institutions. Health departments operate on a philosophical premise and have a mission different from clinics or general hospitals. These varying agencies focus on the following:

1. What health problems they address
2. What ethnic and moral precepts or conditions are imposed by their funding source
3. The realities of the size and categories of their budgets
4. The type of health care provided in their nursing system

These factors dictate many of the service goals of the nursing department.

Another aspect of the setting component is the influence of those factors contributed by the community the agency serves. That community may be the immediate geographic area of the health agency; it may be a state or, in the case of some health agencies such as the National Institutes of Health at Bethesda, Maryland, it may be a nation. In the case of agencies such as the World Health

Organization, it can be global. Factors that must be considered in the conceptual framework of any agency regarding its community or service area are as follows:

1. The politics of the area
2. State and federal regulations about practice and quality control standards
3. Geography of the area (climate, topography)
4. Types of industry and economic basis of the area

A third group of factors to be considered in the setting is the type of nursing care delivery system generally used in a geographic location. The nursing care delivery system is influenced by several factors:

1. The types and qualifications of the nurses available to fill positions
2. The character of nursing practice in the geographic area of the hospital, that is, what is acceptable nursing practice in the area
3. The structure of the health care delivery system within which the nursing department operates

The fourth factor involves the availability of professional nurses. The availability of people prepared as nurse-specialists and nurse-practitioners varies from one geographic area to another. The availability of people with baccalaureate and masters degrees varies from place to place, and the number of people available having special preparation in nursing administration varies, depending on the availability of these special educational programs. It is impossible to plan a nursing care delivery system that calls for many nurse-practitioners, nurse-specialists, or masters-prepared people in nursing administration when these people are not available. In most urban areas, people are available to fill special kinds of jobs requiring special education; however, in many of the rural or remote areas of the United States, nurses who have special training are not always available. Naturally the availability of highly trained people influences the kind of nursing care delivery system that can be implemented in an agency.

The type and kind of nursing practice in the geographic setting constitute a fifth factor. Some modes of nursing care delivery systems are more popular in some areas than in others. The four classical modes of nursing care delivery systems — case, functional, team, and primary nursing — are used in various configurations throughout the country.

The case mode is regaining a measure of popularity because of the increasing popularity in primary nursing. Many agencies that believe they cannot implement primary nursing do implement case method nursing instead and combine some of the aspects of case method nursing with primary nursing. The case mode is also popular in special care units. The team method, used with varying degrees of success throughout the country, is still one of the more popular methods in use. One nurse leads a group in giving care to a group of patients. This mode of care is usually mixed with some form of case and functional nursing and is seldom practiced in its pure state. The functional method of nursing care delivery is probably the most common method in use, as the job-centered or task-oriented system requires the least amount of organization, planning, and professional personnel.

That a particular kind of nursing care is popular in a geographic area does not necessarily mean that this mode of nursing care delivery will be chosen for every agency in that area; it simply means that nurses in the area may be more familiar with one mode than another, and when switching to another mode of nursing care delivery, the degree of familiarity is a factor to be considered. In an area where functional nursing has been in use, a much more extensive educational program must be planned to ensure success if a new delivery system is introduced.

The sixth factor about setting is the structure of the health care delivery system within which the nursing department operates. Some health care delivery systems, by their very nature, rely more heavily on the independence of nurses than do other health care delivery systems. Nurses operating with protocols function with a fair degree of independence in many clinics, health departments, and hospitals. (Protocols or standardized procedures describe actions that may be taken by nurses that are not included or articulated clearly in state nurse practice acts. They are developed by joint committee action including representation from administration, medical, and nursing personnel.) However, if the health care delivery system in an area is not structured to accommodate the degree of independence of practice desired by the nursing service department, plans may be thwarted. Sweeping changes in the health care delivery system may be beyond the energy level of nursing service departments; therefore nursing service departments may have to alter the degree of independence expected of its employees based on the structure of the health care delivery system in that area.

Clients

The Chater model for construction of a conceptual framework considers the character of the clients served. In order to structure the data about clients, one must determine the kind of people who will be or are being served by the agency, their needs, and their expectations and characteristics.

Some of the factors to be considered that will enable a clear statement of commitment to the group to be served are as follows:

1. Ethnicity of the population
2. Educational level—literacy rates
3. English language comprehension or foreign languages usually spoken
4. Cultural mores and folkways
5. Values of the people
6. Economic level of the people

7. Ethnicity of the nursing staff and its ethnic congruency with clientele
8. Employment and unemployment rates
9. Age statistics
10. Health problems of the population

Each of these factors provides critical information that helps an agency determine its service commitments. Each influences the priority of problems, the management of budget, the planning of staff development, and the concentration of effort. These items and their impact on nursing care will not be discussed individually. However, an example of the impact of each of these items can be seen in item 10 above, the health problems of the population served.

Some health service areas have vastly different health problems from others. For instance, the San Francisco Bay area has exceptionally high rates of cirrhosis of the liver whereas the coastal areas of South Carolina and Georgia have exceptionally high rates of stroke. Parts of the Midwest have high rates of tuberculosis. Some agencies address particular health problems with greater vigor because they are special problems peculiar to the community in which the agency is placed.

Knowledge base

The knowledge base is what Waters* calls "the conceptualization of nursing practice." Each nursing service department needs a conceptualization of nursing practice to provide structure to the practitioner's role, the organization, and the client care approach. A conceptualization of nursing practice gives unity and integrity to nursing care. The conceptualization of nursing practice will dictate the way in which the nursing service department wishes nursing to be practiced. It will explain what happens to patients when they are nursed. According to Waters, a conceptualization of nursing practice has six aspects:

1. The goals of care
2. Who the clients are
3. What the nursing problems are
4. The types of nursing interventions that will enacted
5. The settings of practice
6. The work role relationships

The kind of conceptualization of nursing practice chosen or devised by a nursing service agency dictates the content under each of these six areas.

Goals. If Dorothea Orem's framework for nursing practice is chosen, the goals of nursing practice will be self-care or self-help. If Sister Calista Roy's perception of nursing practice is chosen, the goals of nursing will be adaptation. If Dunn is selected as a component of the conceptualization of nursing practice,

---

*Waters, V.: Address: Conceptualization for nursing practice, presented at Workshop: Conceptual frameworks for nursing, Calgary, Canada, July 1975, Institute of Nursing Consultants.

the goals of practice will be high-level wellness. An acute care hospital may have as its goal the return to optimal health possible for each client served, whereas a public health department nursing service may have as its goal attaining the degree of independence considered possible for each client. A hospice for the terminally ill may have goals such as maximum comfort of its patients and death with dignity. Goals will vary according to the agency's philosophy, mission, and perception of nursing practice.

Clients. The kind of clients depends largely on the setting, that is, the kind of institution. Some agencies treat only pediatric clients, or only pregnant women, or only people with eye, ear, nose, and throat conditions. The kind of agency will dictate the selection of clients that nursing service will address. The client's developmental level, ethnicity, and personality characteristics are factors that must be identified and described if the conceptualization of nursing practice is to be functional.

Problems. The kinds of problems nursing will address are an important aspect of the conceptualization of nursing practice and are derived from the mission of the agency as well as the philosophy and intent of the nursing service department. A nursing department that operates on the medical model will probably choose to address those problems centered around the medical diagnosis of the clients, for example, diabetes, fractures, congestive heart failure, strokes, pregnancy, or blindness. Nursing service agencies that are centered on the nursing problems will choose nursing's domain of practice as the area of problems for nursing service to address. These will be problems in mobility, self-help, communications, grief, sexuality, etc. Clarity in the domain of practice and the nursing care diagnoses enables nurses to function as nurses, rather than as "junior doctors," and to provide nursing diagnoses and nursing care prescriptions in keeping with the whole framework of the agency, thereby clarifying such things as evaluation, auditing, and quality control of nursing care. It is extremely important for nursing service managers to be clear about the kinds and types of problems their nurses may legitimately confront. Control can be attained through a committee structure that allows nurses to identify and collaborate on problems and their nursing management.

Intervention. The kinds of interventions legitimized by the conceptualization of nursing practice follow various formats. One is the focus of the intervention. Focus of the intervention may be prevention/care/cure/rehabilitation, or it may go into Leavell and Clark's* three levels of prevention—primary, secondary, and tertiary prevention. Nursing services may choose to look at the divisions of interventions according to the 1965 AMA position paper, that is, care, cure, and coordination, or they may choose to devise a separate category system

---

*Leavell, H., and Clark, E.: Preventive medicine for the doctor and his community, ed. 3, New York, 1965, McGraw-Hill Book Co.

for practice interventions. Whatever the case, some agencies concentrate more on prevention than on care. Some agencies are rehabilitation hospitals and concentrate on rehabilitation interventions. Most general hospitals concentrate on secondary prevention, or the care/cure aspect, with minimal emphasis on prevention and rehabilitation. Thus the emphasis on the kind of care is an important highlight to the conceptualization of nursing practice, since it enables nurses to know where the energy focus lies. Other things pertaining to intervention are the tools of the trade, that is, the processes, techniques, and concepts that nurses use to carry out their interventions. These would include such things as problem solving, systems theory, research, communications, stress theory, role theory, caring, teaching/learning, and maturational theory. These tools and processes tell the nurse which theoretical base will be used in practice to provide the basis for the vocabulary and jargon that will be used in making diagnoses, in writing nursing care prescriptions during charting, during nursing audits, in devising criteria for the evaluation of nursing care, or in any other communication.

Settings. Settings are the fifth item to be considered in conceptualization of nursing practice. Some agencies have a wider variety of settings than others. All settings where nursing will be practiced must be listed and described in the conceptualization of nursing practice. Some agencies send nurses only into homes and clinics; other agencies have them in the structured environment of the hospital. Some hospitals have both clinical and home care follow-up and therefore a wider variety of settings than those offering only acute hospital treatment. Other facilities provide a variety of settings within the agencies themselves. Intensive care, rehabilitation, intermediate care, and ambulatory care are some of the work settings of hospitals. These settings require a wide variety of skills and dictate such prerequisites as orientation programs, in-service education programs, and selection of employees.

Work role relationships. The work role relationship is one of the more difficult areas to deal with in any nursing care agency. Work role relationships are dictated not only by the conceptualization of nursing practice of the agency but also by the culture of the health care provider group in any given community. In some communities, work role relationships between physicians and nurses are easy and collegial; in others they are highly formal, hierarchical, and often patronizing. Nursing service departments that have a clear conceptualization of nursing practice and a clear articulation of the work role relationships expected of their employees can provide the support system necessary to enable nurses to act in colleague relationships with physicians. If the work role relationships of coordinator, collaborator, and colleague are supported by the conceptual framework, in-service programs can teach nurses these roles and how they may be developed in agencies where these roles will be new ones for nurses to assume. Work role relationships are, to some degree, influenced by the degree of independence supported by the nursing service.

· · ·

A conceptual framework gives structure to the practice of nursing, enables it to be carried forward by a whole group in a unified way, and provides a basis for talking about, as well as practicing, nursing care and guidelines for evaluating that care.

Summary

This chapter provides the key hypotheses or theoretical constructs that form the premises on which the rest of the book is based. Management, in the final analysis, has the ability to bring together many areas of knowledge and skill into a unified set of behaviors that facilitate the movement of individuals, families, groups, and communities toward a goal. This role enactment presumes knowledge and skill in role learning and taking, in analyzing and organizing the components of life processes, and in theorizing, problem solving, and decision making. The ability to predict the consequences of a nursing act is one of the key cognitive processes of nursing problem solving. In other words, a predictive principle is a nursing action hypothesis and as such constitutes a limited nursing theory. The following five predictive principles summarize the conceptual framework of this book:

1. A clear operational definition of leadership/management facilitates role definition and enactment.
2. Eclectic selection and synthesis of the many components of the processes of life enable utilization of these components in a unique, effective leadership/management act conducive to an established goal.
3. Conscious role learning, role taking, and role enactment and a large role repertoire facilitate more effective and efficient role adaptation and perception and response to leadership/management role needs.
4. Skill in theory identification, selection, and building enables identification of the level at which individuals and groups are operating and facilitates the use of appropriate behaviors that will complete the theoretical progression toward a desired end.
5. Skill in the use of problem-solving facets and heuristics promotes more effective and appropriate decisions and ease in helping others in participatory decision making.
6. A clear conceptual framework provides cohesion and decision-making guidelines for the management of the nursing enterprise.

BIBLIOGRAPHY
Books

Atkinson, L., Murray, M.: Understanding the nursing process, New York, 1980, Macmillan Publishing Co., Inc.

Bevis, E.: Curriculum building in nursing: a process, ed. 3, St. Louis, 1982, The C.V. Mosby Co.

Bower, F.: The process of planning nursing care: a model for practice, ed. 2, St. Louis, 1982, The C.V. Mosby Co.

Bower, F., and Bevis, E.: Fundamentals of nursing: concepts, roles, and functions, St. Louis, 1979, The C.V. Mosby Co.

Bruner, J., Goodnow, J., and Austin, G.: A study of thinking, New York, 1956, John Wiley & Sons, Inc.

Burton, W., Kimball, R., and Wing, R.: Education for effective thinking, New York, 1960, Appleton-Century-Crofts.

Byers, V.: Nursing observation, Dubuque, Iowa, 1977, Wm. C. Brown Co.

Claus, K.E., and Bailey, J.T.: Power and influence in health care: a new approach to leadership, St. Louis, 1977, The C.V. Mosby Co.

Gagne, R.: The conditions of learning, New York, 1965, Holt, Rinehart & Winston, Inc., pp. 31-61.

Houle, C.: Continuing learning in the professions, San Francisco, 1980, Jossey-Bass.

Huckabay, L., and Dadenian, M.: Conditions of learning and instruction in nursing, St. Louis, 1980, The C.V. Mosby Co.

Johnson, M., Davis, M., and Lowbough, A.: Problem solving in nursing practice, ed. 3, Dubuque, Iowa, 1980, Wm. C. Brown Co.

Leavell, H., and Clark, E.: Preventive medicine for the doctor in his community, ed. 3, New York, 1965, McGraw-Hill Book Co.

Lewis, L.: Planning patient care, ed. 2, Dubuque, Iowa, 1976, Wm. C. Brown Co.

McDonald, F.: Educational psychology, Belmont, Calif., 1966, Wadsworth Publishing Co., Inc.

Pohl, M.: The teaching foundation of the nurse practitioner, ed. 4, Dubuque, Iowa, 1981, Wm. C. Brown Co.

Sarbin, T.R., and Allen, V.L.: Role theory. In Lindzey, G., and Aaronsen, E., editors: The handbook of social psychology, vol. 1, ed. 2, Reading, Mass., 1968, Addison-Wesley Publishing Co., Inc.

Smuts, J.C.: Holism and evolution, New York, 1926, Macmillan Publishing Co., Inc.

Strategy notebook, San Francisco, 1972, Interaction Associates, Inc.

Tools for change, ed. 2, San Francisco, 1971, Interaction Associates, Inc.

Whitehead, A.N.: Process and reality, New York, 1929, Macmillan Publishing Co., Inc.

Periodicals

Advances in Nursing Science, vol. 3, no. 3, 1981 (entire issue). (This periodical is given over to nursing education, professionalism, models and model building in nursing, cognitive learning and affective behaviors.)

Bavaro, J.: Questioning the key to learning, J. Nurs. Leadership and Management: Superv. Nurse, 1980.

Brown, B.: Follow the leader, Nurs. Outlook **28**(6): 357-359, 1980.

Chater, S.: A conceptual framework for curriculum development, Nurs. Outlook **23**(7):428-433, 1975.

Dickoff, J., James, P., and Wiedenbach, E.: Theory in a practice discipline. Part I. Practice oriented theory, Nurs. Res. **17**(5):415-435, Sept.-Oct. 1968.

Glatt, C.: How your hospital library can help you keep up in nursing, Amer. J. Nurs. **78**(4):642-644, 1978.

Hall, J., O'Leary, V., and Williams, M.: The decision-making grid: a model of decision-making styles, Calif. Manag. Rev. **7**(2):43-54, 1964.

Hibbert, J., Craven, R., and Blinski, J.: Instant problem solving, Nurs. Management **12**(12):37-38, 1981.

Katefian, S.: Critical thinking, educational preparation, and development of moral judgment among selected groups of practicing nurses, Nurs. Research **30**(2):98-103, 1981.

Kausch, J., and Rune, D.: Nurses' clinical judgment, Nurs. Manag. **12**(12):24-27, 1981.

Kissinger, J., and Munjas, B.: Nursing process, student attributes, and teaching methodologies, Nurs. Res. **30**(4):242-246, July-Aug. 1981.

Masson, V.: On power and vision in nursing, Nurs. Outlook **27**(12):782-784, 1979.

Mauksch, I.: Nurse-physician collaboration: a changing relationship, J. Nurs. Admin. **11**(6): 35-38, 1981.

Nugent, P.: Management and modes of thought, J. Nurs. Admin. **12**(2):19-25, 1982.

Trussell, P., Brandt, A., and Knapp, S.: Science as a way of knowing, J. Nurs. Admin. **11**(10):37-40, 1981.

Other

American Nurses' Association: Educational preparation for nurse practitioners and assistants to nursing: a position paper. New York, 1965, The Association.

Waters, V.: Address: Conceptualization for nursing practice, presented at Workshop: Conceptual frameworks for nursing, Calgary, Canada, July 1975, Institute of Nursing Consultants.

chapter two

Predictive principles
of management

Definition of terms
Definition of managerial terminology provides the learner with a basis for assimilating the concepts of management.

Organizational structure
Creation of an organizational system compatible with the philosophy, conceptual framework, and goals of the organization provides the means for accomplishment of purpose.

A working knowledge of types of health agencies in which the nurse-manager works determines the amount and degree of authority that can be delegated.

Understanding of the organizational structure as a whole facilitates development of roles and relationships enabling goal achievement.

Knowledge of earlier practices, values, and orientations of hospital nursing directors contributes to a better understanding of the contemporary role of the hospital nursing director.

Assessment of motivation toward management roles assists in selection of nurses who have potential as successful administrators.

The degree of fulfillment of an agency's mission for nursing reflects the nursing service administrator's use of power.

Recognition of a dual pyramid of power between personnel employed by the organization and independent individuals authorized to practice in the agency assists the nurse-manager in coping with the dual forces.

Operational strategies for effective management
Awareness of management theories allows the nurse-manager to determine appropriate management styles for the work setting.

Planning process
A statement of purpose for an agency, department, or group directs the individual involved in planning for achievement of purpose.

Management by policy, objectives, standards, procedures, and control establishes the framework for conformity to preestablished regulations.

The success or failure of plan achievement depends upon the degree of understanding of the system, and commitment and participation in the plan.

Budgetary process

Participation by nursing personnel in planning and controlling the budget leads to cost consciousness, increased awareness of activities, and increased cost effectiveness.

A budgetary process that functions on a planned, continuous, and cyclic basis offers participants an effective way to operate efficiently and to provide information for making future key decisions.

Coordination process

Coordination of personnel and services through intradepartmental and interdepartmental activities brings about a total accomplishment far superior to that possible through fragmentation of individual effort.

The span of control directly affects the size and complexity of the coordinating function.

Activities directed toward regulating, preventing, correcting, and promoting coordination provide a comprehensive and efficient approach to management.

Review of the utilization of the nurse-manager's time provides a means for comparison of role expectation and fulfillment.

The presence or absence of conflict influences a nurse-manager's ability to coordinate activity.

Unresolved conflicts regarding contractual agreements for jobs often requires negotiation of collective bargaining and the reality of a strike.

Controlling process

Contracting for accountability of services rendered identifies the scope and limitations of the nurse-manager's span of control and provides a guide for assessment of the degree to which the nurse-manager's responsibilities are being fulfilled.

Setting standards serves to clarify purpose and provides a gauge for controlling quality and quantity of services.

Governmental control on hospitals encourages and/or constrains patterns of care that patients receive thus requiring nurse-managers to have an understanding of the regulations.

Consideration of structural, process, and outcome standards as interrelational and interdependent serves to keep the management process balanced and in perspective.

Management is considered both an art and a science. It is viewed as an integrated system in which human and technical resources are mobilized to produce desired outcomes. Management is seen as a process that meshes tested theories with findings discovered through trial and error in the work arena. Many health care organizations or components of these organizations managed by nurses do not have preparation in management. Therefore the organization and management of the delivery of health care services are hampered in keeping pace with clinical advances.

The term "nurse-manager" applies at every level in nursing, whether as staff nurse, head nurse, supervisor, or administrator, and varies from direct care of clients to responsibility for those persons providing direct care. Management usually refers to those in some position of authority who direct their energies to manipulating, directing, and coordinating people, environments, finances, time, and materials in ways that will accomplish purposes and goals. Staff nurses often function in lower managerial positions. The most effective managers are those who can use the scientific, technical, and behavioral modes to the best advantages for client, worker, and organization. The best workers are those who know the role of lower and middle managers so that they can better enact the role of the managed.

The purpose of this chapter is to present theories, systems, and predictive principles of management that will enable the nurse functioning at any level of management to confidently and successfully assume responsibility and accountability for the management of quality care. Because of the magnitude of the problem, the staffing process is treated separately in the next chapter.

Definition of terms

A health care delivery agency's primary function is to provide services to the client for disease prevention, health maintenance, diagnosis, treatment, cure, or rehabilitation. These agencies are of many types, with objectives and methodology depending on major purposes of the organization. Although differences do exist, all organizations provide for the managerial role. Labels ascribed in organizations often become blurred for lack of definition. Even with explanation, it becomes apparent that there is much overlap in function between managerial roles. The reader is encouraged to study the terminology so that positions within the work setting can be clearly understood.

PREDICTIVE PRINCIPLE: Definition of managerial terminology provides the learner with a basis for assimilating the concepts of management.

> **Organization:** Efficient integration of subunits for the good of the whole. This purposeful structure and systematic arrangement of elements can be applied to an entity such as a hospital or other health agency or to a process. The administrative and functional structure includes relationships of people, departments, and work to each other and to the whole. Organization enables the health care delivery system, or health agency, to implement its philosophy and achieve its purposes.
>
> **Administration:** Comprehensive executive function; exercising organizational powers and duties, including setting goals, formulating policies, and establishing management procedures.
>
> **Administrator:** One who performs the executive or power-laden role of formulating policy and establishing broad goals for implementation and monitoring the overall process of an organization.
>
> **Management:** Process that takes place within the organization in accomplishing

institutional goals and specific purposes through the use of interpersonal and technical aspects.

Manager: One who has the official authority and responsibility for overseeing and directing the work of others by virtue of his or her position in an organizational structure. A manager gets the work done at the right time by the use of manpower and material resources. Managers implement policy, plans, and directives by motivating and managing themselves and other individuals and groups to obtain the money, materials, and environment to meet successfully both agency goals and worker's needs. Managers have official authority and responsibility but may or may not have the power to establish goals for their immediate territories. Managers create and maintain an environment so that other people can work efficiently in it. In some settings the administrator and manager are one and the same.

Leader: One who uses the processes of life to facilitate the movement of one or more persons toward the establishment and attainment of a goal. Leaders promote a climate of cooperation and respect so that the follower(s) will want to be influenced by them. Leaders usually hold their positions more through characteristics and behavior than through official designation. A leader has some charisma that makes others want to follow. A manager, on the other hand, is official, with a job description, designated responsibility, and a chain of command. A manager may be a leader and a leader a manager, but some managers are not good leaders and not all leaders are managers at all.

Levels of management: Organizational structure in nursing has levels. *Top level management* positions are responsible for overall operation of the organization. These people are directors of nursing services, usually with policy-making power. *Middle level management* positions usually direct the operation of several units within the organization. These people are often called supervisors and have the responsibility for coordinating activities and interpreting and implementing agency policy. *First level management* positions direct the operation of one unit or a part of a unit within a department and are concerned with delivery of care to clients. This could be such persons as the head nurse, team leader, or primary care nurse. They have as their major purpose control of the work environment.

Centralization and decentralization: These terms relate to levels of management and refer to the kind of decision making done at each level. In a *centralized* structure, most major decisions are made at the top level. This system is congruent with the scientific method of bureaucratic control. Large organizations in which nearly every decision must go through many levels are highly centralized. Centralization also results from the design of the organization itself. When operations are highly specialized and departments finely subdivided, decisions must be made by higher levels in the organization and rigid rules and regulations employed. No manager, any more than a single employee, is in a position to be independent. Because only a small part of the total job is done by one member of a unit, upper levels of management must oversee all functions to ensure cooperation and coordination. Alternatively, in a *decentralized structure*, considerable planning and activities take place at the direct care-giving levels under the overall surveillance of the organization. Managers are considered resource persons for striving to achieve results rather than authoritarian decision makers operating at the apex of a hierarchical structure. Through decentralization the interrelated resources of environment, materials, and people are divided into subsystems performing a part of a task, and all efforts are integrated to achieve the goals of the subgroup.

Decentralization is dedicated to the concept that management belongs at the ground level. This grass roots approach is checked closely against policies and regulations of the total organization. Emphasis on decentralization places a high value on the assertion of independence and the willingness to make decisions and to act without constant consultation with superiors. Decentralization generates a sense of local control and encourages initiative and change. There is a danger in decentralization because it may lead to fragmentation of effort. Unless controlled, each unit could operate primarily in terms of its own subsystem rather than in terms of the needs of the organization as a whole. The ideal situation is for an agency to combine the best of the two systems, which allows for orderly fulfillment of an agency's overall mission and provides for individual initiative and creativity among the personnel.

Organizational structure

What the employer expects from an employee is based on the policies or objectives that guide the enterprise as determined by the philosophy, or conceptual framework, and standards set by the organization. Most health institutions possess a common basis for existence: to serve the health needs of the public. This goal is reached in accordance with the type of health requirements of the agency's clients. Inherent in meeting health needs are (1) administering patient care, (2) educating health agency personnel and the public, (3) engaging in research, and (4) protecting the health of the public and employees. The type of nursing agency determines the major emphasis, for each kind of agency shapes or sets limits to the types of goals likely to prevail, although there will be much variation among agencies, even of the same type.

PREDICTIVE PRINCIPLE: Creation of an organizational system compatible with the philosophy, conceptual framework, and goals of the organization provides the means for accomplishment of purpose.

Organization comprises structure and process, which allow the health care delivery system to enact its philosophy and utilize its conceptual framework to achieve its goals. Organization refers to a body of persons, methods, policies, and procedures arranged into systematic process through the delegation of functions and responsibilities for the accomplishment of purpose. Organizations involved in health care delivery are many and varied. Most common are the hospital, which is the center of health care delivery in the United States, and health maintenance organizations. The latter are commonly referred to as

HMOs and have been in existence for a number of years. The Kaiser-Permanente Plan in California and the Health Insurance Plan of New York are examples. The federal government gave backing to this system of care in the 1970s by appropriating monies and formulating guidelines to provide for an HMO option in public and private health insurance plans throughout the United States. With cutbacks in funding in the 1980s, government support is drastically curtailed.

There are also nursing homes offering skilled, intermediate, and custodial care as well as group medical and nursing practices and clinics.

The degree of organization in health care delivery systems ranges from highly structured systems to loosely knit organizations bound by contractual and professional agreements. One of the more controversial aspects of leadership common to business, industry, government, education, and health care systems is the creation of the most effective organizational system for the enterprise.

Some behavioral scientists suggest that the simpler the structure in the organization, the better the outcome. They postulate that too much organization inhibits growth, creativity, and flexibility and often results in an authoritarian style of leadership. At the other extreme are countless organizations that have failed through too little rather than too much structure. The obvious goal is to develop an organizational policy that will allow structure to be designed to fit each particular setting, the unique clients served, and the type of care provided—in other words, the conceptual framework must be congruent with the organizational structure. This means the least structure possible to efficiently achieve goals.

PREDICTIVE PRINCIPLE: A working knowledge of types of health agencies in which the nurse-manager works determines the amount and degree of authority that can be delegated.

There are basically three types of health agencies—official, voluntary, and proprietary. Conceptual frameworks for nursing practice are influenced by the type of agency in which nursing is practiced.

Official agencies operate under federal, state, county, or city direction to provide health benefits for the large segment of the population covered in some way by legislation. Tax monies are the primary source of income. Examples of these agencies are Veterans Administration hospitals, city and county hospitals, city and county health departments, and the U.S. Public Health Service clinics.

Voluntary agencies are nonprofit groups that serve the public according to some special interest group or according to the availability of services to the public through other means. Voluntary agencies depend on monetary gifts for an important part of their capital and operating budget. Since money flows through a special interest group, voluntary agencies may be oriented toward service for a religious, ethnic, economic, or age group. Such orientations have goals that affect standards and techniques of care, priority of services, access to care, relations with other organizations, and directions and rate of development. Examples of these agencies are the Red Cross, Benevolent and Protective Order of Elks hospitals, and the Salvation Army.

Proprietary agencies are privately owned corporations operated for profit by independent owners. Many proprietary agencies receive supplementary funds through private and public funding for provision of health care, research, and special services and are in a position to provide financial assistance to eligible clients. The transplanting of human organs is an example of a service that is financially out of reach for the average citizen but can be made available by special grants or fundings.

The type of agency—official, voluntary, or proprietary—influences the following data:

1. Source of funds
2. Cost scales to clients
3. Organizational complexity
4. Number of constraints
   a. Legal
   b. Policy
5. Managerial flexibility and autonomy

PREDICTIVE PRINCIPLE: Understanding of the organizational structure as a whole facilitates development of roles and relationships enabling goal achievement.

Organizational structure refers to the process or way a group is formed, its channels of authority, span of control, and lines of communication. The establishment of formal organizational patterns through departmentalization and division of work is an attempt to provide orderliness in administration. A well-organized enterprise results in effective functioning through a breakdown of tasks so that each individual is responsible for and performs a specified set of activities. The successful accomplishment of organizational structure, then, makes it possible for an organization to achieve its purposes: (1) It lets members of the organization know what their responsibilities are so that they can carry them out, (2) it frees managers and workers to concentrate on their individual roles and responsibilities, (3) it coordinates all organizational activities so that there is minimal duplication of effort or conflict, and (4) it reduces the chances of doubt and confusion concerning assignments.

In small organizations with only a few employees the manager can verbally explain organizational relationships and changes in these relationships to employees as needed. In larger, more formally structured organizations, the chain of command is too complex for verbal communication alone; therefore an organizational chart is set up in which each position, department, or function is diagrammed and the relationships between them shown. The separate units of the organization usually appear in boxes, which are connected to each other by solid lines that indicate the official chain of command, or by broken lines to indicate an unofficial relationship.

Organizational charts have five major characteristics: (1) division of work, where each box represents an individual or subunit responsible for a given part of the organization's work load, (2) chain of command, with lines indicating who reports to whom and by what authority, (3) the type of work performed, indicated by the labels or descriptions for the boxes, (4) the grouping of work segments, shown by the clusters of work groups (departments, single units), and (5) the levels of management, which indicate individual and entire management hierarchy regardless of where an individual appears on the chart. While horizontal and circular charts may be used, the most common format for a large health facility to describe relationships is the vertical chart, constructed to reflect the hierarchical chain of command from the top down. *Hierarchy* refers to a body of persons or things organized or classified in pyramidal fashion according to rank, capacity, or authority, with authority assigned to vertical levels with offices ranked in grades, orders, or classes, one above the other. Those having the greatest decision-making authorization are at the top, and those with the least authority are at the bottom.

Fig. 2-1 is a typical agency organizational chart showing channels of authority and communication that progress downward from trustees or board of directors, through a chief administrative officer, to the directors of the various services performed in a health agency. The structure is designed to define the levels of management and to show the degree of centralization and decentralization of control for the coordination of all activities of the organization. The nursing services segment follows the same pattern of organizational structure as that established for the agency. Fig. 2-2 is a typical nursing organizational chart showing the lines of authority and the channels of communication from the director, chief executive officer of nursing, who is the top nursing administrative officer, through the various associate directors and supervision or middle management group, to the lower management or head nurses.

An organizational chart is meaningful only to the extent the system represented on paper is a reality. Its precision sometimes masks what is actually taking place in an institution. Hierarchies are far more complex than the average description would indicate. Most observers agree the dynamic levels throughout the hospital organization are those that occur through informal day-to-day interactions, not by periodic maneuvering of structural arrangements. Questions need to be addressed as to what degree is the formal organization consistent with what actually takes place, and to what degree does hierarchy obstruct or serve organizational purpose? Understanding of the organizational structure in which the nurse-manager works is vital in developing roles and relationships for goal achievement.

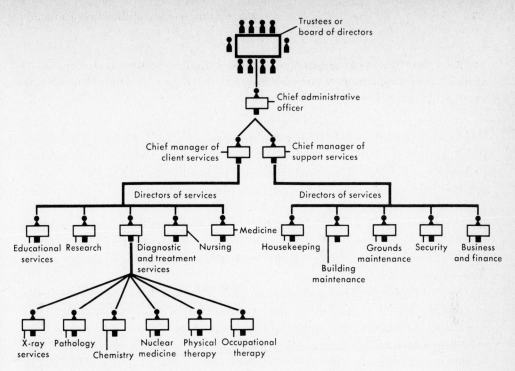

Fig. 2-1. Typical agency organizational chart with one example (diagnostic and treatment services) of complete hierarchy.

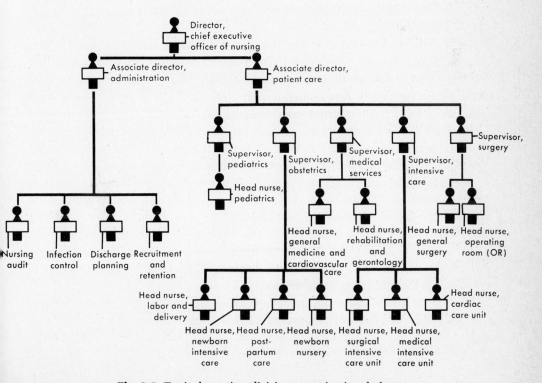

Fig. 2-2. Typical nursing division organizational chart.

PREDICTIVE PRINCIPLE: Knowledge of earlier practices, values, and orientations of hospital nursing directors contributes to a better understanding of the contemporary role of the hospital nursing director.

Directors of nursing service have held many titles over the years, with "superintendent of nurses" being the most popular. Eva Erickson,* professor emeritus from the University of Iowa College of Nursing, surveyed the literature pertaining to the role of the nursing service director from 1880 to 1980. She discovered that descriptions of the position of superintendent of nurses placed greatest emphasis on personal characteristics of the position holder (e.g., purity of character, a just and equitable temper). Isabel Hampton Robb (1907) remarked that a superintendent of nurses was expected to be a woman of executive ability, education, tact, refinement, and keen perception, with training in theory and in every practical detail of nursing.

Until the 1930s, most superintendents of nurses were managing schools of nursing as well as nursing service without benefit of formal training. They were held responsible for obtaining and training personnel, monitoring their activities, and meeting emergency needs and budget. Most nursing staff was comprised of students. The superintendent was on call 24 hours a day and in some institutions was expected to give nursing care to patients. Nursing superintendents functioned without direct input into organizational structure or management policy. In the 1920s and 1930s the superintendent of nurses had access to the board only through the superintendent of the hospital, to whom she was subordinate.

With the depression in the 1930s many training schools closed, leaving nursing administrators with more time to spend directing nursing service. On-the-job training was all that most administrators had as preparation for their roles, which obviously was inadequate to cope with the complexities of large and increasingly sophisticated organizations. In 1951 the Kellogg Foundation recognized the grave problems of nursing directors and provided funds for planning and implementing curriculum for their benefit in fourteen universities. Principles of general administration within nursing were studied. The Kellogg project identified criteria for the position of nursing administrator: (1) meeting people's total health needs, (2) developing co-workers' leadership abilities, (3) employing research methods in problem solving, and (4) continually evaluating the effectiveness of nursing care in relation to the objectives of the health agency and the nursing department. Even with formal preparation for their roles (fewer than 50% received this training), many nursing administrators had difficulty in coping with the demands of their jobs.

In the 1960s leadership behaviors were analyzed. Effective and ineffective behaviors in directors of nursing service were studied. The director was

---

*Erickson, E.: The nursing service director, 1880-1980, J. Nurs. Admin. **10**(4):6-13, 1980.

viewed as a person rarely seen by staff, but as one who provided leadership for the total administration of nursing service. She had little to do with direct patient care, professional organizations, or long-range planning. In 1964 the National League for Nursing (NLN) studied nursing services in more than 600 hospitals of over 200 beds. The directors had a median age of 48, with varied levels of preparation, many having diploma school as their basic preparation. Activities included coordination, communication, personnel and departmental planning, policies, formal reporting, and budget. In larger hospitals more of the nursing director's activities was executive, concerned with meetings, formal reports, organizational planning, and budget. About half the directors listed staffing problems as consuming most of their time, as well as those relating to standards, policies, and procedures for nursing care.

In 1970, Erickson, while at Teacher's College, Columbia University, polled almost 900 administrators of 200 to 2000 bed hospitals in the United States. He found that in small hospitals high priority was given to daily operations and activities. In hospitals of greater size, directors valued independence of action and creativity while under the continual pressure of deadlines. These administrators placed their priorities in order of: (1) budget, (2) philosophy, (3) objectives of nursing care, (4) organizational structure, (5) facilities and supplies, (6) personnel management, (7) policies and procedures, and (8) nursing care delivery. They listed nursing research and participation in professional organizations as important also.

Nurse administrators have come a long way since 1880. It is interesting to note the contrast in priority setting between those issues itemized by the Kellogg project in 1951 (meeting total health needs was number one), and those itemized by Erickson in 1970 (budget was number one with nursing care delivery last). Nursing administrators are working hard to establish and maintain quality nursing care but are often forced to limit their activities in favor of budget constraints. As the United States moves through recession in the 1980s, with drastic cuts in health, education, and welfare budgets affecting all levels of care, administrators are expected to have sufficient skill to meet the challenge. They need the administrative talent to protect the client as well as to maintain the integrity of the nursing profession, no small task.

PREDICTIVE PRINCIPLE: Assessment of motivation toward management roles assists in selection of nurses who have potential as successful administrators.

Although there is need for management skills in nursing, tools for selection of nurse-managers are inadequate. While all nurses are leaders, there is a distinct difference between the role of nurse-manager (head nurse, supervisor, coordinator, director of nursing services) and that of staff nurse. It cannot be assumed that a nurse who is highly skilled as a staff nurse and enjoys the role will be equally skilled as a manager or will enjoy that role.

Miner, a psychologist interested in management, has developed a theoretical framework based on six specific role prescriptions identified as essential for managing within a hierarchical organizational setting.*

1. A manager has positive feelings toward those in authority and works toward gaining their support.
2. A manager accepts challenge and competition.
3. A manager takes charge and behaves in an active and assertive manner.
4. A manager uses power over individuals under his or her direction.
5. A manager is willing to be in the spotlight to invite attention and dialogue with workers.
6. A manager accepts responsibility for accomplishing routine administrative functions.

These items identified as predictive factors for successful management should be of interest to administrators who are responsible for selecting nurse-managers. Determination of a nurse's attitude concerning these role prescriptions prior to appointment could be one means of assuring managerial success.

PREDICTIVE PRINCIPLE: The degree of fulfillment of an agency's mission for nursing reflects the nursing service administrator's use of power.

PREDICTIVE PRINCIPLE: Recognition of a dual pyramid of power between personnel employed by the organization and independent individuals authorized to practice in the agency assists the nurse-manager in coping with the dual forces.

Power is a dynamic element of human behavior in all organizations, even those that are committed to healing and preventing illness. Power is defined as one (or more) person's degree of influence over others, to the extent that obedience or conformity is assumed to follow. To be powerful one must have strength, force, and influence. Wieland and Ullrich† describe five categories of power: (1) *legitimate power*, which is authority to act by reason of one's role (e.g., "director of nurses," "head nurse," or "team leader"); (2) *reward power*, which occurs when an administrator uses positive reinforcers, such as behaviors (e.g., smiles, pats on the back, compliments) or money (bonuses or salary increases); (3) *coercive power*, which is the use of negative force, such as withholding benefits, punishing, or making threats; (4) *expert power*, which is based on specific knowledge or information (e.g., management expert, computer analyst, nurse-specialist); and (5) *referent power*, which relies upon appealing personal characteristics to make others want to be like the leader or to seek his/her approval. All

*Miner, J.: Twenty years of research on role-motivation theory of managerial effectiveness, Pers. Psychol. **31**(8):740, 1978.
†Wieland, G., and Ullrich, R.: Organizations: behavior, design, and change, Homewood, Ill., 1976, Richard D. Irwin, Inc.

of these types of power are acceptable and available to the nurse-administrator of a hospital.

Another form of power not as clearly defined is *associative power*. Wieland and Ullrich describe this power as coming from close alliance with a powerful influence or group. Perhaps the association of nurses with physicians best describes this relationship in hospitals. Nurses' salaries are paid by the hospital, and they are subject to the controlling governing board. Most physicians, on the other hand, have authorization to practice in the agency, but primarily control their own functions. The independent nature of this arrangement creates some problems, as the organizational pattern is literally a dual pyramid, sometimes with conflicting goals. Results of interaction in associative interrelationships are more uncertain than in clearly defined roles. The two groups interacting must utilize all types of power in reaching desirable decisions.

Qualified nursing administrators have position, knowledge, professional backing, and an organizational structure in which to carry forth their mission. Directors of nursing are in a unique place in the organizational structure of their hospitals. They are executives in some institutions, having the full title of "administrator of nursing services." In many other agencies the presiding nurse is an "assistant administrator," or "assistant," or "chief." It is how the administrator utilizes the institution's mission in planning, establishing communication networks, exercising power, and guiding the nursing staff in the delivery of patient care that spells success or failure. Doris England,* a nursing service administrator for several years, suggests four recommendations for nursing administrators:

1. *Set priorities of quality and patient needs first and staff numbers second.* Select the right nurses, give them appropriate orientation, set expectations at their level of expertise and allow them to use creativity and judgment in meeting individualized patient needs, and support continuing education.
2. *Take risks.* Try new methods and ideas; then incorporate them into formal job descriptions later if they work. Nursing in hierarchical structures more often than not fosters dependence and mediocrity. The nursing administrator needs to seek ways to reward innovation, creativity, and the independent spirit, for it is through this avenue that many beneficial changes are made. The administrator must take risks when negotiating additions, deletions, or changes in nursing services with board members, hospital administrators, medical personnel, and other power figures.

---

*England, D.: The strengths and weaknesses in nursing service administration, Nurs. Outlook **28**(9): 555-556, 1980.

3. *Develop an organizational style that is supportive and caring.* A demonstration of respect, honesty, and acceptance of individual differences reflects this humanistic approach.
4. *Lay biases to rest,* or at least recognize them and do not allow them to hinder progress and creativity. The nursing administrator may have feelings regarding styles of dress, conduct, preparation for nursing roles, etc., but unless they bear relationship to fulfillment of the agency's mission for nursing, recognize them for what they are and set them aside.

Nursing administrators without power or the willingness to use it lose the confidence and respect of nursing staff. Administrative nurses use their professional knowledge and skill to promote nursing goals in their respective settings.

Operational strategies for effective management

PREDICTIVE PRINCIPLE: Awareness of management theories allows the nurse-manager to determine appropriate management styles for the work setting.

Organizational theory emerged in the literature just before the turn of the twentieth century. Scientific and technical theories were studied first, followed by a focus on behavioral management.

Scientific approach. Most literature dealing with scientific management focuses on management in the general industrial setting.

Frederick Taylor and the Gilbreths were the first to attempt the study of management on a scientific basis. In the early 1900s, these scientists studied industry at the worker's level to prove that methods could be used to identify the best ways to accomplish a task and that people in work situations were important factors in the search for efficiency. Taylor looked on workers as automatons, but he did recognize that individual differences existed and needed to be considered in the total work situation.

The basic criterion of the scientific approach is to achieve maximum output with resources available through *planning, directing,* and *controlling.* The four pillars of classical organization used in the scientific approach are (1) *division of labor,* almost always occurring where there are numbers of people attempting to provide a service; (2) *span of control,* referring to the number of people who can effectively be managed; (3) the *scalar process,* separating tasks vertically into managerial levels, recognizing that with more decentralized span of control, more levels are required; and (4) *structure,* referring to the basic orderly arrangement of functions between management and staff personnel.

All theories of scientific management present their major goals as that of organizing to produce maximal output. Certain common elements appear: (1)

assumption of a hierarchical, bureaucratic model; (2) identification of the power structure with designated decision makers; (3) development of separate rules and regulations with detailed job specifications; (4) clear communication channels; (5) management by objectives providing the baseline for evaluation of outcomes; (6) equal treatment of all employees, with reliance on expertise relevant to each position; (7) a complete record-keeping system; and (8) a means for accountability.

Scientific theories provide excellent guidelines for general management in any organization. However, because of the nature of the product in health care systems, there is need for adaptation. For example, delivery of care must always take into account the total needs of the client, an area that presents difficulties in terms of maximal output with the least amount of services.

Behavioral approach. Behavioral science was begun seriously in 1927 with the Hawthorne studies. The first major attempt to understand the motivational processes of workers, it was geared toward the nonhuman element of work and was conducted by Elton Mayo,* then at the Harvard Business School. Experimenters found that workers worked harder and increased their productivity when supervisory pressure was reduced and they had no one watching their every move.

Douglas McGregor produced *The Human Side of Enterprise* in 1957, having thirty years of behavioral science progress as a resource. He proposed a set of assumptions about the nature of people, labeling them "theory X" and "theory Y."

Theory X contained traditional assumptions that people (1) consider work as a job to be done with no thought of pleasure; (2) are naturally lazy and prefer to do nothing; (3) work mostly for money and status rewards; (4) are productive in their field because they fear being demoted or fired; (5) are children grown larger and are naturally dependent on leaders; (6) expect and depend on direction from above and do not want to think for themselves; (7) need prodding and praise; and (8) believe adults remain static and resist change.

Theory Y proposed that workers are emerging individuals who are dynamic, flexible, and adaptive. Assumptions included in this theory were that people (1) are naturally active and enjoy setting goals and striving for their achievement; (2) seek many satisfactions in work other than money and status, in that they take personal pride in a job well done, enjoy the people and process, and are stimulated to new challenges; (3) produce in their desire to achieve their personal and social goals; (4) are normally mature beyond childhood and aspire to independence, self-fulfillment, and responsibility; (5) need understanding of the work scene and are capable of assessing what needs to be done and are able

*Mayo, E.: The social problems of an industrial civilization, Cambridge, Mass.: 1945, Harvard University Press.

to be self-directive; (6) understand and care about what they are doing and therefore can devise and improve their own methods of work; and (7) seek self-realization and are constantly striving to grow.

McGregor sought to prove the inherent complexity of human behavior and that people are not motivated by a single driving force. Instead, people move in and out of categories, seeking many satisfactions, and their needs change as they grow and develop.

In 1943 Abraham Maslow* outlined the elements of his overall theory of human motivation. It was not until 1962 that he personally began to study industrial relations. According to Maslow, although external forces or incentives can have an effect on motivation, real motivation is not something that is externally produced or imposed on human beings. Motivation is the state of being stimulated to take action in order to achieve some kind of goal or to satisfy some kind of need.

Maslow's theory of personality and motivation classifies human goals according to a conceptual hierarchy of needs. He bases his theory on the following basic concepts about human behavior:

1. Humans are wanting creatures; as soon as one need is met, another need will emerge to take its place.
2. Satisfied needs do not motivate or cause behavior; only unsatisfied needs cause an individual to move.
3. Needs of individuals can be thought of in a hierarchy of importance, each with its own rank and level of importance to the individual.

Maslow defines five levels in the need hierarchy:

1. Physiologic, the most important, taking precedence over all other needs if unsatisfied. Needs such as air, food, water, sex, and sleep are examples.
2. Safety, which includes physical as well as emotional needs and reflecting the need to feel secure from harm at home, at work, or in any other activity.
3. Social, which includes a desire to belong, to be loved, and to be accepted in all environments.
4. Esteem, representing the desire for achievement and status, with the needs to feel good about one's self and to gain esteem from others.
5. Self-actualization, reaching the point realizing all one's potential.

Relating Maslow's theory to the work environment can be done as follows: physiologic needs are satisfied by remuneration earned from working; security and social needs are met through a feeling of belonging, friendships, and status. Organizations recognize that most people who work are no longer trying

---

*Maslow, A.: Motivation and personality, New York, 1954, Harper & Row.

to satisfy primary or lower level needs. It is hoped that the work arena will provide opportunities for self-esteem and self-actualization.

In summary, the behavioral science approach stresses (1) the characteristics of a leader as a facilitator with respect to productivity and good management, (2) building morale and team spirit, and (3) motivation and self-development of employees through promoting work cooperation and communication. The premise is that when the employee is satisfied, the organizational goals will be met.

Although the behavioral approach contains many fine elements, some limitations are present in the system. Not all employees respond well to the individualistic approach and therefore they may not produce the desired results. Assuming that each participant will exhibit initiative and creativity, there is no means provided for the manager to deal with noncompliance.

Technical approach. Technology calls attention to the need for tools and techniques that link the whole organization together. All approaches to management incorporate a degree of this element. The tools and techniques of management planning, budgeting, control systems, information systems, and even management by objectives are examples of linking technologies. The pragmatic approach views the content of the work as the most important aspect. Attention is devoted primarily to quality and quantity of nursing care, with little focus on organizational structure and behavioral concerns of the staff. With the technical or functional approach, job descriptions and procedure manuals are highly in evidence. The nurse-manager serves as a practicing role model and may be highly esteemed because of demonstrated competence.

Although there are definite advantages to a skill-oriented approach, there is danger in substituting the practical "how to do it" method for basic understanding of why these techniques are successful or unsuccessful. In addition, the technical approach assumes that every problem can be clearly defined and solved. A problem arises if the defined technique or skill does not have the right variables or if the formula for work production proves ineffectual.

Modified technical-behavioral approach. There is no one best way to organize and manage a health care facility or any part of it. Management is a process, with organizational, technical, and interpersonal aspects. Selection of an organizational structure and management system that is right for an agency is crucial to efficiency and effectiveness of the organization. The structure and system selected must match the purposes and goals of the organization and be compatible with the needs of those charged with fulfillment of those purposes and goals. The consequences of an inappropriate structure and management system can be inefficiency, high cost, unrest, dissatisfaction, or even outright failure of the organization. Rarely is one structure or system used exclusively, and after selection there can be many changes, for organization is a dynamic

Table 1

Comparison of characteristics of bureaucratic and human relations approaches to organizational structure and management systems*

Bureaucratic approach (conservative, technical, scientific)	Human relations approach (democratic, participative, liberal)
Organizational control	Democratic or participatory control
Assures formal leadership appointed by head(s) of hierarchy	Leaders are approved by followers
One-way directions; nonquestioning obedience	Open, multidirectional communication system
Organization manipulates needs of employer and serves its goals; loyalty to organizational goals	Goals are consistent with individual goals; otherwise workers' first loyalty is to profession; second to organization
Workers at each level are viewed mechanically as objects to be used interchangeably to get work done	Workers are matched carefully with work assignment; value given to individualism, self-control, initiative, and creativity
Manager is a controller	Manager is a facilitator
Personnel are manipulated; management defines objectives	Natural work groups define own objectives
Class and class status structure leads to job satisfaction	Acceptance as part of a stable group leads to satisfaction
Physiologic factors (strength, speed, skill, etc.) produce fluctuations in production	Social conditions (acceptance, common interests, etc.) determine level of production
Workers relate to organization individually	Members of small groups relate to one another and then to the organization
Job fragmentation and specialization	Individual behavior is subject to the group
Economic factors are primary motivation; emphasis on quantity output within least amount of time	Social forces and quality of service are more important than economic factors

*One can readily see that parts of each system are present in any organized structure and management system.

process with continuous need for appraisal and adaptation. Table 1 compares the major characteristics of the bureaucratic and human relations approaches; each system is represented in the extreme.

Planning process

Health care facilities are in a particularly vulnerable position with respect to planning because they operate in an environment subject to social, economic, political, and technologic forces demanding almost continuous adaptation and change. Predictions cannot be made with assurance; however, planning must go forward. Planning can be defined as deciding in advance what needs to be done and how to do it. Planning includes the aspects of duration, function, and scope of operation. Planning involves analyzing relevant information from the past and present and using it to outline a course of action that enables goal achievement. The question facing the planner is "What has to be done today to be ready for tomorrow?" Planning in the simplest sense is a control system exerted before an action is taken. Planning is crisis prevention and is performed by all levels of management. Top level administrators engage chiefly in long-range planning to achieve organizational objectives. This usually includes comprehensive planning that will take one or more years to achieve. For example, an agency may decide to plan for the opening of a kidney dialysis center or to add an entire floor to the building for treating geriatric clients. Plans at this level are usually broad in nature and general in terms. Any long-term plan must be flexible, permitting change as conditions dictate. Influencing factors might be financial implications, new knowledge, or a change in the law or regulations.

Concomitant with top level management's concern for long-term planning is an interest in short-term goals. A well-run agency attends to policy, goals, and programs for implementation with a control system that sets target dates for assessment and accountability for both long- and short-range plans. Short-term objectives need to be replaced with new ones as soon as they are accomplished to ensure that efficiency and forward motion of the organization will occur. Similarly, the long-term plan cannot be alive, vibrant, and realistic except in account with the current progress. All objectives must fit into the overall philosophy, mission, and goals of the organization.

Planning is also engaged in at the middle and first (lower) levels of management within health care facilities. At these levels planning is more operationally oriented, aimed at achieving specific tasks effectively and efficiently. Appropriate planning provides nurse-managers with the tools necessary to control rather than to react to change. It enables nurse-managers to avoid routinely making crisis or stopgap decisions. Planning also enables the nurse-manager to manage with efficiency rather than with fear.

PREDICTIVE PRINCIPLE: A statement of purpose for an agency, department, or group directs the individual involved in planning for achievement of purpose.

The statement of purpose, mission statement, or philosophy describes the reason for being. It is an explanation of the system of beliefs that determines the way the purpose is achieved. A philosophy addresses those issues about which the group is concerned and decisions are required. A good mission statement is formulated when the nurse can supply positive demonstrations as to how the statement is actualized in the clinical setting. For example, if the statement is written "We believe that all persons should be admitted for treatment regardless of color or economic status," and it is discovered that delays occur with blacks and nonpaying clients, the philosophy as written has little meaning. If it is apparent that all eligible clients are admitted and treatment begun regardless of either of these contingencies, the stated philosophy has been put into practice.

A well-written philosophy stated in meaningful terms leads to the development of a conceptual framework, which in turn is a necessity for planning, organizing, implementing, and evaluating any operation. A philosophy for a health agency, department, or group is a statement or system of beliefs about their collective concerns for people and their responsibility to serve them.

A philosophy can be defined as a system of values or beliefs. All individuals have a personal philosophy that motivates their actions and determines how they manage their lives. Likewise, a nurse-manager of an organization or any part of it serves as a guideline for determining the quality of service to be rendered. The manager's patterns of beliefs, attitudes, and values set the tone for all relationships with clients, personnel, physicians, and community.

It is the manager's responsibility to get in touch with his or her own feelings, to guide the staff in understanding the purpose and philosophy of the agency in which they function, and to help them identify what it is they believe about the provision of nursing services in their respective settings. The conceptual framework commits the agency to respond to setting, clients, and professional factors and provides decision-making guidelines for all agency operations. These commitments need to be periodically reviewed to determine what is worth preserving and what is not and to be sure the staff members adhere to what they believe in their everyday organizational life and service to the clients. The following statements reflect purposes that are typical of voluntary agencies:

Patient services. The hospital is dedicated to provide high quality patient care economically. It will strive toward the ultimate objective of total service of the quantity, quality, and the types required to serve the best interests of the citizens of this community.

Education and research. The hospital provides qualified personnel to assure adequate patient care. Skilled educators recruit and educate (or reeducate) persons in specific work skills in order to meet and maintain hospital standards. The director of medical education, in conjunction with the various medical and nursing staff audit committees, constantly evaluates the quality of care and presents various educational programs to improve certain areas of patient care, as well as presents programs of emerging new methods of care. The hospital cooperates with educational institutions in making available its facilities for the clinical part of training health personnel. The hospital recognizes the need for scientific research and spearheads or participates in projects appropriate to this institution.

Community involvement. The hospital cooperates with health agencies within the community in offering programs emphasizing prevention, early detection, and treatment of illness. The hospital makes its auditorium and other such facilities available for those various health programs.

Responsibility to government. The hospital recognizes the increasing government involvement in health care and keeps abreast of their implications as they affect this hospital.

PREDICTIVE PRINCIPLE: Management by policy, objectives, standards, procedures, and control establishes the framework for conformity to preestablished regulations.

Some agencies operate under the simple plan of establishment of policy, objectives, standards, procedures, and methods. This plan is found primarily in hierarchical, bureaucratic structures. It is utilized in an effort to ensure consistency throughout the organization and to avoid the time and cost of constant review of management at the lower levels of operation.

Policy is formed at the top level and guides managerial thinking and action during the process of achieving objectives. Policy establishes broad limits and provides direction, but permits some initiative and individuality.

Objectives clarify what is to happen in behavioral terms. Often the people who are responsible for carrying them out become involved in their formulation. Objectives outline who, what, where, when, and often why an action is to occur.

Standards indicate the minimal level of achievement acceptable to meet the objectives. Standards are compiled by middle and lower levels of management primarily. For example, standards of care for a medical or surgical area are stated with input from nurse-coordinators, head nurses, their assistants, and staff, using quality assurance resources as a guide.

Procedures provide the direction for carrying out policy, standards, and objectives. They give guidelines for taking care of commonly occurring events. Procedures establish customary ways of handling specific, recurring activities, involving individual or group effort (e.g., committees, activities such as irrigations, instillations). For each procedure, a sequence of steps or operation is established.

Control serves as a regulating mechanism, with comparison of achievement made against standards and regulations. Control measures are usually established by the same persons or groups involved in the formulation of objectives, standards, and procedures.

An example is given below illustrating how policy, objectives, standards, procedure, and control are carried out for committee activity.

For committee activity: Patient Care Evaluation Program; Nursing Services Audit Committee*

Policy: Appropriate nursing committees shall be formed to assist in monitoring professional activities within the hospital.

Objectives: 1. To identify the patient's response (affect) to nursing intervention (cause) based on objective, predetermined criteria.

2. To obtain information indicating that current nursing practice standards are effective.

3. To communicate findings that indicate a need for change in existing practice through educational programs, procedure/policy changes, or development of practice standards.

4. To establish that current nursing practice is based on sound rationale that is capable of interpretation to the consumer.

5. To assist the practicing nurse to actively participate in setting care standards for improved patient care when necessary.

Standards: The committee shall adhere to quality assurance guidelines accepted by the hospital's Quality Assurance Committee.

Procedure: 1. One registered nurse from each patient care unit will be selected by the staff with the approval of the Head Nurse to represent the staff. An alternate representative also will be selected.

2. The Nursing Audit Coordinator for the Nursing Education Department will function as the liaison between the Nursing Services Department and the Medical Education Department.

3. Written patient responses and other data will be reviewed using the objective, predetermined criteria.

4. Achievements, failures, omissions, or need for improvement will be identified and action taken as deemed appropriate to improve patient care.

Control: Objective, predetermined criteria for evaluation will be employed in all committee activity.

PREDICTIVE PRINCIPLE: The success or failure of plan achievement depends upon the degree of understanding of the system, and commitment and participation in the plan.

Problems with plan achievement are generally caused by weaknesses in the participants and are not inherent in the system. The system most commonly fails because of lack of participation or commitment, poor monitoring, ignored feedback, too little coaching and assistance, insufficient planning to reach objec-

---

*Adapted from manuals of The Good Samaritan Hospital of Santa Clara Valley, San Jose, California.

tives, overemphasis on objectives rather than perspective of the whole system, omission of review, and inability to delegate. There are, however, several assumptions made concerning management by policy, objectives, standards, procedures, and control that are significant to success:

1. The system presumes that policies, objectives, standards, procedures, and control measures are in the best interest of the institution it serves.
2. Better planning occurs, in that the entire organization focuses attention on goal setting and plans to achieve those goals.
3. There is individual commitment and participation.
4. There are provisions for establishing motivation toward organization objectives, self-fulfillment, internal satisfaction, and successful accomplishment.
5. There is common ground and feelings of acceptance and security for widely different personalities.
6. There is recognition of the need to change traditional power structures through definition of the individual's authority, delegation, and self-control.
7. Authority is delegated along with responsibility.
8. Self-control replaces control imposed by outside forces.
9. Interaction among all branches of the organization is aided upward, downward, and laterally through a more effective communication system.
10. The organization maintains a clear identity under constant change, as objectives serve as a compass to properly direct effort and to offer standards for measuring progress.

Health organizations that have successfully implemented a sound, workable system agree that the benefits are many. The system allows for setting specific goals for a given time period by the persons engaged in the tasks, assessment, coordination, and collaboration between agency and personnel and affords a high-level sense of accomplishment by the membership.

Budgetary process

A budget is a plan that expresses the activities of a health care facility or unit in terms of dollars and covers a specific period of time. A budget is a forecast of anticipated operations. As such, it can never be definitive or absolute. The purpose of the budget is to set operating cost limits. It is a guide to performance, for although the budget includes costs of personnel, supplies, support services, travel, and buildings, it is essentially a commitment to the people who utilize the resources offered.

PREDICTIVE PRINCIPLE: Participation by nursing personnel in planning and controlling the budget leads to cost consciousness, increased awareness of activities, and increased cost effectiveness.

Operation of the nursing department or unit represents a large portion of a health agency's total expenses. Hospital management is becoming acutely aware of the importance of effective planning and the use of greater control in providing a sufficient number of appropriately prepared personnel and adequate facilities at minimum cost.

The effective nurse-manager recognizes that producing good nursing care can be strongly affected by the nurse's concept and practice of fiscal management. Nurse-managers who are aware of the procedure for budget planning and control can participate intelligently and can compete for the share of the budget necessary for their anticipated client care operation.

Successful planning for control of budget requires top level management participation and approval. But all levels of management should understand and participate in both the planning and control phases as well, and a clear report system must be established, with specific target dates for accountability.

There are several advantages in involving nurse-managers in preparation of the budget. By looking intensively at activities and results from past expenditures, they are better able to modify future plans and objectives to increase cost effectiveness. Also, personnel who operate within a budget become cost conscious and begin to assign different priorities to the use of resources. They look for better and more efficient ways of delivering health care services to clients. In management by objectives, both setting of realistic objectives and the ability to obtain them are closely tied to budgets.

Nurse-managers who want to learn how to prepare and control budgets well may do so within the agency through guidance from experts, reading about budgeting process in material geared toward health care delivery system management, and taking courses of instruction concerned with budgetary planning. When nurses demonstrate their interest and competence in fiscal matters, they will have a better chance to be included in all aspects of the budgetary process, thereby becoming more efficient at realizing dreams and ideas about improved nursing services.

PREDICTIVE PRINCIPLE: A budgetary process that functions on a planned, continuous, and cyclic basis offers participants an effective way to operate efficiently and to provide information for making future key decisions.

The usual method for budget planning and monitoring the system is as follows: (1) determine requirements, (2) develop a plan, (3) analyze and control the operation, and (4) review the plan. The entire process functions on a continuous and cyclic basis, usually over a calendar year.

Determine requirements. Top level managers usually assume responsibility for forecasting the needs for a new fiscal year. They do this by looking at major factors such as past experience and records, considering any changes such as closing or opening facilities or services, and studying anticipated population changes, needs for services, and any regulating changes that might occur as a result of policy change or legislation.

Ideally, these projections are reviewed with middle and first level managers to determine what the effect will be on departmental activity. It is at this time that needs for staffing, equipment, supplies, and facilities are scrutinized and requested. Once needs are assessed, cost studies of these needs are done; for example, the costs of supplies, manpower, equipment, and support services are estimated and allowances provided for the rate of inflation.

Develop a plan. Each manager, usually at the middle level, develops a budget for his or her area of responsibility, for each quarter of the ensuing year, with the first quarter broken down into months. The established objectives are an integral part of the budget plan. The nurse-manager can set up simple graphs and charts to help control expenses on a day-to-day basis and contribute to cost containment. Business personnel are usually available to provide assistance in the formulation of such plans as needed. There is an increasing use of computer printouts to apprise the nurse-manager of cost appropriations, expenditures, and whether or not the budget is on target or over or under projections. The astute nurse-manager will utilize this resource. Use of the support system of the budgetary department not only offers educational benefits, but the nurse increases credibility in the eyes of the budgetary personnel, making routine inclusion of the nurse in the planning stage more feasible.

The items most common to health care budgets are personnel and operating expenses. Unfortunately, many nurse-managers deal only with the category of operating expenses. The significance of this matter is discussed in Chapter 3 on staffing.

Numbers and kinds of *personnel* and salaries and wages for each job classification reflect any anticipated changes in the upcoming year. These costs include employee payroll, provision for overtime, taxes, and fringe benefits. In order to accurately calculate these costs, the number of clients and the level and skill of the workers necessary to provide care for them must be determined. For example, for coverage to be sufficient it must be recognized that nurse, practical nurse, nursing assistant, and orderly ratios are directly related to the kind of care required by clients.

For *operating expenses*, each department or unit lists supplies by major types, determined on the basis of usage anticipated through the coming year rather than on purchases. Examples of items that may be included in the operating budget are medical and surgical supplies, repairs and maintenance, provision for depreciation and replacement, office equipment and supplies, reference books and periodicals, and appropriation for in-service education. Most budgets

MONTHLY RESPONSIBILITY SUMMARY
[computer print-out]

Area of service	Month	Year	Nurse manager							
				Current period			Year-to-date			Prior year		
Items budgeted	Actual	Budget	Variance	Actual	Budget	Variance	Actual	Budget	Variance	
Salaries										
Management										
R.N.										
L.V.N.										
Aides										
Orderlies										
Clerical										
Total wages										
F.I.C.A. taxes										
Vacation pay										
Group health insurance										
Group life insurance										
Pension and retirement										
Workman's compensation insurance										
Holiday pay										
Sick leave										
Surgical packs; CSS sterilizer										
Surgical supplies, general										
IV solutions										
Pharmaceuticals										
Other medical care supplies										
Office/administration supplies										
Instruments/minor equipment										
Repairs and maintenance										
Depreciation/equipment										
Equipment rental										
Telephone										
Training sessions; books										
Travel										
Dues and subscriptions										
Other expense										
TOTAL EXPENSE										

Fig. 2-3. Example of a form in which monthly expenditures for an area of responsibility can be logged.

do not include consideration of utilities and housekeeping, since they are considered part of the indirect expenses. However, an accounting is shared with the nursing department or unit so that its members may be aware of the cost and assist with the control of these items to reduce waste and unnecessary expenditure.

Analyze and control the operation. Each level of management is held accountable for performance and corrective action. This accountability extends only to the costs the nurse-manager directly controls. The reporting system is based on the organizational structure of the individual agency.

The most effective system is to have a two-way flow of information between middle and top management with material distributed on a monthly basis for use in analyzing actual activity. Fig. 2-3 illustrates how budgetary responsibility can be assumed. Nurse-managers are provided computerized statements each month indicating the items for which they are responsible, the current period of budget, and how much has been spent, with an indication of variance (over or under the budget). They are also given the year-to-date analysis, along with a comparison of the previous year's budget.

Review the plan. As the health agency and various components within the facility move through the fiscal plan for the year, each succeeding quarter is evaluated on the basis of current results. As each current quarter comes to a close, it is necessary to formulate a definitive plan for the upcoming quarter. Minor modifications are made in comparison with projections and actual occurrences. No major changes are made without going through the entire budgetary process.

Toward the end of the year the budgetary cycle is begun again. As the nurse-manager gains more experience with the planning cycle, more accurate forecasting results. An effective system of planning and controlling results in benefits of efficiency and cost savings, with provision of vital information necessary for making future key decisions. With such a plan the goal of providing quality care at minimum cost can be attained.

The nurse-manager who has sufficient information can identify problem areas and unfavorable trends concisely and can initiate corrective action where necessary. If there are significant variations from the plan, an explanation indicating the nurse-manager's assessment as to possible causes of the expense variances needs to accompany the report. Of course, any noticeable deviation will be discussed with appropriate controllers at the time of the expenditure to determine if on-the-spot remedial steps are needed.

Coordination process

Coordinating is an essential part of managing. It is the orderly synchronization of individual efforts with respect to their amount, time, and directions, so that unified action is channeled toward the attainment of stated goals. The coordinating function helps the nurse-manager to ensure that all important activities are accounted for and assists in the identification of overlap, duplication, or omissions of function. Coordination pulls together all activities to make possible both their working and their success. In health care facilities, there is great diversity among workers and activities. To achieve coordination with minimal friction and maximal effectiveness, each member is helped to see how his or her work benefits the total enterprise.

It is important to keep in mind that the fundamental principles of management are interrelated. Mission, goals, policies, and standards affect planning, and planning affects organizational structure. Coordinating activities becomes a natural outgrowth of all these functions, for they are inextricably interwoven.

PREDICTIVE PRINCIPLE: Coordination of personnel and services through intradepartmental and interdepartmental activities brings about a total accomplishment far superior to that possible through fragmentation of individual effort.

Coordination of personnel and services within a health agency cannot be confined to a single area or a particular function. Overall collaboration must occur vertically and horizontally among departments to keep the viewpoint of management broad and to foster a desired balance among various interrelated efforts. These controls provide a better means for (1) keeping the coordinating efforts adapted to the goals of the institution, (2) appreciating functions of other departments in order to better understand individual operations, (3) measuring the total effort of nurse-managers rather than assessing the work of a single manager, and (4) maintaining a control system for assessing the delivery of care to decentralized units.

Coordinated efforts at all levels can offer many benefits through planned and informal contact. Help can be forthcoming for problems with planning, staffing, and other aspects of nursing management. Greater knowledge and appreciation of the work of other nurses in the agency can be realized. Meeting with representatives from allied services on a regular basis can help to apprise the nurse-manager of the comprehensive range of services available that might better be utilized in coordinating work at the operational level.

By reaching out to others for information and support the nurse-manager becomes a more effective coordinator. Ongoing efforts can be improved. Accumulation of new knowledge will stimulate innovation of techniques. Behaviors will be changed, creating environments where work can be accomplished with efficiency and satisfaction never before thought possible.

PREDICTIVE PRINCIPLE: The span of control directly affects the size and complexity of the coordinating function.

Span of control is a major concern in coordination because of the impact on how many and what categories of personnel are required to achieve the desired goals. There are some nurse-managers who have a centralized or wide span of supervision, ranging from coordination of all nursing services in an agency (nursing director) to responsibility for entire floors or clusters of units (clinical coordinators or supervisors). Others manage groups of specialty areas, such as coronary care or maternal-child care.

An organizational approach that has received much attention, with varied results, is unit management. Unit management programs appoint a nonnurse unit or ward manager to relieve nursing personnel of many of their nonnursing activities and free them to provide client care. This concept, properly adapted to a hospital or agency setting, has been shown to be an effective productivity improvement technique for nursing, although it has not proved to be cost beneficial for the hospital or agency as a whole. Unfortunately, if not properly implemented, the program can easily fail. In the majority of cases, unit management has been successfully implemented and its nursing benefits realized.

Decentralization in large-, small-, and medium-sized agencies is a valuable tool that allows nurse-managers to fulfill their responsibility for providing personalized, competent care to clients through coordinated efforts. For best results, coordinating efforts should be made by a person at the lowest organizational level who possesses ability, desire, and access to relevant information and who is in a position to impartially weigh all factors. When a nurse-manager coordinates the unit within his or her realm of specific responsibility, all personnel can be supervised and are accountable to the manager.

PREDICTIVE PRINCIPLE: Activities directed toward regulating, preventing, correcting, and promoting coordination provide a comprehensive and efficient approach to management.

Managerial activities are varied and complex. The effective nurse-manager wants to (1) use planning strategies that will ensure smooth operations on the job while looking to the future, (2) organize the unit or department for maximum productivity, (3) utilize staff in a way that matches the tasks with talent, (4) delegate functions intelligently, (5) attend to employee needs and development, (6) motivate staff to perform to their maximum potential, (7) use leadership behaviors appropriate for the situation, and (8) adopt control methods that continually compare actual results with previously determined goals.

Skill and experience in problem solving and decision making are required for successful coordination. The heart and quality of operation are found in the nurse-manager's ability to assess needs for nursing service and to set in motion the activities that will meet those needs. In the decision-making process the nurse-manager recognizes the importance of assembling available information. The magnitude of data flowing through most agencies defies description, but it must be reviewed and processed. Provision of health care requires attention to the needs of daily living as well as the voluminous services necessary to prevent illness, promote and maintain health, and restore and rehabilitate the client. Data processing systems have had a definite effect on decision-making responsibilities. Computers can relieve nurse-managers of making decisions concerning staffing, budget, and some personal assignments, allowing the capabilities of the nurse to be used for more client-centered activities.

Another major approach in decision making is concerned with the communication system and the maintenance and improvement of human relations. The average nurse-manager spends about 80% of the time speaking, writing, reading, or listening. The ability or inability to communicate well with others and to determine which person or group should take part in the activities experts a powerful influence on whether or not coordinative efforts are successful.

Although information gathering and communication are important, underlying the entire effort is a need to understand the policy-making and policy-implementing systems of the organization. The nurse-manager will understand how influence is exerted and will have a frame of reference for coordinating activities.

Georgopoulos and Mann* have identified four types of coordination: (1) corrective, defined as those activities that correct an error or repair a malfunctioning or dysfunctioning system (this includes equipment or personnel); (2) preventive, which anticipates problems and coordinates efforts to prevent or reduce the impact of the problem; (3) regulative, defined as those coordinative activities that maintain the ongoing, day-to-day activities; and (4) promotive, interpreted as functions directed toward improving existing circumstances irrespective of identified problems. The basic premise is that there is a constant need for improvement. The most effective manager views coordination as an integrated system. If one phase of activity is weak or nonfunctioning, the output of the whole unit or department suffers. A successful coordinator translates this knowledge into practice.

Inclusion of preventive and promotional aspects in coordinating efforts provides higher quality care more efficiently and with greater cost effectiveness than if reliance is solely on coordination through regulatory and corrective activities.

PREDICTIVE PRINCIPLE: Review of the utilization of the nurse-manager's time provides a means for comparison of role expectation and fulfillment.

Using time effectively is a challenge to every manager. Nurse-managers in a health care facility are very often under pressure and are so involved in the day-to-day operation that they sometimes fail to see the relevant issues. Managers who have a heavy work load find it difficult or impossible to stop what they are doing and take stock of the work process. They often complain that time is

---

*Georgopoulos, B.S., and Mann, F.C.: The community general hospital, New York, 1962, Macmillan Publishing Co., Inc., pp. 277-278.

wasted on telephone calls and myriad other interruptions that keep them from doing their job. Surprisingly few nurse-managers can explain what their job is and how they spend their days. They move about exclaiming, "There never is enough time," or "I can't seem to get everything done." Each day they leave their jobs feeling frustrated that their work is unfinished. In contrast, observers might describe the manager as frittering away time on trivial details.

For effective control, it is essential for a nurse-manager to recognize the importance of time-use control. Four approaches to improved time-use control by the nurse-manager can be employed: (1) use of assistants to protect against time wasters, (2) primary use of the manager's time for major decision-making efforts, (3) collection of time data on current activities and evaluation, and (4) improvement of methods of time utilization.

A good assistant (ward clerk or secretary) can help the nurse-manager save time. This assistant can take care of the endless paper work, deal with the public, help in working out problems of other health professionals and ancillary personnel, and screen telephone calls. The key to relief through this avenue is in employing a capable person, training the person well for the job, and then vesting the authority to do the job without need for sanction from the nurse-manager concerning every detail.

The concept of using the major share of the nurse-manager's time for major decision making is sound in that the manager is employed for expertise in managing nursing services and for clinical expertise. It is logical to assume that the nurse-manager can better forecast the effect of alternatives in decision making when the major considerations are the care of clients and the implications of those decisions.

For nurse-managers to recognize time-use controls in their work, they need to collect facts concerning present time utilization. Keeping a daily log by 15-minute intervals is recommended for this purpose. The log should show what activity is performed, whether or not it is basic to the manager's role, and the significance in terms of priority. Recording such information for a period of one month provides a reasonable sample. Study of such data could reveal that, in fact, the nurse-manager's time is put to good use and that there is an overload of responsibility. The data could also reveal what the time robbers are, what nonessentials should be eliminated, and what improvement can be made. Sharing the findings with other nurse-managers can prove beneficial as well.

PREDICTIVE PRINCIPLE: The presence or absence of conflict influences a nurse-manager's ability to coordinate activity.

Conflict occurs where there is a struggle between interdependent forces. A controversy or disagreement exists in desires or opinions. Organizational conflict is both desirable and useful if maintained at a functional level. Most health care organizations experience a high level of conflict because there is much interfacing of roles and function, each dependent on the other. Clients are becoming very aware of their "rights" and of ways to achieve them. Nurses are giving more attention to such matters as patient advocacy, systems of care, salary, and benefits. Administrators, medical and nursing staff, and ancillary personnel are encountering an increasing amount of conflict as they seek to understand and to meet the expectations of the others. How conflicts in these kinds of interactions are managed determines positive or negative outcome. The good manager seeks to identify potential and actual points of friction in the organization and to determine whether they are the result of poor organizational design, personality problems, or problems with delegation and follow-up procedures.

Prior to the mid-1940s almost all management people looked on conflict as destructive and something to be avoided. Managers were trained to establish and maintain predictable patterns, with little or no allowance for individual reaction to the system. This traditional approach to social interaction has gradually given way to a recognition and acceptance of conflict as a way of life. The behavioral approach calls for rationalizing the existence of conflict, looking to the reasons why individuals and groups behave negatively, and focusing on the development of resolution techniques through which positive action can emerge.

Interactionists carry the behavioral approach even further. They recognize the absolute necessity of conflict to stimulate the search for new methods or solutions. They believe that conflicts are usually distributed along the continuum between a level of conflict that may be too high and require reduction and a level of conflict that may be too low and need stimulation before the individual or group becomes inept with regard to performance.

Human conflict arises at the intrapersonal, interpersonal, and intergroup levels. *Intrapersonal* conflict is that dissention within one's self regarding a troubling issue. Examples are a nurse who has seen a peer give a wrong medication and who has not reported the incident or one who consistently gives less than adequate care to clients for lack of sufficient staff and supplies.

Interpersonal conflict happens between two or more persons. Common examples are those differences of opinion between nurse-managers and members of the work force. The group, for instance, may believe it necessary to meet a client's need by assigning someone to be at his side constantly; the nurse-manager may think this action unnecessary. Or several members in the work group may perceive that one member is failing to carry her load.

Intergroup conflict takes many forms, depending on the interdepartmental interaction. Dissention commonly occurs between caregivers and servicing units such as the dietary department, laundry, pharmacy, or x-ray department. Conflict is also an ever-present possibility between nursing units or nurse and physician groups within the organization.

Sources of conflict usually focus on role expectations, value systems, and communications. Characteristics of social relationships that are associated with various kinds or degrees of conflictive behavior are as follows:

1. Unclear boundaries of responsibility (job descriptions, assignments)
2. Conflicts of interest (nurse-manager interested in providing comprehensive care to the clients through primary care system and staff preferring functional system)
3. Communication barriers causing misunderstandings (evening versus night shift; language problem)
4. Dependency of one party or group on another (client at the mercy of staff for positioning; nurses waiting for housekeeping services)
5. Organizational structure related to the number of organizational levels and the number of job specialties represented (aide, LPN/LVN, ADRN, BSRN, nurse-specialists, or nurse-practitioners) and the degree to which labor is divided in the organization
6. Decision-making process (nurse-manager "tells" staff what they will and will not do about all activities)
7. Need for consensus (all parties believe they must agree on all decisions)
8. Behavior regulation (arrive at work on time, take breaks on schedule, adhere to a dress code)
9. Unresolved prior conflicts (resentful RN member who was not chosen to become nurse-manager; attitudes about what kind of care should be given versus what care is given)

These situations need not lead directly to conflict, but they have a high potential for doing so, thus influencing the coordination of activities. The direction taken depends on the perception of the conditions that exist and the attitude of the persons involved.

Not all conflicts are the same kind. There are basically those forms of conflict that follow definite rules (competitive) and those that are typically associated with angry feelings (disruptive). A third kind of conflict (constructive) uses open and honest dialogue to examine ideas until decisions are produced that are satisfying to all the participants.

American society generally subscribes to *competitive* behavior. A misinterpretation of Darwin's notion of survival of the fittest has led to individuals and groups competing with each other from the time they are able to react until life ends. Successful people, or "winners," receive the prize, and failures, or "losers," suffer the pain of defeat. It is argued that competition strengthens performance and increases cohesiveness within each individual group, and this does happen. After the competition is over, however, only one person or group is the winner and likely to remain satisfied and cohesive. The defeated individual or group may seek an opportunity for retaliation.

Consider the following situation. Two nurse-managers share a concern about a more than usual degree of dissatisfaction expressed by clients on their evaluation of care received during hospitalization. A plan was formulated and put into effect by the nurse-managers whereby evaluation forms would be tabulated, compared, and posted publicly in the agency's newsletter. Each group was presented the plan and agreed to work hard to "win." But the competitive scheme backfired. The winning group enjoyed having their achievements published as being the "best" caregivers and felt cohesive and positive about their efforts. The "losers" were saddled with a label of failure and inadequacy, when in fact they believed they had provided excellent care that was not recognized for a number of legitimate reasons. This competitive situation ceased to be motivating and moved into disruptive conflict.

In *disruptive* conflict the intent is on reducing, defeating, harming, or doing away with the opponent. In the foregoing situation, members of the "losing" group shared their disgruntled feelings with each other interdepartmentally, during breaks, and in their daily on-the-job contacts. They used such tactics as rationalization ("If they had as difficult patients as we had to cope with, the results would have been different"), accusation ("They must have set the patients up to responding well for them"), and blame ("If so-and-so had worked harder, we would have gotten higher marks," or "If the administration had sent us enough help, we would have won").

In both competitive and disruptive conflict, there exists a win-lose situation, for only one person or group can emerge the victor.

There is a great deal of consistent evidence to suggest that cooperative effort results in reduction of conflict and therefore becomes *constructive*. When interdependent individuals cooperate in working toward the goal of quality client care, there is greater interest in the task, production is increased, and the clients and workers are more satisfied.

Strategies used by nurse-managers to handle conflict are either restrictive or constructive. The *restrictive* procedure is aimed at creating a situation where there are as few differences as possible or, if differences exist, they are not recognized. Soothing platitudes are offered: "We don't need to worry about that; it doesn't matter." The staff are picked because they agree to be followers of direction. "Whatever you say" depicts the general attitude. Were this situation totally possible, individual and group actions would be quite predictable. One danger of smoothing over conflicts is that individuals and groups could fall into complacency. If everyone agrees to the same thing with no challenge, little thinking is going on, and quality of service rapidly deteriorates. More important, the soothing strategy is short lived, as strife will emerge in one form or another and must be handled.

Repression is another restrictive strategy. It is a "put-the-lid-on" approach. Leadership is aimed at punishing those who disagree and rewarding those who comply. The repressive climate overly stresses the organizational values of cooperation and framework, facing the danger of stifling individuality and creativity. "Those are the rules," "Do it because I say so," and "What you think doesn't matter" describe the prevailing attitude. The environment is so tightly controlled that latent ideas are curtailed. One problem with repression is that resentments are generated, and the workers punish or retaliate in ways such as procrastinating, doing a poor job, or taking sick leave.

The use of confrontation can also be restrictive in nature if the competitive "win-lose" approach is taken in which the individual or group seeks to gain as much as possible. Reaching a solution to a problem by an arbitrary decision, compromise, or majority vote results in losses for both sides. With this "lose-lose" strategy, differences are not dealt with and may fester again at other places, at other times, and in other forms.

Facilitating dispute resolution through the strategy of participative or integrative decision making takes a *constructive* approach. Participative effort implies the expectation of a "win-win" outcome or acceptable gain to both parties or groups.

Thomas Jefferson articulated the notion that power can be participated in by all the people in the social system. In 1820 he said, "The only safe depositor . . . is in people themselves." In the participative model, employers and workers try to produce the best result for all. It is a "both/and" system rather than an "either/or" system, thus creating a "win-win" possibility. The participative group requires (1) clear definition of values, purpose, and goals; (2) open and honest communication of information; (3) a sense of responsibility shared by all who participate; and (4) an environment of trust and commitment of all to the success of the process.

Suppose for a moment that conflict has arisen among a care-giving group. They meet together in the conference room. The problem is introduced. Two points of view are offered in the form of a thesis and an antithesis. Through open and honest dialogue the ideas for and against possible solutions are listened to and synthesized until they become integrated. The answer to the problem is one of higher quality than any one person could possibly have arrived at alone, the wisdom of the group becoming greater than that of the individual.

In the decision-making process, a constant effort exists at all levels to treat conflict and conflict situations as problems subject to the problem-solving methods. A clash of ideas is encouraged and little energy is spent in conflict over interpersonal difficulties because they will have been generally worked through as they have arisen.

Basic beliefs are necessary for integrative decision making to occur. Those in conflict must believe that (1) there is a mutually acceptable solution to the problem, (2) the mutually acceptable solution is desirable, (3) others' statements are legitimate and truthful, and (4) differences of opinion are helpful.

A constructive format for the nurse-manager to implement when conflict is present or anticipated is as follows:

1. Program a special time for meeting all persons involved in the disagreement, making sure that there will be time to discuss the issue and that there will be no interruptions.
2. Present the problem and have people give full expression to both positive and negative feelings. (As this happens more often, positive feelings will increase and negative ones will decrease.)
3. Use a paraphrasing ground rule, that is, when A says something to B, B cannot respond until A is satisfied. State what is heard and the feeling generated by the words. If done on every response, it can become very tedious, but the process forces hearing and promotes understanding. Often after two or three exchanges, B will say, "Oh, if *that* is what you are saying or feeling then we don't really have an argument."
4. Keep the focus on the problem.
5. Do not stop the meeting until a mutually satisfactory solution is reached.

PREDICTIVE PRINCIPLE: Unresolved conflicts regarding contractual agreements for jobs often requires negotiation of collective bargaining, and the reality of a strike.

With the emergence of professionals in labor unions, nurses have adopted collective bargaining strategies, often through an arm of their nurses' association. Management is obliged to see that representation is not forced upon nurses and to ensure that they have free choice in the matter of union representation. Nursing management's basic position should be to protect each professional's rights. Legal points to be aware of are first, under Public Law 93-360 enacted in 1974, professional nurses along with other health care facility employees in nonprofit hospitals have the legal right to organize as one hospital or a group of hospitals and seek representation for the purpose of collective bargaining. However, these same professionals also have the right to refrain from organizing or seeking representation. Second, both the employer and the union are under strict limitations with respect to communications during an organization period.

Nursing administrators have an additional responsibility of becoming knowledgeable and prepared in all aspects of collective bargaining. Robert Claus,* an attorney interested in nursing problems, states that the key negotiation factors for nursing administrators are: (1) composition of both bargaining

---

*Claus, R.: The ins and outs of collective bargaining, J. Nurs. Admin. **10**(9):18-21, 1980.

teams, (2) timing of negotiations, (3) content of negotiations, and (4) selection of negotiating site.

Composition of both bargaining teams. Administrative people from the general administration, personnel, business, and nursing departments should be present. The number of negotiators on the employer's bargaining team should be equal to and never less than that in the negotiating team. Top administrative people, such as board members, hospital administrator, and nursing service director, should never sit on the bargaining team. The team must be able to defer a decision in order to seek counsel with the highest levels of management. One person from each side is selected as the spokesperson for the group. The remaining members provide facts and serve as consultants to their leader. The nurses' group usually select team members for their political clout. These individuals may not have the necessary skills to bargain, but their involvement promotes acceptance of the agreement by the membership at large. Nurses also give negotiating power to a person from their labor organization, for example, the nurses' association union representative.

Timing of negotiations. Negotiations begin soon after the nurses' bargaining team has been accepted by the nurses and administration. Common practice is to begin talking approximately 90 days prior to the contract's expiration. The number of meetings depends upon the number of items to be negotiated and the dedication of the members to reach agreement. Usually, as the contract expiration date draws closer, the momentum of negotiations increases, particularly if there is a threat of strike.

Content of negotiations. The National Labor Relations Act defines items for negotiation as (1) rates of pay, (2) wages, (3) hours of employment, and (4) other conditions of employment. Some states have statutes placing limitations on what points are subject to bargaining, for example, Iowa excludes negotiation of patient care issues. It is wise, before discussing issues, to validate their legality. An important item to consider is the need to include all issues that are important to the negotiations in the proposed contract before the meetings begin. One group of nurses, for example, served notice and struck a hospital primarily for an increase in wages. In the process of negotiating, the nurses' representatives added the issue of "pay equal to that of other comparable professionals, such as pharmacists." Hospital administrators balked and filed suit against them, claiming that this issue was never a part of the original demands and therefore could not be a part of the content for negotiation. The decision went in favor of the administrators.

Selection of a negotiating site. The place of meeting should be arranged by mutual agreement. A location outside the hospital is best, as it allows freedom from interruption of work-related problems and establishes neutral ground.

Preparation for bargaining. Once the content for negotiations is established, each team meets for assignment such as acquisition of copies of contracts of other similar organizations, gathering facts, assessing feelings, and deciding the parameters for acceptance of possible offers made. Avenues for obtaining additional information not previously considered are set up to prevent delay.

Procedures for collective bargaining. The first session usually consists of (1) introductions, (2) a statement of issues and proposals (without argument), and (3) establishment of future meeting dates. At subsequent sessions issues are considered item by item. When agreement is reached on one item, the provisions are listed and signed, indicating tentative accord. Final acceptance depends on agreement on all items. Noneconomic negotiations are considered first, as they usually create the least amount of friction. Emotionally charged issues such as salaries and fringe benefits are commonly agreed upon last. Matters of overtime; differential pay for P.M.s, nights, or special services; insurance; vacations; and pay for education are often considered. The general practice is for nurses to ask for much more than they expect to receive, then bargain downward.

Careful negotiations. Nursing management should negotiate the contract carefully or the terms of the contract can be used as a vice to press each other for power. Some of the most typical general errors in drafting agreements resulting in loss of nursing management rights and the broadening of management liabilities are: (1) making statements too general and vague (e.g., "All nurses will have their needs considered."), (2) having too many restrictions with little room for exception (e.g., "Nurses with at least a baccalaureate degree shall be assigned to the intensive care units."), (3) giving too much power to the other side (e.g., 'All nursing management decisions must have the approval of the union." "All major committees must have representation from nursing management and the union."), (4) drafting promotion policies without proper consideration to preparation, ability, or availability of staff, (5) formulating guidelines in such a way as to disallow any room for change, (6) shifting employee privileges to employee rights. Strict attention to language in the contract at the time of negotiation and before signing into agreement can protect nursing administrators and staff. Otherwise, much unnecessary time and energy will be spent attempting to live with the agreement or to bring about changes that are more acceptable.

Impasses in the bargaining process. When agreement of certain issues becomes impossible, an informal third party is often sought to advise whether or not resolution is possible. If, after discussion with both parties, it is decided that nothing further can be accomplished, there are four actions that can be taken for resolution: (1) mediation, (2) fact-finding, (3) arbitration, and (4) strike. The *mediation* process includes outside source persons to aid in reaching an agreement. Typically, mediators are provided by federal or state governments or from organizations such as the American Arbitration Association. The mediator has no authority, but uses skills in conflict resolution to move the parties out of impasse toward positive action. *Fact-finding* is a more formal situation, requiring a third person to hear facts from both sides represented and to make recommendations. The fact-finder is provided through federal, state, or private sources and has no power; however, it is hoped that his or her recommendations will influence a settlement. Sometimes the matters are solved, but often the members return to the bargaining table to argue from other points. *Arbitration* occurs when administration and workers relinquish their responsibility for establishing the terms of a contract to a third party from federal, state, or private associations. The arbitrator has the power to say what the terms will be and the parties involved have no further right to participate. There is high risk in this procedure for both parties, but it can avoid a strike.

Strike. When nurses feel they are not being listened to by the administration and their requests are not being taken seriously through proper negotiation channels, a strike is likely to occur. The civil rights movement of the 1960s and the women's rights movement of the 1970s have influenced American nurses to become more outspoken about their rights. Assertiveness training also has equipped them with skills necessary to effect change. In addition, labor laws have given hospital workers the legal right to organize and to strike. Notice provisions for a strike are provided under Section 8(d) of Public Law 93-360, a 1974 amendment of the National Labor Relations Act (NLRA) of 1947. Unions are required to give written notice to the respective private health care institution (HCI), whether operated for profit or not, and the Federal Mediation and Conciliation Services (FMC) ten days in advance of a strike, picketing, or other concerted refusal to work. This notice is given whether action is for wages, working conditions, recognition, area standards, or sympathy. Its purpose is to protect the public's interest in continuity of care and patient welfare. Ten days' notice allows the health care institution to make arrangements for their in-patients and to restrict admission to those numbers and kinds of patients they can handle during a strike.

Strike action is designed to accelerate negotiations. Sometimes the plan backfires, especially if hospital administrators believe it to be to their advantage to wait it out. A grave danger for the complainants is for some of their membership to become so discouraged and disenchanted with the strike that they give up and return to work. Some nurses are the sole support of themselves and their families, and their paycheck pays the rent. Having no income becomes frightening and unbearable. A significant break in the ranks erodes the strength of the nurses, a domino effect occurs, and the nurses settle for far less than they had hoped for. Conversely, if nurses maintain the strike until a desirable outcome is reached, the hospital suffers losses. Some regular nurse employees will have gone on to jobs in other health agencies and will not return, physicians may have found other facilities more to their liking, and considerable income has been lost irreparably as a result of curtailed services.

Economic factors are only a part of a strike. Emotions run high characterized by anger, suspicion, distrust, confusion, bitterness, guilt, ambivalence, sadness, and pain. Fearful nurses listen to grape-vine communication and accept distorted messages as fact. Some striking nurses may turn their backs upon those who break the strike and return to work. Others vacillate from support of the cause to inaction or withdrawal. Many suffer from lack of income, creating family problems. Public harrassment may loom large in the situation. Video and newspaper coverage can be sympathetic or accusing. Patients and their families speak of nurses deserting them in their time of need, and nurses feel guilty because they are not available to provide the care desired. Physicians become angry that nurses disrupt their practices. Trust between administration and staff is broken. Sorting out feelings and repairing relationships is a time-consuming job, requiring commitment, perhaps long in coming.

Strikes are a no-win situation, to be avoided if at all possible. A strike creates greater differences between employer and employee than ever before. Patients are caught in the middle. The remedy for both parties is to maintain an open two-way communication system between administration and staff that invites collaboration about any employment issue, and to solve problems as they are identified.

Controlling process

Controlling is a process designed to bring about an orderly and desired flow of activities in accordance with the requirements of plans. Controlling is like a checkup to make sure that what is done is what is intended. Purposes of control in nursing services are as follows: (1) to have sufficient quantities of staff and supplies available where they are needed, (2) to know whether the operation is economical, and (3) to determine if desired performance has been achieved. Fundamental questions as to what, when, where, how, and why are addressed in each phase of the controlling process. The basic steps in control are to (1) establish standards, (2) measure performance and compare results with standards, and (3) make corrections or adjustments in the care-giving operations to obtain results compatible with expectancies.

PREDICTIVE PRINCIPLE: Contracting for accountability of services rendered identifies the scope and limitations of the nurse-manager's span of control and provides a guide for assessment of the degree to which the nurse-manager's responsibilities are being fulfilled.

Accountability for the nurse-manager is blurred. By definition, accountability means answering to authority or becoming responsible or liable for one's actions. The accountable individual is prepared to explain and to receive credit for the results of his or her actions.

Multiple roles are often thrust on nurse-managers by the very nature of the organizational system. The nurse-manager may be expected to (1) set standards for quality of care and ensure their implementation; (2) manage staff

through selection, staffing patterns and assignments, development, and evaluation; (3) be adept in communication and interrelational skills; (4) be an effective
decision maker; (5) know how to plan, implement, coordinate, and control; (6)
be involved with budgetary planning and control; and (7) serve as a role model
for personnel and clients.

In accepting administrative responsibility the nurse-managers assume
accountability for management tasks and clinical outcomes. As controllers, it is
their job to secure, formulate, and prepare information that makes possible effective control. The manager cannot be all things to all people. Before accepting the
position nurse-managers need to know to whom they are responsible and the
mutual areas of accountability. They need to know to what degree the administration shares responsibility, because accountability depends on the authority of
the position and the responsibilities inherent in the role. This function takes
place between the nurse-manager and the immediate supervisor.

Unfortunately, most health care organizations are basically bureaucratic,
with maintenance of the administrative hierarchy given greater importance than
organizational goals. In a bureaucratic organization, authority and accountability
are well defined for all employees, with rules and routine. Where decentralization is present, nurse-managers have more freedom and can become involved in
developing standards and objectives more congruent with their priorities for
professional practice, but with a strong feeling of accountability for hospital and
medical procedures.

Independent practice is another matter. Medical personnel have made
inroads within health facilities by practicing on a collegial basis with autonomy
for their profession, allowing each physician to maintain control for the care of
clients.

Nurses have not kept pace in developing a system in which they can
function autonomously as independent nurse-practitioners. Typically, nurses
are employed in a department of nursing within an institutional hierarchy. The
nurse-manager is delegated administrative authority and accountability but has
not been granted major responsibility for the control of nursing care to the
clients from the time of admission through discharge. There are some beginnings in transferring more accountability to professional nurses through the
avenue of primary care, which incorporates the strong components of responsibility and accountability. There is need for the development of a nursing model
that will define innovative roles for nurses within organizational conditions and
that will allow for improved services to be given with greater professional nurse
autonomy and accountability.

Wade* suggests a neoteric model for professional autonomy that can be
adapted for hospitals, nursing homes, and similar institutions. He provides a set

---

*Wade, L.L.: Professionals in organizations: A neoteric model, Hum. Organization, pp. 40-66, Spring-
Summer 1967.

of conditions that, if present in an organization, are conducive to a high level of autonomy for the professional in the organization, as follows: (1) decisions made at the operational level in terms of the needs of clientele, (2) systems for services that will best meet objectives, (3) a climate that is open and receptive to new ideas and change, (4) effective interpersonal relationships among the organization's professionals and between workers and clients, (5) equal distribution of supplies and services, (6) allowance for expressions of individuality, (7) belief that authority arises from knowledge and expertise and not hierarchy, (8) congruence among organizational professionals, and (9) goal setting and evaluation of professional behavior only by fellow professionals.

Irrespective of organizational system, contracting for accountability allows each party to see the other's perception of the role. In the process, each is helped to see if their expectations are realistic or unrealistic. Furthermore, agreement to assume specific responsibilities provides criteria for assessment of the degree to which the nurse-manager's obligations are being accomplished.

PREDICTIVE PRINCIPLE: Setting standards serves to clarify purpose and provides a gauge for controlling quality and quantity of services.

Quality control is a foremost consideration in nursing management. The goal is assurance of a satisfactory quality for the intended purpose. Specifically the goal sought is that which is best in terms of consistency with the standards set and satisfactory and dependable results being provided. Standards are the yardstick for gauging the quality and quantity of services. They serve to clarify purpose.

As much as possible, standards are stated clearly, objectively, and quantitatively so that they may be seen, measured, and judged and thereby become useful in the control function. There are some qualitative standards such as attitudes, morale, or relationships that are difficult to measure, but even these variables can be assessed with some degree of confidence.

It has been pointed out that there is no one set of standards used by all health care agencies for quality assurance, but that it is the task of each caregiving group to develop standards and objectives to guide the actions of individual personnel into purposeful, safe, and effective client care. Standards that have been developed by many people and organizations such as joint commissions, the American Nurses' Association *Standards for Nursing Services* and *Standards for Nursing Practice*, and the National League for Nursing's *Criteria for Evaluating a Hospital Department of Nursing* are broadly stated but can be drawn on to develop appropriate standards for individual nursing care settings against which quality of care can be compared.

Standards of practice may be stated in terms of minimal or optimal activity, or any place in between. They describe the level or degree of quality considered appropriate and adequate for a single purpose.

The agency's philosophy, purpose, budget, and organizational structure influence specific standard settings. Written policies, objectives, and procedures are then formulated to assist personnel in making correct decisions in the performance of nursing care, organizational function, and personnel development. These guidelines serve as a tool for the management of nursing care and become the department or unit's official guide. They serve as evidence that standards have been set up reflective of the value system and beliefs of the organization and the individual caregivers.

A committee of nursing personnel can be appointed to develop, review, and revise performance standards as necessary. Representatives from other concerned groups such as physicians and consumers may be included.

PREDICTIVE PRINCIPLE: Governmental control on hospitals encourages and/or constrains patterns of care that patients receive thus requiring nurse-managers to have an understanding of the regulations.

In response to consumers' expressed concern, the Social Security Amendments of 1972 mandated the development of professional standards review organizations (PSROs), directing health care professionals to change their concept of accountability for nursing care from one of private to public accountability. Criteria and mechanisms for accounting are published in PSRO manuals annually. Also, the Joint Commission on Accreditation of Hospitals (JCAH) directs physicians, nurses, and other professionals to formulate criteria and to implement mechanisms to assure quality in those aspects of care provided by them. As a result, evaluation and review programs have developed throughout the nation in response to both official and voluntary direction.

Prior to 1980, the PSRO and JCAH manuals were quite general, leaving implementation up to individual agencies. Between 1980 and 1982, criteria have become very specific. The Joint Commission required each hospital to implement a quality assurance program by January 1, 1981. Consequently, administrators, medical staffs, and trustees are now mandated to establish a program that examines the types and patterns of care that patients receive. State regulatory programs set limits on hospital reimbursements based upon compliance with quality assurance criteria.

The new JCAH standard requires hospitals to: (1) implement a comprehensive quality assurance program that reviews the care that is provided by all clinical departments, disciplines, and practitioners, (2) coordinate and integrate the findings of quality assessment activities, and (3) devote special attention to known or suspected patient problems. Each hospital must have a written plan that explains its quality assurance program. The program must be formalized by the governing body and put into operation through a central coordinating unit. It must include mechanisms aimed at assessing and correcting problems and at ensuring sound clinical performance. Corrective policies are to be implemented,

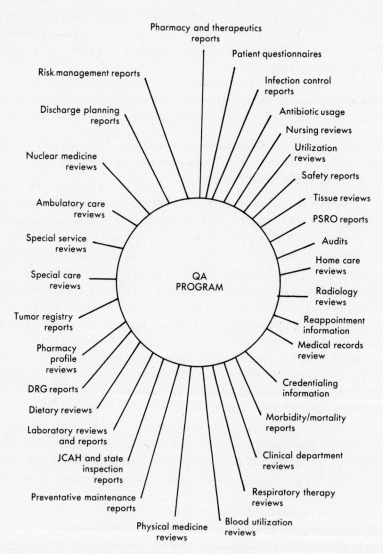

Fig. 2-4. Information needed for an effective quality assurance program. (From Miccio, B.: Rate setting promotes interdepartmental cooperation in QA, Hospitals **55**(11):84, 1981.)

and unlike past practice, the program must be monitored continuously and evaluated at least annually.

Because of the flexibility allowed by the Joint Commission, different hospitals will implement different quality assurance programs. Nevertheless, hospitals' objectives are likely to be the same: (1) to maintain an ongoing program, (2) to integrate reviews and evaluations of patient care, (3) to establish priorities to resolve problems, and (4) to improve cost-effectiveness by using resources more effectively.*

The strength of a quality assurance program depends heavily on the acquisition and use of appropriate data for utilization review, as illustrated in Fig. 2-4, and in establishing committees and functions throughout the hospital that will accomplish their purposes. A common plan is for creation of a hospital-wide quality assurance coordinating body comprised of representatives from medical, nursing, and allied service groups. This body sets hospital-wide goals in accordance with JCAH standards and establishes a committee structure to meet them, outlining what committees perform the functions and who is primarily responsible for such functions on each committee. Examples of committees are medical quality assurance, nursing quality assurance, medical records, and safety. Examples of functions are performance review (medical and nursing audits), examination of unusual incidents, reports, recommendations, action, and evaluation.

Nursing administrators are responsible for quality assurance in areas such as staffing, policies, procedures, standardized procedures, skills, staff development, and continuing education. An example of a formalized quality assurance program for nursing follows:†

Goal: To provide a well-defined quality assurance program within Nursing Services Department that is designed to enhance patient care through (a) ongoing objective assessment of patient care, (b) correction of identified problems, and (c) coordinated and integrated with hospital's Quality Assurance review program.
Nursing Services' responsibilities for review of quality assurance:
1. Quarterly review of nursing process/patient outcomes.
2. Regular, ongoing review of quality-based care, on preestablished criteria.
3. When possible, integrated with medical/ancillary services.
4. Activities coordinated by committee/chairperson.
5. Findings reported to Nursing Administration and Quality Assurance Coordinator.
6. Documentation of: problem source (how identified), patient impact, who assessed, method used, resolution/action, reporting mechanism, and follow-up (monitoring, effectiveness).
7. Integration with hospital Quality Assurance program, including staff support.

---

*New Jersey Hospital Association. Quality Assurance Manual. Princeton, New Jersey Hospital Association, 1980.
†From the Quality Assurance Manual of The Good Samaritan Hospital of Santa Clara Valley, San Jose, California, 1981.

Review processes: The Nursing Services Department will use, but is not limited to, the following review activities:

1. Hospital and/or individual unit standards of care compliance studies.
2. Concurrent and/or retrospective patient outcome studies.
3. Medical record reviews for relationship between process and outcome of nursing activities.
4. Continuous monitoring of patient events, e.g., medication/patient event pattern, infection control systems, blood transfusion reactions, cardiac arrests/CPR, patient injury patterns. (Items one through three may be identified by data generated from Patient Notification Form system)
5. Immediate problem search of important patient events documented.

Communications systems: The Nursing Quality Assurance Committee will have both written and verbal communications with Nursing Administration, Head Nurses, the nursing staff, and the hospital Quality Assurance Coordinator. Communications with other hospital departments will be as the direct/indirect results of a problem search, problem identification, or problem resolution action. Interdepartmental activities will be coordinated through the hospital's Quality Assurance Coordinator. There will be frequent communications between hospital Quality Assurance Coordinator and Nursing's Quality Assurance program.

With a sound quality assurance plan, the response of hospital staff to the program will be positive, partially because of the involvement in the process by staff throughout the hospital, and partially because of the outcome. And in the process, the hospital has met governmental controls, necessary for on-going operation.

PREDICTIVE PRINCIPLE: Consideration of structural, process, and outcome standards as interrelational and interdependent serves to keep the management process balanced and in perspective.

Methods for measuring the quality of nursing care can be classified into structural approaches, focusing on the organization and management of the client care system, process approaches, emphasizing the actual delivery of care, and outcome approaches, concentrating on client welfare.

Structure of the setting in which care is given might include the scope of services, functions engaged in, education level of those providing the services, budgetary allotment, staff development programs, and specific conditions of the environment. Structural criteria evaluate the administrative processes that arrange the flow of work. Various tools are used to make a systematic analysis of activities. Questions and checklists are typical of this style. Such audits can yield results that lead to cost control as well as general improvements in departmental operations.

Performance appraisals are a necessary part of the control process, as they provide back-up data for management decisions concerning salary, retention, promotion, transfer, or dismissal; pinpoint strengths and areas that need improvement; establish standards of job performance; and help the nurse-manager to determine if goals are being met. Methods of performance appraisal are discussed in detail in Chapter 8.

Professionals and nonprofessionals may be involved in controlling the structural aspects, for there are many facets included that could bear scrutiny from individuals who are prepared in other fields, such as business and management. The objectives of structural review are to bring into focus the activities and operations of the department and to allow a careful appraisal of the effectiveness and efficiency of work performance.

The *process* approach measures the delivery of nursing care to clients within the providing structure. In this process of quality control a comparison is made between standards set and specific nursing activities and interactions utilized to achieve them. They judge the adequacy with which the activities are performed. This is accomplished through formal and informal methods using direct observation and review of data. Whereas nonnursing personnel can engage in controlling the structural areas of nursing practice, only professional nurses should participate in determining whether or not nursing plans are adequate for the client.

The nurse-manager uses the process approach informally every day by observing work, checking on personnel, and reviewing input relating to provision of care. Comparing information obtained in these ways with existing standards is a continuous daily function of managers as they control their areas of responsibility. This on-the-job surveillance permits each nurse-manager to remain current and accurate in assessment and to reinforce or make necessary adjustments.

Numerous formal devices for evaluating quality of nursing care are available for use or adaptation. The most beneficial systems are set up in such a way that the evaluation can be recorded as objectively as possible. Instruments such as quality patient care scales, appraisal guides, and audits on charts and records while the client is hospitalized provide criteria that are broken down into categories and items reflecting the authors' perception of quality care. In the controlling process, data are gathered, reviewed, and acted on.

The *outcome* approach takes a retrospective look at the state or condition of the client after services have been delivered. Some define the parameters of outcome as when care is initiated and when the client is discharged. Others consider outcome as the effects of nursing care on the client after discharge. Outcome is the most difficult variable in nursing to measure, as it cannot be determined precisely how much of the outcome of client care has resulted from nursing intervention. Provision, or the lack of provision, for care through organizational design, physician control, or personal or social involvements with any number of contacts could influence the client's health outcome. One of the things that greatly increases the problems surrounding the measurement of quality nursing care is the fact that few specific nursing actions are linked to specific client outcome. This means that whichever method is selected to focus on outcome, assumptions will have to be made about its relation to the nursing process. Nursing must proceed with an attempt to develop precise definitions, criteria, and instruments that can be applied to test the quality of outcome for the client.

In using a quality control system, it is important for the staff to know how the findings will be used. There may be mixed purposes, as follows: (1) to provide information to the nurse-manager for reporting results and evaluating personnel, (2) to assist the staff in assessing their effectiveness and to guide their development, (3) to obtain feedback from the client, and (4) to increase the quality of care delivered.

A determination is made by the governing group at the centralized or decentralized level as to the format that will be used for quality control. Then the group needs to know the logistics of the plan. Stevens* suggests that the following guidelines have been found useful in some organizations for the study of process and outcome:

1. Schedule evaluation sessions at regular but unannounced intervals to reflect a more normal pattern of nursing care.
2. Use a sample of the clients.
3. Select clients at random or study those who require or required challenging nursing care.
4. Appoint only those people who are familiar with the evaluation process.
5. If nurses divide the work of evaluation, each member should grade the same portion of the evaluation tool on all clients or units evaluated.

Application of predictive principles of management

Mrs. Langley is nurse-coordinator of six medical-surgical units. Six months ago a decision was made by the head nurses of these units to adopt primary nursing as their system for delivery of care for one year. Now three of the head nurses indicate they plan to drop primary nursing in favor of the team plan, because "the system is not working."

Problem	Predictive principle	Prescription
Three head nurses propose action that is contrary to group decision.	Coordination of personnel and services through intradepartmental and interdepartmental activities brings about a total accomplishment far superior to that possible through fragmentation of individual effort.	Nurse-coordinator schedules meeting with all of the head nurses to ascertain the status of primary nursing in their units.

*Stevens, B.: First-line patient care management, Wakefield, Mass., 1976, Contemporary Publishing, Inc., p. 121.

Problem	Predictive principle	Prescription
	The span of control directly affects the size and complexity of the coordinating function.	Meet in a conference room on one of the units.
	Activities directed toward regulating, preventing, correcting, and promoting coordination provide a comprehensive and efficient approach to management.	At the meeting, discuss reasons for the dysfunctioning primary nursing system.
		Identify potential and actual points of friction and determine whether they are the result of poor organizational design, personality problems, or problems with delegation and follow-up procedures.
The presence or absence of conflict influences a nurse-manager's ability to coordinate activity.		Reaffirm and nurture trusting relationships that encourage free and open communication.
		Review the decision made by the group to adopt primary nursing in each unit for 1 year. Hold them to their decision and give time for progress reports at each subsequent meeting.

BIBLIOGRAPHY
Books

Boyer, J.L., Westerhaus, C.M., and Coggeshall, J.H.: Employee relations and collective bargaining in health care facilities, ed. 2, St. Louis, 1975, The C.V. Mosby Co.

DiVincenti, M.: Administering nursing service, Boston, 1972, Little, Brown & Co.

Davis, C., Oakley, D., and Sochalski, J.: Leadership for expanding influence on health policy, J. Nurs. Admin. **12**(1):15-21, 1982.

Donovan, H.M.: Nursing service administration: managing the enterprise, St. Louis, 1975, The C.V. Mosby Co.

Drucker, P.F.: Managing for results, New York, 1964, Harper & Row, Publishers, Inc.

Drucker, P.F.: Management tasks, responsibilities, practices, New York, 1974, Harper & Row, Publishers, Inc.

Filley, A.: Interpersonal conflict resolution, Palo Alto, Calif., 1975, Scott, Foresman & Co.

Ganong, J., and Ganong, W.: Nursing management, Germantown, Md., 1976, Aspen Systems Corporation.

Georgopoulos, B.S., and Mann, F.C.: The community general hospital, New York, 1962, Macmillan Publishing Co., Inc.

Glueck, W.: Management, Hinsdale, Ill., 1977, The Dryden Press.

Henning, M., and Jardim, R.: The managerial woman, Garden City, N.Y., 1977, Anchor Press/Doubleday.

Longest, B., Jr.: Management practices for the health professional, Reston, Va., 1976, Reston Publishing Co.

Lysaught, J.: Action in affirmation: toward an unambiguous profession of nursing, New York, 1981, McGraw-Hill Book Co.

Marriner, A.: Contemporary nursing management: issues and practice, St. Louis, 1982, The C.V. Mosby Co.

Maslow, A.: Motivation and personality, New York, 1954, Harper & Row.

Mayo, E.: The social problems of an industrial civilization, Cambridge, Mass., 1945, Harvard University Press.

Stevens, B.: First-line patient care management, Wakefield, Mass., 1976, Contemporary Publishing, Inc.

Stone, S., et al., editors: Management for nurses: a multidisciplinary approach, St. Louis, 1976, The C.V. Mosby Co.

Wieland, G., and Ullrich, R.: Organizations: behavior, design, and change, Homewood, Ill., 1976, Richard D. Irwin, Inc.

Periodicals

Adkins, R.: Responsibility and authority must match in nursing management, Hospitals **53**(3): 69-71, 1979.

Aiken, L., Blendon, R., and Rogers, D.: The shortage of hospital nurses: a new perspective, Am. J. Nurs. **81**(9):1612-1619, 1981.

Araujo, M.: Creative nursing administration sets climate for retention, Hospitals **54**(9):72-76, 1980.

Archer, S., and Goehner, P.: Acquiring political clout: guidelines for nurse administrators, J. Nurs. Admin. **11**(11,12):49-55, 1981.

Atkinson, P., and Goodwin, L.: The role of the nurse administrator in collective-bargaining. Nurs. Clin. North Am. **13**(1):111-128, 1978.

Bell, M.: Management by objectives, J. Nurs. Admin. **10**(5):19-26, 1980.

Bloch, D.: Criteria, standards, norms—crucial terms in quality assurance, J. Nurs. Admin. **7**(9):20-30, 1977.

Bryant, Y.: Labor relations in health care institutions: an analysis of Public Law 93-360, J. Nurs. Admin. **13**(3):28-37, 1978.

Cain, C., and Luchsinger, V.: Management by objectives: applications to nursing, J. Nurs. Admin. **8**(1):35-38, 1978.

Cannon, P.: Administering the contract, J. Nurs. Admin. **10**(10):13-19, 1980.

Carral, M.: Education must adapt to changing health care system, Am. Nurse, March 1980, pp. 5-6.

Castrey, B., and Castrey, R.: Mediation—what it is, what it does, J. Nurs. Admin. **10**(11):24-32, 1980.

Chism, S.: The nurse administrator: a long distance runner, Superv. Nurse **12**(1):36-37, 1981.

Claus, R.: The ins and outs of collective bargaining, J. Nurs. Admin. **10**(9):18-21, 1980.

Council, J., and Plachy, R.: Performance appraisal is not enough, J. Nurs. Admin. **10**(10):20-26, 1980.

Daines, E.: Participative management, Nurs. Manag. **12**(11):50-54, 1981.

Doerr, B., and Hutchins, E.: Health risk appraisal: process, problems, and prospects for nursing practice and research, Nurs. Res. **30**(5):299-306, 1981.

Donnelly, L.: Patient classification, Nurs. Manag. **12**(11):42-43, 1981.

Duffy, M., and Gold, N.: Education for nursing administration: what investment yields highest returns? J. Nurs. Admin. **10**(9):31-38, 1980.

Duldt, B.: Anger: an alienating communication hazard for nurses, Nurs. Outlook **29**(11):640-644, 1981.

Ellis, B.: Winds of change sweep nursing profession, Hospitals **54**(1):94-95, 1980.

England, D.: The strengths and weaknesses in nursing service administration, Nurs. Outlook **28**(9):551-556, 1980.

Erickson, E.: Collective bargaining: an inappropriate technique for professionals, J. Nurs. Admin. **3**(4):355, 1973.

Erickson, E.: The nursing service director, 1880-1980, J. Nurs. Admin., **10**(4):6-13, 1980.

Fisher, D.: A review of organizational development, J. Nurs. Admin. **10**(10):31-36, 1980.

Friesen, L., and Conahan, B.: A clinical preceptor program: strategy for new graduate orientation, J. Nurs. Admin. **10**(4):18-23, 1980.

Fuller, M.: The budget: standard V, J. Nurs. Admin. **8**(5):36-38, 1976.

Ginzberg, E.: The economics of health care and the future of nursing, J. Nurs. Admin. **11**(3): 28-36, 1981.

Gugenheim, A.: Health care leaders examine role of nursing service administrator, Hospitals **53**(3):109-111, 1979.

Haar, L., and Hicks, J.: Performance appraisal: derivation of effective assessment tools, J. Nurs. Admin. **8**(9):20-29, 1976.

Hegyvary, S., and Haussmann, D.: Monitoring nursing care quality, J. Nurs. Admin. **8**(11):3-9, 1976.

Hitt, D., and Harristhal, M.: Financing health care in the 1980s, Hospitals **54**(1):71-74, 1980.

Holland, M.: Can managerial performance be predicted? J. Nurs. Admin. **11**(6):17-21, 1981.

Kinzer, D.: Cost reduction remains goal of federal regs, Hospitals **54**(1):91-94, 1980.

Krueger, J.: Women in management: an assessment, Nurs. Outlook **28**(6):374-378, 1980.

Laser, R.: I win—you win negotiating, J. Nurs. Admin. **11**(11,12):24-29, 1981.

Leatt, P., Bay, K., and Stinson, S.: An instrument for assessing and classifying patients by type of care, Nurs. Res. **30**(3):145-150, 1981.

Lewis, J.: Conflict management, J. Nurs. Admin. **8**(12):18-22, 1976.

Little, K., and Matthews, L.: Staffing function and management techniques, Nurs. Admin. Q., Summer 1977, pp. 27-30.

Lynaugh, J.: The "entry into practice" conflict: how we got where we are and what will happen next, Am. J. Nurs. **(2)**:266-270, 1980.

Marshik-Gustafson, J., Kopher, S., and Terze, M.:

Planning is the key to successful QA programs, Hospitals **55**(11):67-76, 1981.

Masson, V.: On power and vision in nursing, Nurs. Outlook **27**(12):782-784, 1979.

Mayers, M., and Watson, A.: Evaluating the quality of patient care through retrospective chart review, J. Nurs. Admin. **8**(4):17-21, March-Apr. 1976.

McClure, M.: The long road to accountability, Nurs. Outlook **26**(1):47-50, 1978.

Melum, M.: Hospitals must change: control is the issue, Hospitals **54**(5):67-74, 1980.

Melum, M.: 10 lessons point the way toward successful hospital planning, Hospitals **55**(23):58-64, 1981.

Metzger, N.: Hospital labor scene marked by union issues, Hospitals **54**(7):105-116, 1980.

Miner, J.: Twenty years of research on role-motivation theory of managerial effectiveness, Pers. Psychol. **31**(8):740, 1978.

Murray, M.: The nursing service administrators, Nurs. Manag. **12**(11):59, 1981.

Nichols, B.: An open letter from the ANA president, Am. J. Nurs. **81**(7):1335, 1981.

Nugent, P.: Management and modes of thought, J. Nurs. Admin. **12**(2):19-25, 1982.

Pilous, B.: The advantage of part-time nursing, Am. J. Nurs. **81**(5):981-982, 1981.

Public Law 93-360, 29 U.S.C., Section 8(d).

Reineri, P., and Grant, D.: A classification system to meet today's needs, J. Nurs. Admin. **11**(1):21-25, 1981.

Rinaldi, L.: Quality assurance '81—satisfying JCAH, Nurs. Manag. **12**(9):23-24, 1981.

Rogatz, P.: Directions of health system for new decade, Hospitals **54**(1):67-70, 1980.

Rothman, N., and Tothman, D.: Equal pay for comparable work, Nurs. Outlook **28**(12):728-729, 1980.

Rotkovitch, R.: The nursing director's role in money management, J. Nurs. Admin. **11**(11,12):13-16, Nov.-Dec., 1981.

Schmied, E.: Living with cost containment, J. Nurs. Admin. **10**(5):11-18, 1980.

Schmied, E.: Allocation of resources: preparation of the nursing department budget, J. Nurs. Admin. **9**(9):31-36, 1977.

Shaffer, K., Lindenstein, J., and Jennings, T.: Successful QA program incorporates new JCAH standards, Hospitals **55**(16):117-122, 1981.

Shapiro, E., Haseltine, F., and Rowe, M.: Moving up: role models, mentors, and the patron system, Sloan Management Review **19**(3):51, 1978.

Shiflett, N., and McFarland, D.: Power and the nursing administrator, J. Nurs. Admin. **13**(3):19-23, 1978.

Silber, M.: Nurse power—projecting self and ideas, Superv. Nurse **12**(7):65-68, 1981.

Sovie, M.: The role of staff development in hospital cost control, J. Nurs. Admin. **10**(11):38-42, 1980.

Swansburg, R.: Planning—a function of nursing administration: Part 1, Superv. Nurse **9**(4):25-28, 1978.

Taylor, V.: The dynamics of a strike, Superv. Nurse **12**(7):51-52, 1981.

Turner, G., and Mapa, J.: Board takes action in quality assurance role, Hospitals **54**(9):109-114, 1980.

Watson, J.: Professional identity crisis—is nursing finally growing up? Amer. J. Nurs. **81**(8):1488-1490, 1981.

Wade, L.L.: Professionals in organizations: A neoteric model, Hum. Organization, pp. 40-66, Spring-Summer, 1967.

Wilkinson, R.: Effective management, Superv. Nurse **12**(1):44-45, 1981.

Zaleznik, A.: Managers and leaders: are they different? Harvard Business Review **55**(3):75-78, 1977.

chapter three

Predictive principles of staffing

Goals and standards

A statement of nursing service goals gives direction to the number and kinds of nursing services that will be provided in performing the mission of the institution.

Standards of care, clearly defined, allow for descriptions of personnel necessary for implementation.

Job satisfaction and dissatisfaction

Identification of factors that contribute to nurses' job dissatisfaction and a high rate of turnover allows administrators to analyze and respond to the nurses' concerns.

Congruence among personal, professional, and organizational goals reduces nurse turnover and shortages.

Staffing process

Provision of sufficient numbers and qualifications of personnel to meet the expectations of the institution depends upon an accurate staffing system.

Circumstances peripheral to client needs and qualified personnel to meet those needs influence the staffing process.

Assignment of staff for continuity of service and economical use of personnel promotes client satisfaction and results in cost effectiveness.

Flexibility in staffing patterns increases the recruitment and retention of nursing staff needed.

Criteria established for supplemental or temporary staffing helps support continuity of care.

Establishment of policies and programs that ensure fairness, consistency, and professional development of human resources enables recruitment and maintenance of a sufficient number of qualified nurses.

Staffing may be defined as the process of assigning competent people to fill the roles designated for the organizational structure through selection and development of personnel. Staffing is the most critical issue of administration because the quality of the participants' effort determines the degree of goal achievement. The issue of staffing is further complicated because it takes place in an ever-changing environment in which practices, task assignments, and responsibilities fluctuate.

An institution whose concern is the delivery of quality health care is presented with the problem of supplying sufficient human resources for the administration of that care. For most health care agencies, staffing constitutes 70% to 80% of the total budget, with nurses providing the major share of the personnel. When a nurse-manager is given responsibility over a particular part of an organization, staffing is one of the central aspects of this responsibility. Because there is limited research on the relationship between numbers and kinds of nursing staff and quality care, it is difficult to predict with assurance that whatever is done will produce desired results. However, there is enough sharing of theories and practice relating to matters of staffing to provide the nurse-manager with predictive principles that can be applied to the issue of staffing with a high degree of confidence.

Several factors are considered when designing staffing patterns. The first, of course, is the goals of the agency. Goals always are the most influential factor, followed very closely by the standards of care established by the various regulatory agencies such as the Joint Commission on Accreditation for Hospitals, the American Nurses' Association, and the National League for Nursing. After these come other factors equally important for their effect on the agency, staff, and clients. These are factors such as job satisfaction of employees and the nursing care of clients.

Goals and standards

Goals serve as criteria against which staffing decisions are made and evaluated. The task of translating broad goals, such as the hospital's mission, into more concrete, measurable objectives for staffing is difficult but necessary. When selecting more specific aims, it becomes easy to lose sight of the true meaning and intention of the organization's broad goals. Once managers have selected their goals for staffing, they must determine what factors will aid or hinder them in pursuit of these goals. Often the resources of the organization (its finances, equipment, and personnel) will be the main influences in establishing which direction nursing staffing will take. Standards provide baseline or minimal criteria for goal achievement and are an important consideration in the staffing process.

PREDICTIVE PRINCIPLE: A statement of nursing service goals gives direction to the number and kinds of nursing services that will be provided in performing the mission of the institution.

Before the numbers, kinds, and patterns of care can be established, the operational objectives of the nursing service department must be known. Ideally, the director of nursing services and nurse-managers at all levels participate in their formulation. Interaction and interrelationship among personnel within the organizational structure vertically and horizontally strengthen the probability that beliefs and values pertaining to the delivery of care will be carried out at all levels. Following is a set of objectives adapted from the Good Samaritan Hospital of Santa Clara Valley, California.

Nursing service department operational objectives

To assist in achieving the hospital's objectives on the care of the sick and injured by:

1. Providing preventive, curative, restorative nursing care
2. Providing a safe, efficient, and therapeutically effective environment for the care of the sick
3. Fulfilling the state and local public health standards and requirements for patient care services
4. Providing and implementing a program of continuing education for all nursing personnel to increase professional, technical, and psychosocial skills
5. Participating in the formulation, implementation, and evaluation of personnel policies
6. Coordinating the functions of the Department of Nursing Service with the functions of all other departments and services of the hospital
7. Developing and maintaining a working rapport and communication system with other hospital departments that are conducive to mutual respect and cooperative planning
8. Recommending and implementing policies and procedures to maintain an adequate and competent nursing staff based on methodical estimates of personnel requirements of the Department of Nursing Service
9. Providing the means and methods by which the nursing personnel can work with other groups in interpreting the objectives of the hospital and Nursing Service to the patient and community
10. Developing and maintaining an effective system of clinical and administrative nursing records and reports
11. Estimating needs for facilities, supplies, and equipment
12. Initiating, utilizing, and participating in studies or research projects designed for the improvement of patient care and the improvement of other administrative and hospital services

A written statement of nursing service goals such as this provides the blueprint for all that follows in the effective management of an operation. For example, objective No. 8 addresses staffing, giving attention to definitive goals and standards of care of the agency, a natural outgrowth when the proper framework for management has been provided.

PREDICTIVE PRINCIPLE: Standards of care, clearly defined, allow for descriptions of personnel necessary for implementation.

Although each health care agency is charged with the responsibility for determining the level of service for their individual operation, there are many factors and constraints to be considered that influence the decision-making process.

In 1972 the U.S. Congress amended the Social Security Act and mandated the establishment of Professional Standard Review Organizations to review the quality and cost of care paid by Medicare, Medicaid, and Maternal-Child Health programs. The American Hospital Association and the Joint Commission on Accreditation of Hospitals have established comparable programs for the evaluation of patient care.

In response to concern about the acceleration of programs and the problem of control, the U.S. Department of Health, Education and Welfare issued a report entitled "Forward Plan for Health, Fiscal Years 1977-81." This was a quality assurance plan discussing a framework for integrating the many different health functions of the federal government into a coherent program and thus improving health services throughout the United States. One action is highly significant to nurses. Under Part B, Title XI, of the Social Security amendment, a Professional Standards Review Organization was established in each state and locale by July 1, 1978. Each separate organization is responsible for defining its own standards. Each facility providing services meets minimal legal standards established by authoritative bodies. There is no legal requirement that a hospital or any other type of health care facility aspire to reach beyond minimal standards. But many agencies are not satisfied with meeting minimal standards prepared by licensing agencies and look for more criteria that denote quality. Examples are the Joint Commission on Accreditation for Hospitals (JCAH), the American Nurses' Association (ANA), and the National League for Nursing (NLN), who have prepared five standards that are recommended for use in planning nursing service in hospitals, public health agencies, nursing care homes, industries, and clinics.*

>   **Standard 1:** Nursing service shall be under the direction of a legally and professionally qualified registered nurse. There shall be a stable staffing program with a sufficient number of duly licensed nurses on duty at all times to plan, assign, supervise, and evaluate nursing care, as well as to give nursing care.
>
>   **Standard 2:** Nursing service shall have a current, written organizational plan that spells out the decision-making structure and methods for cooperative planning. Development of nursing personnel and management of nursing care are the primary considerations.

---

*American Nurses' Association: Standards for organized nursing services in hospitals, industries, and clinics, Kansas City, Mo., 1973, The Association.

Standard 3: There shall be written policies and procedures for nursing administration and provision of nursing care.

Standard 4: Each patient served shall have a nursing care plan that provides for safety, efficiency, and a therapeutic approach.

Standard 5: Opportunities shall be provided nursing personnel for continuing and advanced education.

Although standards of practice are either imposed or suggested by many bodies, nursing standards for the total enterprise for each level of operation need to be developed and tailored to fulfill the specific philosophy and purposes of the individual work setting, irrespective of any mandatory body. Standards of nursing practice have been established by the American Nurses' Association Congress for Nursing Practice and are available to any interested individual or group. They define nursing practice and provide models against which nurses can measure their practice. The American Nurses' Association has published standards of nursing practice, a general statement, and specific standards in each of the following areas: medical-surgical nursing, orthopedic nursing, maternal-child nursing, geriatric nursing, community health nursing, operating room nursing, cardiovascular nursing, emergency nursing, and psychiatric–mental health nursing. Guidelines such as these provide much help in facilitating the promotion of quality care because institutions can compare and contrast their own views and standards with those established by authorities to make sure that all important issues pertaining to the delivery of care have been included.

Nurses in an institution or agency can work through a nursing practice commission to set standards for practice and to plan for peer review. Everyone who is directly affected should be involved in the standard setting. Other knowledgable, talented, and experienced people should be sought to provide a foundation on which to build nursing standards. Setting of standards is a crucial matter, as everything that is done from the planning through the evaluation stage stems from these statements. When standards for the agency have been determined, nurses in each work setting can develop standards of care that relate directly to the needs of their particular kind of client.

Job satisfaction and dissatisfaction

Job satisfaction is feeling good about one's work assignment and having a desire to continue in that role. Increased specialization in nursing makes more demands upon the nurse. When nurses are asked to fulfill a highly skilled role and to continue with many unspecialized work tasks, satisfaction may be replaced by dissatisfaction. These factors, along with others, lead to problems that must be addressed. Recognition of the degree of satisfaction and dissatisfaction among nurses is the first step. This section discusses attitudes of nurses and offers solutions to dissatisfaction.

PREDICTIVE PRINCIPLE: Identification of factors that contribute to nurses' job dissatisfaction and a high rate of turnover allows administrators to analyze and respond to the nurses' concerns.

PREDICTIVE PRINCIPLE: Congruence among personal, professional, and organizational goals reduces nurse turnover and shortages.

Even though there are more nurses than ever before (500 per 100,000 population today compared to 250 per 100,000 population in the 1950s) the shortage of nurses in the health care system has reached a critical stage. Agencies not only have difficulty in recruiting nurses but also have problems retaining them. Evidence that a scarcity exists is given by the National League for Nursing: (1) a low unemployment rate for newly licensed registered nurses (1.9% compared with the 6% national average), (2) a zero growth rate in basic nursing education programs, (3) declining applications to registered nurse programs, (4) an increase in budgeted but vacant nursing service positions, (5) an increase in budgeted but vacant nursing faculty positions, and (6) greatly expanded advertising and recruitment activities that address the professional nurse.

Possible reasons why the larger nurse population is unable to meet demands include: expansion of nursing into an increasing variety of settings, an increase in the older population, many of whom require nursing care, increased need for nurse-specialists who are trained in the use of current technologic equipment and in giving intensified nursing care, and the many options open to nurses in health-related fields.

The national turnover rate for registered nurses in the United States averages from 32% to 40%, depending on the source.* It often reaches 70% during any one year. The highest turnover rate is in metropolitan areas. The outcome of this problem affects quality of care provided and increases costs to the agencies affected. The National Association of Nurse Recruiters reports the cost of recruiting one nurse in 1980 was $866. With the added expense of orientation, physical work-up, processing, and pay for supplemental staff while the nurse is being prepared, a hospital may spend from $2,500 to $4,000 to replace one nurse who resigns.

Discovering why nurses leave their jobs is difficult at best (see chapter 10). Some agencies fail to conduct exit interviews, and even when interviews are required honest answers may not be forthcoming. Nurses may fear repercussions affecting their next job if they state their true reasons for quitting. Some agencies are hesitant to release nurse turnover information, as they believe that doing so would hamper recruiting efforts.

---

*National Association of Nurse Recruiters; American Nurses' Association.

As the turnover problem magnifies, several researchers are taking an interest in identifying factors that influence nurses to vacate one job for another.

Studies show *job dissatisfaction* as the primary reason for nurses leaving their employ. Problems identified focus on these complexities:

1. Unrealistic job expectations, a problem particularly applicable to new graduates, many of whom leave their jobs in the first six months
2. Salary, a primary job condition with which employed nurses are dissatisfied
3. Too many responsibilities outside the hospital, for example, child care, social commitments, or educational pursuits
4. Feeling of inadequacy for the job
5. Unreasonable demands on the job because of either too heavy an assignment or an inadequately prepared staff
6. Worry that quality care is not being provided
7. Being floated to units other than those originally assigned, shift rotation, or overtime
8. Lack of support from the nurse in charge of the unit
9. Poor physician-nurse relationships, such as lack of professional respect and indifference to what the nurse has to offer in client care
10. Lack of nursing autonomy and professional recognition
11. Lack of opportunity for advancement except through administrative positions

Each health care institution must examine the reasons given by the nurse for exiting their facility and must be proactive rather than reactive. Nursing administrators must be intensely involved in the discussions and decision making that address the immediate crisis, while seeking long-term solutions to the problem. Resolutions to the turnover problem become the responsibility of individual agencies; nevertheless, there are generalizations to be made that may prove helpful.

Unrealistic job expectations can be offset by a more reality-focused orientation. New graduates, for example, enter the job market having different levels of preparation. Baccalaureate programs prepare "professional" nurses and associate degree programs "technical" nurses; yet in many health care settings, graduates from all schools are treated alike concerning placement. Nurses from four-year programs find they are unable to find positions that will allow them opportunities to practice in the manner for which they were prepared. Graduates from all programs often state they are not ready to assume responsibilities required of a staff nurse until they have had adequate orientation. Nurse-educators concur, believing it impossible to prepare students for all situations, given constraints on budget, time, and experiences in clinical settings. Employers agree that new graduates are not ready to function independently, yet counter that the cost of orienting inexperienced new graduates is great. The management of a 310-bed hospital estimated the direct cost for orienting one nurse to be $2,500.*

The need for an extended orientation period for new graduates or for orientation to special programs has been accepted by most administrators as the best answer to the problem of excessive turnover. Chapter 4 presents nurse preceptor programs as one response to the problem.

Staffing process

Matching client need with personnel who are able to meet that need requires a proper framework. After the preliminary work of developing the purpose, goals, standards of care, and method of control has been accomplished, an appropriate staffing pattern can be determined. The organizational structure will show the line of staff relationship of the personnel in the various departments. Also needed for successful staffing efforts are job descriptions that list the function and the various types and levels of personnel. Given this framework the nurse-manager will consider the following factors in the process of staffing: (1) the numbers and qualifications of personnel to meet the expectations of the institution, (2) circumstances peripheral to client needs and qualified personnel to meet those needs, (3) assignment of staff for continuity of service and economical use of personnel, (4) flexibility in staffing patterns, and (5) effective recruitment, orientation, and maintenance programs.

PREDICTIVE PRINCIPLE: Provision of sufficient numbers and qualifications of personnel to meet the expectations of the institution depends upon an accurate staffing system.

Researchers estimate that hospitals spend $15,000,000 yearly on nurse staffing studies.† It is their belief that much of this investment is used to rediscover old methods. The recommendation is that terminology for nurse staffing systems be standardized so that directors of nursing can better assess their organizations and make meaningful comparisons with other institutions.

Traditionally, nursing administrators have used one or more assessment methods for determining staffing patterns. These may consist of a tactical or flexible method of assessing the total client population of an agency or concentrating on a particular segment of services and dividing this number among the nursing staff available. Using the tactical system the staff needed is compared with what staff one has, with a final determination as to the number of nursing personnel required to provide care. This system allows a shift-by-shift analysis,

---

*Vaughan, R., and MacLeod, V.: Nurse staffing studies: no need to reinvent the wheel, J. Nurs. Admin. **10**(3):9, Mar. 1980.
†Hofmann, P.: Accurate measurement of nursing turnover: the first steps in its reduction, J. Nurs. Admin. **11**(11-12):37, 1981.

but also builds in a bi-weekly report that can be fed into an annual productivity report for long-range planning. The tactical or flexible plan has the disadvantage of working nurses at maximum capacity all of the time. Nurses have little opportunity to reflect on the care given or means for improvement.

Another assessment method concentrates on activities or task performance. The number of direct and indirect nursing tasks is correlated with the amount of time spent on these tasks. This method is borrowed from business, where the study of work focuses on identification of tasks, work flow, work reorganization, reassignment, and work simplification. Task analysis is particularly useful in work of a repetitive nature, where conditions are standard and predictable. Although specific data are provided with the task analysis approach, there are issues left unanswered for nursing. Cases in point are qualitative matters such as individual needs of clients, nurses fulfilling their roles to optimal capacity, and whether these tasks could be done better or equally as well by individuals with less preparation.

Attempts to overcome these shortcomings in staffing have been made fairly widely by many nurse-managers through client care classification methods to determine the client's needs and then to match these needs with qualified personnel.

A *client care classification system* is used by most hospitals in an effort to quantify the nursing work load in terms of categories that are broadly identifiable. The classification system is based on the premise that better staffing patterns will be realized by adjusting staffing according to the number of clients needing certain levels of care. Client care classification may encompass any number of categories or levels of care, such as clients who need self-care, partial care, and complete care. Other terms used are essential nursing care, progressive nursing care, and comprehensive care, or minimal, moderate, extensive, and intensive care. Specific criteria are described for each category or level of care, and a specific level of personnel is assigned for each category.

The problem of client classification is difficult because much overlap between classifications occurs, and all methods involve a degree of subjectivity. Many tools are used for data collection: direct observation, nursing audit, interviews with clients and staff, incident reports, and audit of charts. Descriptions of care include activities associated with daily living, treatments, and psychosocial needs.

Some methods for classifying patients are based on the point system. Values are ascribed to work required to fill a particular care need. For example, vital signs q.i.d. might have a value of 1 point, while a dressing change is given 2 points, and a bed bath and change of linen might be given a value of 5 points. Prepared charts are used to simplify the process. The point values for all activities required for each client are totaled and staff numbers decided. Obviously, this is a time-consuming task and it is impossible to account for every client need. Another method used is a system in which the acuity level for each client is classified according to numbers. Number 1, for example, might require minimal care and be assigned 3 hours. Class 2 may call for moderate care and is given 4 hours. Class 3 requires extensive care and is allotted 5 hours. Class 4 needs intensive care and therefore is given 6.5 hours.

Standardizing classification systems would be helpful in many ways. Patient classification data could be shared from agency to agency and comparisons made so that administrators can begin to evaluate productivity realistically.

The ratio of registered nurses to nonprofessionals and proportions of staff on the various shifts are also considered in staffing. When careful attention is given to matching client need with personnel who are capable of supplying that need, efforts will be made to staff accordingly. With increased focus on classification of services, the nursing profession has been able to demonstrate the need to move toward greater involvement of registered nurses in client care by all levels of nurses, including nurse-managers.

Both the American Nurses' Association *Standards for Nursing Services* and the Joint Commission on Accreditation of Hospitals emphasize the importance of the total concept of staffing. They call for sufficient numbers of registered nurses on duty at all times to provide clients with the nursing care that requires the judgment and specialized skills of the registered nurse. This standard is interpreted to mean that a determination of nursing personnel can be made only by evaluating the needs of the clients and the capabilities of the nursing staff assigned to a special area.

The goal of utilizing the professional nurse as fully as possible in performing only nursing functions has led to a reorganization of structure in nursing services to increase the proportion of personnel giving direct care to the client. Smaller spans of control through decentralization of services have helped to return the registered nurse to the bedside, planning and giving the care or directly supervising it.

A further delineation is needed between the registered nurses. If there is built into the system slots of various levels of nurses, for example, associate degree RN, baccalaureate RN, clinical specialists, or nurse-practitioner, and various values are assigned to these differing classifications of personnel, then one may expect greater efficiency, more job satisfaction, and higher levels of productivity. The possible contribution and competency levels of personnel with different educational backgrounds vary greatly. The best approach is to review the classifications or levels needed by reviewing the job descriptions. This helps determine how much and what duties can be performed by one worker as compared to another. In agencies where workers other than registered nurses are utilized, the nurse-manager will look to see which activities can be performed best by licensed practical or vocational nurses and will determine those tasks that can well be assigned to a nurse's aide.

PREDICTIVE PRINCIPLE: Circumstances peripheral to client needs and qualified personnel to meet those needs influence the staffing process.

There are many circumstances relating to the provision of quality care that may not have direct bearing on the individual need of the client or necessarily pertain to the competency of the nursing personnel but need to be taken into account when the staffing pattern is determined. The consistency of census is one problem. In some services, particularly where the birth and care of children are concerned, there is a great fluctuation in the census. Another issue is that of the physical layout of the area where excessive time and energy are required to cover the territory. Other circumstances that require consideration are use of automation through intercommunication systems and computerized control; use of reusable versus disposable equipment; centralized or decentralized services; support staff; utilization of part-time nurses, students, or private duty nurses; and the size and involvement of the medical staff.

PREDICTIVE PRINCIPLE: Assignment of staff for continuity of service and economical use of personnel promotes client satisfaction and results in cost effectiveness.

PREDICTIVE PRINCIPLE: Flexibility in staffing patterns increases the recruitment and retention of nursing staff needed.

Basically a schedule for nursing staff needs to (1) adhere to the policies of the employing agency regarding utilization of professional nurse personnel and workers in different categories while ensuring appropriate balance of professional and nonprofessional staff, (2) provide for continuity of services, (3) seek to make effective and economical use of personnel, (4) consider vacations and other scheduled time off, (5) allow for adjustments in case of illness, emergencies, or changes in care needs, and (6) protect the rights of individuals against discriminating action because of sex, ethnic differences, or religious beliefs.

Scheduling may be performed centrally or at the departmental or unit level, or through combined effort. There are advantages and disadvantages to each system. With *centralized control* the personnel can be distributed objectively in a more balanced manner among the nursing units, and understaffing or overstaffing can be handled to some degree. Centralized staffing is less time consuming than other methods. The one who determines the master schedule is in a position to know the overall staffing situation; thus it is easier to make adaptations to unforeseen circumstances. Requests for special privileges are likely to be fewer than with the decentralized system.

Disadvantages of the centralized system are that opportunities for personal contact with employees is reduced, causing the one who plans the schedule to know little or nothing about the person scheduled on the time sheet. The maker of schedules may not have a true picture of the needs within each departmental unit.

With *decentralization* of schedules the nurse-manager at the middle or first level has opportunity to base the scheduling plan on knowledge of the clients and of the personnel assigned to that unit. The nurse-manager is more in control of the activities on the unit. The decentralized system poses some problems in that it is time consuming and sometimes provides inadequate coverage, as when there are not enough staff members on hand to cover unexpected absences or there is the need for additional help and individual employees are subjected to inequities in rotation and days off.

A common staffing pattern utilized by the nurse-manager is to plan a staffing schedule using the personnel assigned to a unit and to depend on additional help from a centralized source such as the nursing service offices for unexpected absences or emergencies. This staffing method works well if each nurse is expected to work a fair share of weekends, holidays, and unpopular work hours, such as evenings or nights. The approach to developing a time schedule often focuses on consideration of preferences of individual staff and the matter of seniority. Resultant inequities occur, with the newer or less experienced personnel being assigned to the undesirable shifts and most of the weekends and holidays. With this approach, little attention is given to the development of a schedule that is directed toward adequate and qualified nursing services on a twenty-four hour basis.

The traditional *5-40 pattern*, or five eight-hour days, still meets with approval from the majority of nurses; however, staffing experiments around the country suggest there is interest in alternate plans. The *4-40 pattern* of four ten-hour days (Fig. 3-1) was first tried in 1972. Advantages are that overlapping shifts provide for better coverage and client care, staff members have weekends off

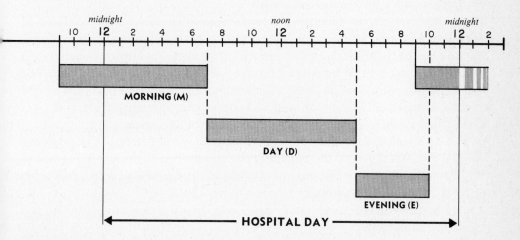

Fig. 3-1. Example of schedule for 40-hour, 4-day workweek. (From Fraser, L.P.: The reconstructed workweek: one answer to the scheduling dilemma, J. Nurs. Admin. **2:**12-16, Sept.-Oct. 1972.)

more frequently, there are decreases in absenteeism and in expenses related to overtime, and the system is cost effective. The main problems with the ten-hour day are fatigue and difficulty finding relief personnel to work an extended day. A number of variations of the 4-40 workweek have been tried. A popular approach has been to use this schedule on the night shift to attract staff with three days off per week.

Cyclic scheduling is one method of staffing that probably is the most valid and workable system for numbers of personnel. It involves the development of schedule patterns that are repeated at regular intervals. Schedule patterns for days and time off are established at a centralized level for a certain number of weeks, ranging from two to twelve, and are repeated within the given cycle period, while giving attention to the need for appropriate numbers and categories of personnel, continuity of client care, and establishment of work groups. Examples are given in Figs. 3-2 and 3-3.

In cyclic scheduling with a ten-hour day, four-day workweek, one plan is to provide every other weekend off, with single days off added to weekends (Fig. 3-4). No employee is scheduled for more than four consecutive ten-hour shifts in a row. All have at least fourteen hours free between any two shifts. Those who "float" are given a four-day weekend every six weeks. Likewise, it is possible to rotate shifts on a regular basis, usually every three months, if the staff is in accordance with the plan.

Cyclic scheduling of an eight-hour shift for a twelve-week cycle is particularly useful, because twelve weeks is easily divisible for days off and can be adapted uniformly to both large and small units. Each nurse has four weekends off, two of which are three-day weekends. The period also includes six single days off and five workweeks of six days each. The plan presented in Fig. 3-3 can be duplicated for the twelve-week span.

The cyclic scheduling system lends itself well to the computer, thus saving manpower and providing for early printouts of the schedule. With the cyclic method a pool system of floating personnel is necessary to ensure assignment of an adequate number of personnel during each shift to any unit insufficiently staffed because of illness, absence, or emergency. If computers are not available, cyclic staffing sheets can be printed and names can be recorded manually.

The cyclic staffing system has a number of advantages:

1. A stabilized work force is provided, allowing personnel to synergize their efforts for the benefit of the clients.
2. A correct number and mix of personnel are provided with a minimum of floating personnel.
3. Time off is known well in advance so that workers can plan their personal lives.
4. "Good" and "bad" days off are shared by all.
5. A controlled maximum number of work periods before a day off is provided.

Elements:

Every third weekend off	Number of "split" days off each period = 2
Maximum days worked: 4	Operates in multiples of 3, 6, 9, ...
Minimum days worked: 3	Schedule repeats every 3 weeks

▢ Scheduled day off

Position	Name	Week I							Week II							Week III							
		S	M	T	W	T	F	S	S	M	T	W	T	F	S	S	M	T	W	T	F	S
Full time	R.N. 1																					
Full time	R.N. 2																					
Full time	R.N. 3																					
Total R.N.s on duty each day		2	2	3	2	2	2	2	2	3	2	2	2	2	2	2	3	2	2	2	2	2
Full time	R.N. 1																					
Full time	R.N. 2																					
Part time	32 hrs/week R.N. 3																					
Total R.N.s on duty each day		2	2	2	2	2	2	2	2	2	2	2	2	2	2	2	2	2	2	2	2	2
Full time	R.N. 1																					
Full time	R.N. 2																					
Full time	R.N. 3																					
Full time	R.N. 4																					
Full time	R.N. 5																					
Full time	R.N. 6																					
Total R.N.s on duty each day		4	4	5	4	5	4	4	4	5	4	4	5	4	4	4	5	5	4	4	4	4
Full time	R.N. 1																					
Full time	R.N. 2																					
Part time	32 hrs/week R.N. 3																					
Full time	R.N. 4																					
Full time	R.N. 5																					
Part time	32 hrs/week R.N. 6																					
Total R.N.s on duty each day		4	4	4	4	4	4	4	4	4	4	4	4	4	4	4	4	4	4	4	4	4

Note: 8 hrs. of R.N. time saved per week by using part time R.N.s

Note: 16 hrs. of R.N. time saved per week by using part time R.N.s

Fig. 3-2. Example of cyclic scheduling using 8-hour day, 40-hour workweek. Master time schedule for 3-week cycle. (From Eusanio, P.L.: Effective scheduling—the foundation for quality care. J. Nurs. Admin. **8:**12-17, Jan. 1978.)

Nursing management and leadership in action

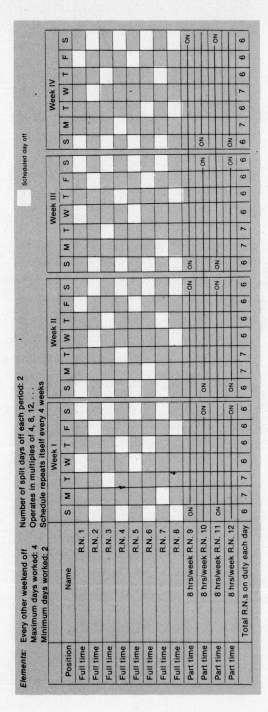

Fig. 3-3. Example of cyclic scheduling. Master time schedule for 4-week cycle. (From Eusanio, P.L.: Effective scheduling—the foundation for quality care, J. Nurs. Admin. **8:** 12-17, Jan. 1978.)

	S	M	T	W	TH	F	S	S	M	T	W	TH	F	S
Employee A	-	on	on	-	-	on	on	on	-	-	on	on	-	-
Employee B	on	-	-	on	on	-	-	-	on	on	-	-	on	on

Fig. 3-4. Example of basic 10-hour schedule for 2-week cycle. (From Fraser, L.P.: The reconstructed workweek: one answer to the scheduling dilemma, J. Nurs. Admin. **2:**12-16, Sept.-Oct. 1972.)

An added benefit to the nurse-manager is that the time spent on scheduling can be significantly reduced. Once the master plan has been developed, a person with less training can prepare and maintain schedules, freeing the nurse-manager for more direct contact with personnel and clients.

The *7-70 approach* utilizes the ten-hour workday with seven ten-hour days on, followed by seven days off. One administrator reports a dramatic decrease in overtime and sick time and a decrease in staff turnover since the initiation of the 7-70 plan. Also, with the increased importance of written communication when staff change every week, documentation of nursing assessments and care plans improved.

The *7-56 plan* calls for night nurses to work seven consecutive eight-hour shifts and then have seven nights off. The intensive care unit at Baptist Medical Center—Montclair in Birmingham, Alabama instituted this system in 1980. It is now extending the plan to all night nurses in their hospital. Nurses are paid at a time-and-a-half rate for the sixteen hours worked in excess of forty hours per week. Instead of accruing time off, workers are paid for approximately 7.5 hours of earned time off weekly.

The *2-days alternative* was introduced at Baylor University Medical Center in Dallas, Texas. RNs can work either two twelve-hour weekend shifts or five eight-hour Monday-through-Friday shifts. Nurses who choose the two twelve-hour day option are paid for 36 hours of work. If they work the night shift, they are paid for 40 hours. This program requires a larger nursing staff, which increases the budget, but Baylor has solved their staffing problem.

The *3-40 plan* was begun in 1975 at Valley Medical Center in Fresno, California on a twenty-seven—bed unit. Six years later the staff have elected to continue with the system. Nurses work a three-day week of two thirteen- and one fourteen-hour days with four days off. Fatigue was a factor at first, but nurses at Fresno report that after several months it diminishes. Under the 3-40 plan, mistakes, turnover, and absenteeism have all decreased. Conversely, retention of nurses has increased, thus making the plan cost effective.

The *two- versus three-day weekend incentive* is employed at Women's Hospital of Texas. The nurse can opt for a traditional five-day forty-hour week, Monday through Friday or can work a two- or three-day weekend. On the two-day weekend, the nurse works two sixteen-hour shifts and is paid for 40 hours. The ICU staff begins at 7:00 A.M. and ends at 11:00 P.M.; on all other units the sixteen-hour shift starts at 3:00 P.M. and finishes at 7:00 A.M. The three-day weekend plan requires twelve-hour shifts with at least one shift on the weekend, running Thursday through Tuesday. The nurse works thirty-six hours and is paid for forty.

Combination shifts are useful for some institutions. Virginia Hospital in Richmond offers a *2-8s plus 2-12s plan* whereby the nurse works eight hours for two shifts and twelve hours for two others. The hospital attempts to simplify the plan by designating Monday, Wednesday, and Friday as eight-hour days and Sunday, Tuesday, Thursday, and Saturday as twelve-hour days. This plan seems particularly appealing to women with small children, as they can adjust their schedule around that of their family.

Another alternative plan used at Doctor's Hospital in Phoenix, Arizona is the *4-6s plus 1-12*. All staff, including unit clerks, work a pattern of either three twelve-hour shifts or a combination of four six-hour shifts with one 12-hour shift.

Whatever the plan, flexibility is the key. Agencies that have chosen to experiment with staffing patterns have found their staffing problems greatly diminished or eliminated.

PREDICTIVE PRINCIPLE: Criteria established for supplemental or temporary staffing helps support continuity of care.

Because there are more nurses prepared and in active practice than ever before (1.4 million) with a higher ratio of nurses per population, one would think there would be an oversupply. However, there is an acute shortage of professional nurses in the United States, the greatest since the 1940s. Perhaps one reason is that the demand for nurses has not remained constant. Budget constraints require more attention to be given to staffing according to patient population and acuity levels, leaving some nurses insecure concerning their jobs. Another cause may be a reaction among today's nurses to traditionally rigid hospital environments.

Strategies are needed to provide for a safe level of nursing care with fewer available RNs employed as permanent employees. Although 60% of all active nurses work in hospitals, significant numbers among them work through agencies established outside the institutional structure. Many agencies make attractive offers of higher pay and flexible schedules, allowing the nurse the option of picking and choosing hours according to home responsibilities and outside interests.

The more common philosophy of contracting for "agency nurses" is to use them in emergencies or until the vacancies can be filled. This approach tends to create a negative attitude toward temporary nurses, as they serve as an irritating reminder of the staffing shortage, further compounding the problem.

Use of temporary nurses needs to be well planned. With a haphazard use of supplemental staff several outcomes can be expected: increased absenteeism and tardiness among both temporary and permanent staff, problems with payroll, orientation of temporary staff requiring more time from already overburdened regular employees, and a lack of continuity of nursing care.

One nursing department at the Rush-Presbyterian—St. Luke's Medical Center in Chicago developed a predictable and consistent system in 1979 to make better use of supplemental staff.* The system has proved highly successful. A statement of the criteria for a temporary staffing system was fundamental to its development. The planners decided the system would have to: (1) be controlled and predictable, (2) support the unit leader as first-line manager, and (3) support continuity of care.

Their strategies included giving one person in the hospital responsibility for developing the temporary staffing program (the assistant to the chairman of the nursing department). She established a close communication with the supplying agencies, asking that the same agency person work with the hospital scheduler. Forms were developed that allowed for control and predictability. Each temporary nurse who worked in the hospital provided information as to which days and shifts she was available. Using this availability sheet and the projected needs of the hospital, a temporary staff request sheet was sent to the agency on a monthly basis, which achieved more balanced scheduling. The hospital used a computerized printout of both regular and temporary staff. It was discovered that the information provided enhanced continuity, because a temporary nurse's time for an entire month could be planned for a given unit at the time of computer scheduling. More balanced schedules were produced because of the increased pool of nurses, making it possible for a more equitable distribution of days and weekends off.

Another advantage to the system was being able to assign a temporary nurse to the same unit and the same clients. This resulted in continuity of care and development of teamwork among the regular and temporary staff, bringing more job satisfaction. Policies relevant to temporary staffing were formulated:

1. Each unit is responsible for using temporary nurses in a supplemental capacity or in "hot spots" (units that become suddenly very active) and not as core staff for that unit.
2. Temporary staff are not used to replace vacancies created by poor permanent staff scheduling decisions.
3. Temporary staff do not replace vacancies caused by unit absenteeism.
4. If staffing should become critically low because of absenteeism on a unit, temporary staff will be asked to float to that unit.

---

*Shanks, K., and Potempa, K.: A system for using supplemental staff, J. Nurs. Admin. **11**(10):42-46, 1981.

5. One standard of performance is expected of all staff members, both permanent and temporary.
6. Verbal and written evaluations are regularly completed on each agency nurse by a designated hospital employee.
7. Each agency nurse receives an orientation.

A well-planned, coordinated, and executed plan for use of supplemental staff can fulfill needs with gratifying rewards. The work force can be stabilized and quality of care improved, thereby providing safe nursing care for every client, with increased job satisfaction for hospital employees and supplemental staff as well.

PREDICTIVE PRINCIPLE: Establishment of policies and programs that ensure fairness, consistency, and professional development of human resources enables recruitment and maintenance of a sufficient number of qualified nurses.

There is really no beginning or ending to the staffing process. A stream of qualified personnel must be kept flowing into the health organization and through the various channels designed to develop and allocate human resources. No organization is static. At any given time one can find employees leaving, and shortages occur at certain points and surpluses at others. Staffing is a composite of dynamic and persistent activities with which the manager must be concerned. Adequate attention to recruitment and maintenance of nurses will pay off in rewards to the agency and retention and satisfaction among the staff employed, as well as being cost effective. However, before staffing efforts can be successful, guidelines need to be established that provide a thorough and honest description of duties, responsibilities, and limits of authority of the position.

Prior to employing a nurse an open exchange of information occurs that will promote an equitable match between the nurse and the job. This can be done through interview, observation, and exposure to the work setting. The manager arranges a time for the prospective employee to tour the work area and to talk freely with the staff. Again, job descriptions are all important. Detailed information about the duties involved in the job and the qualifications an employee must have to perform them are reviewed.

Formal induction of the employee is an important matter. This is the time when policies pertaining to salary, fringe benefits, retention, promotion, and tenure are discussed. The *wage and salary program* is the responsibility of the organization as a whole. However, the manager often plays a key part in making decisions about salary increases and about promotion for employees under his or her jurisdiction. Policies pertaining to the wage and salary program should address (1) differences in pay for various classifications of work, (2) a level of wage that is in reasonable alignment with the prevailing scale for institutions of similar nature in the same geographic location, (3) differences in preparation and experience of employees, (4) means for rewarding individual expertise and contribution through salary increment or promotion, and (5) a clearly defined procedure for offering complaints and grievances.

The *orientation period* is crucial to the retention and satisfaction of the employee. Progressive companies in industry have long recognized the need for properly introducing a new employee to the job. It has been well documented in nursing that a thorough orientation and time to adapt to the new work setting increase the level of performance of employees.

Orientation is the formal process of familiarizing new employees with the organization and their part in it. Not only does the program familiarize new workers with the tasks they will be expected to perform, but also it provides them with information about the overall philosophy, conceptual framework, and objectives of the organization. A carefully planned orientation program helps new employees to identify with the organization and its procedures, enables them to learn the unique ways the agency wants nursing roles and functions fulfilled, and gives some feeling for the significance of the work they will be doing. The new employee is helped to overcome the fears and anxieties that are bound to arise in a new job. A well-run orientation program has the further benefit of helping the new worker gain acceptance by fellow employees. Chapter 4 on teaching and learning presents guidelines for orientation programs and follow-up of new employees.

Application of predictive principles on staffing

Kathy had been functioning at a high professional level as a staff nurse on a medical unit until six months ago when she resigned to have a baby. Now she wants to return to work, but on her terms. She tells the employer (head nurse) that she will work only the day shift, on Tuesdays and Wednesdays, each month.

Problem	Predictive principle	Prescription
Kathy's return to work is desired, but her terms are too restrictive for the needs of the medical unit.	Standards of care, clearly defined, allow for descriptions of personnel necessary for implementation.	Head nurse affirms with Kathy her competency and the head nurse's desire to have her return as an employee.
	Circumstances peripheral to client needs and qualified personnel to meet those needs influence the staffing process.	Head nurse listens to Kathy's rationale for the restrictive work schedule.
	Establishment of policies and procedures that ensure fairness, consistency, and professional development enables recruitment and maintenance of a sufficient number of qualified nurses.	Head nurse states that the timeframe presented is unreasonable; that compliance with her request would require other nurses to be deprived of their preferences, etc.

Problem	*Predictive principle*	*Prescription*
	Congruence among personal, professional, and organizational goals reduces nurse turnover and shortages.	Head nurse presents an alternative plan whereby Kathy is granted Tuesday and Wednesday for three weeks, but must work one weekend a month. The decision rests with Kathy whether or not to accept the offer.

BIBLIOGRAPHY
Books

Donovan, H.: Nursing service administration: managing the enterprise, St. Louis, 1975, The C.V. Mosby Co.

Williams, J.: Human behavior in organizations, Palo Alto, Calif., 1978, South-Western Publishing Co.

Periodicals

Aiken, L., Blendon, R., and Rogers, D.: The shortage of hospital nurses: a new perspective, Am. J. Nurs. **81**(9):1612-1619, 1981.

Alrvizatos, M.: A new concept in scheduling for nurses, Superv. Nurse **12**(2):20-24, 1981.

Bell, M.: Management by objectives, J. Nurs. Admin. **10**(5):19-26, 1980.

Benziger, K.: The powerful woman, Hosp. Forum **25**(3):6-14, May-June 1982.

Bloch, D.: Criteria, standards, norms—crucial terms in quality assurance, J. Nurs. Admin. **7**(9):20-30, 1977.

Calabrese, R.: Interaction skills for nurse managers, Nurs. Management **13**(5):29-35, 1982.

Clark, E.: A model of nurse staffing for effective patient care, J. Nurs. Admin. **7**(2):23-27, 1977.

Eusanio, P.: Effective scheduling—the foundation for quality care, J. Nurs. Admin. **13**(1): 12-17, 1978.

Everly, G., and Falcione, R.: Perceived dimensions of job satisfaction for staff registered nurses, Nurs. Res. **25**(9):346-348, 1976.

Fralic, M.: Nursing shortage: coping today and planning for tomorrow, Hospitals **54**(9):65-67, 1980.

Fredericks, C.: Reversing the turnover trend, Nurs. Manag. **12**(12):42-44, 1981.

Hofman, P.: Accurate measurement of nursing turnover: the first step in its reduction, J. Nurs. Admin. **11**(11,12):37-39, 1981.

Kay, G., and Krol, S.: The nursing shortage: this time traditional responses won't work, Superv. Nurse **12**(7):13-17, 1981.

Kelly, L.: A celebration of nursing, Nurs. Outlook **30**(5):322, 1982.

Pilous, B.: The advantage of part-time nursing, Amer. J. Nurs. **81**(5):981-982, 1981.

Price, E.: The demise of the traditional workweek, Amer. J. Nurs. **81**(6):1138-1141, 1981.

Rose, M.A.: Factors affecting nurse supply and demand: an exploration, J. Nurs. Admin. **12**(2): 31-34, 1982.

Shanks, K., and Potempa, K.: A system for using supplemental staff, J. Nurs. Admin. **11**(10):41-46, 1981.

Silber, M.: The motivation pyramid in nurse retention, Superv. Nurse **12**(4):45-46, 1981.

Smith, M.: Resource team: a staffing solution, Nurs. Manag. **12**(11):39-41, 1981.

Vaughan, R., and MacLeod, V.: Nurse staffing studies: no need to reinvent the wheel, J. Nurs. Admin. **10**(3):9-15, 1980.

Wandelt, M., Pierce, P., and Widdowson, R.: Why nurses leave nursing and what can be done about it, Amer. J. Nurs. **81**(1):72-77, 1981.

White, C.: Where have all the nurses gone—and why? Hospitals **54**(9):68-71, 1980.

Wolf, G.: Nursing turnover: some causes and solutions, Nurs. Outlook **29**(4):233-236, 1981.

chapter four

Predictive principles of teaching and learning

Assessment
The learner's developmental stage, personal characteristics, and prior experiences influence learning potential and dictate content.

The learner's sociocultural and religious group determines the nature, content, and acceptability of learnings.

The learner's prevalent life needs determine what he or she will learn.

Formulation of objectives
Participation of the learner in setting learning goals increases the number of learning activities meaningful and useful to the learner.

The more congruent and relevant that goals are to life needs of the learner-client, the more likely the goals are to be achieved.

Realistic behavioral goal setting enables selection of appropriate and meaningful content.

Setting goals that specify the precise degree of attainment required provides the learner with guidelines that can be followed.

Objectives that describe outcomes in small increments enable successful fulfillment.

Motivation and reinforcement
Use of motivation theories enables the development of guidelines for understanding and assessing behaviors.

An obvious relationship between learning activities and stated goals increases the motivational value of the activity.

Accomplishment of beginning objectives reinforces belief in ability and motivates to greater effort for greater accomplishment.

Closely monitoring the level and source of anxiety and excitement in the learner enables the teacher to adapt the learning plan to learner needs.

Teaching in times of crisis about how to handle the crisis increases the opportunity for reinforcement and retention of learned behaviors.

Rewards consistent with the value system of the learner, such as recognition, praise, peer status, or valued gains, are motivating and reinforcing influences and thus facilitate learning rate, amount of retention, and degree of behavior change.

Practice of learned activities in a variety of ways reinforces learned behaviors and promotes the ability to generalize and discriminate.

Establishing the learning environment

A reciprocal relationship of trust and security facilitates teacher-learner communication and allows accurate assessment, learner participation in goal setting, and better utilization of resources.

Recognition of the effect environment has on learning enables the nurse-teacher to mobilize environmental factors for the reinforcement of content.

Accountability for learning that rests with the learner enables him to meet his own learning needs and goals and enables the teacher to act as resource person, facilitator, validator, conferee, and consultant.

Verbal or written contracts with client-learners for attainment of specific learner needs enable the nurse-teacher to enact the teaching role more precisely.

Structure, limits, and feedback provide an environment that promotes security and trust.

Awareness of legal aspects of client education provides the nurse with the scope and limitations of content to be taught.

Learning activities

Ability to use a varied number of learning theories increases the probability that varied strategies will be used in the nurse-teacher's teaching repertoire.

Learning episodes that contain input, operations, and feedback increase retention and utility of learning.

Varied teaching strategies and operations available to and usable by the nurse-teacher, increase the nurse-teacher's selection of strategy based on learner and situational needs.

Utilization of problem-solving processes promotes continuity and ease of learning.

Increasing the difficulty of learning material in small increments promotes learning success.

Evaluation

Objectives expressed as learner behaviors enable the teacher and learner to know the limits of expected outcomes and to evaluate in meaningful, specific terms.

Criteria by which to measure success, established through collaboration between teacher and learner, provide motivation, reinforcement, and guides for determining achievement.

Staff development

In-service education programs structured to separate orientation, clinical experience, and management aspects promote clarity of content and staff growth.

Effective orientation programs contribute to retention of personnel and promote job satisfaction.

Establishment of preceptor training programs for new nurses bridges the gap between education and service and reduces turnover rate.

Vaccines are helpless to prevent diseases unless people use them; heart patients live longer if they learn how to cope with their disabilities; people with diabetes live fairly normal lives if they learn how to balance their body needs, food, and insulin; cancer can be diagnosed and treated early if people learn to watch for the signs and symptoms; contagion can be stopped when people learn how to intervene in the transmission and resistance systems. The health status of any individual, family, community, or country is directly related to that individual's or group's ability to learn to prevent disease and to maintain health, to get well and to stay well. Medical science is helpless against ignorance, and information is useless without changes in behaviors that translate the information into healthful activities.

All nurses function as teachers. Nurses teach clients, families, ancillary personnel, and one another. Teaching is inherent in the nurse role whether or not the nurse consciously cultivates and exhibits teacher behaviors.

The teaching role in nursing usually is the responsibility of lower and middle level management. It seldom is assumed by upper level management. Upper level management people usually delegate their teaching functions to others—the staff development director, the client education coordinator, the clinical specialist, the clinical coordinator, the supervisor, the head nurse, the team leader, or other staff nurses. Middle and lower management people find teaching one of their major responsibilities. The formal classroom setting, where clearly delineated teacher-learner roles are established, is increasingly common in practice settings. However, more commonly, because of the nature of nursing practice, the nurse-leader serves as teacher in a wide variety of everyday activities. These activities range in scope from role modeling to tutorial one-to-one methods for solving nursing problems to preplanning and teaching small and large groups using a formal structure.

The nurse who assumes responsibility for assessing problems and for seeking ways to teach will be concerned with principles and methodology of the teaching-learning process. The problem facing all nurses is how to develop structures and relationships in which learning can occur.

Nurses are the single largest health worker force in the world. They teach health to people and in so doing prevent disease, maintain health, facilitate coping, and enable individuals to learn to reestablish healthful living patterns. Several factors influence the teaching-learning process. These factors include the following:

1. A value need, problem, or dilemma that will motivate people to learn
2. Information that will enable people to make realistic decisions about behaviors
3. Support, structure, and direction that will enable people to alter behaviors to conform to decisions that have been made
4. Reinforcement, which will ensure the continuation of changes in behavior

Teaching is often considered to be primarily a process of giving information to others; however, information alone will not enable the learner to change behavior. As T.S. Eliot wrote in "The Hollow Men,"

> Between the idea
> And the reality
> Between the motion
> And the act
> Falls the Shadow.

The nurse, whether leader or manager, teaches individuals and groups to ensure that applicable information is available and, additionally, helps the learner translate that information into behaviors so that no "shadow" falls between the idea and the behavior.

A nurse-teacher is a catalyst who can bring knowledge and learner together and stimulate a reaction. The teacher can engage in activity that either facilitates or inhibits the reaction and can function in ways that make the reaction either transient or more stable. Teaching causes learning to take place. Learning is the acquisition of knowledge with subsequent changes in the behavior of the learner. Behavior, as used here, means anything a person does in response to an internal or external stimulus. This response can take the form of overt physical activity, emotions, or mental processes. Teaching and learning are inseparably linked in a cause-and-effect relationship and are consequently treated here as a single topic.

Teachers work with feelings just as often as with information because teaching involves human beings. It is a popular misconception that if the teacher is dealing with feelings, the activity is not teaching but psychotherapy. There is conflict and disagreement among authorities about the similarities and differences between psychotherapy and teaching. Teachers are anxious not to blunder into areas that should be handled by a skilled therapist and are eager to establish some way to discriminate between the two. Basically, both psychiatric therapy and teaching have as their purpose behavioral changes, and this is what generates much of the confusion. In both teaching and therapy the client or learner must rearrange relationships between himself and other people, himself and a task, or himself and the environment. One of the key differences between the person needing therapy and the person needing teaching is the degree to which society has difficulty with the person. The person who needs psychotherapy is perceived either by himself or by others as behaving in a socially unacceptable manner. The person who needs teaching may not be using his fullest potential, but he is neither ostracized by society nor a danger to it. The difference is essentially a matter of degree.

Nurses must exercise considerable judgment in determining the differences between teaching and psychotherapy. There are few definite rules, but there are some guidelines that will help the nurse-teacher to determine if the teaching role is appropriate. Following are some of these guidelines:

1. Does the learner have the mental and physical potential to learn (can he or she alter present behavior to the desired behavior)?
2. Does the learner have a behavioral or thought disorder?
3. Can changes in behavior be brought about by:
   a. increased self-awareness and sensitivity to others?
   b. additional information?
   c. additional physical or cognitive skills?
   d. additional choices or alternatives?
   e. change in habit patterns?
   f. encouragement, reinforcement, or evaluative feedback?

The following example illustrates the use of the foregoing criteria:

Mr. Nesbit, a 38-year-old man, was suffering his first episode of duodenal ulcers. The nurse making the initial hospital admission contact with Mr. Nesbit asked him if he had any idea why he had ulcers. Mr. Nesbit replied that he thought he knew. He stated that there were times when he could feel his "stomach tighten up and the acid just pour in." When the nurse reported this to the team, the group asked, "Why not teach this man a different way to handle his feelings so that he need not jeopardize his health?" The nurse-leader replied, "I can't do that, I'm not a psychiatrist!"

The group decided to apply the criteria to determine if they could teach Mr. Nesbit and thus change his behavior response to feelings.

The following illustrates use of the criteria and the group's findings. No effort is made to discuss clinical content. The focus of the discussion is on the methodology of using the criteria given for the preparation of client teaching plans.

Criteria	*Group conclusions*
1. Has the mental and physical potential to learn	Mr. Nesbit is of normal intelligence, has no physical handicaps, and has held a stable job for many years.
2. Does not have a behavior or thought disorder	The client has socially acceptable behavior, can carry through in ordinary conversation, and makes appropriate responses to interview questions.
3. Changes in behavior can be brought about by	
a. increased self-awareness and sensitivity to others	Mr. Nesbit indicated an honest and well-developed sense of self-awareness as early as the first contact.
b. additional information	Additional information about stress, ulcers, and his behavior was available that would provide further data on which the patient could base changes of behavior.
c. additional physical or mental skills	Earlier awareness of rising stress would enable him to perceive impending situations that would elicit gastric responses.

Criteria	Group conclusions
d. additional choices or alternatives	Mr. Nesbit could participate with the nurse-teacher in exploring helpful ways to deal with stressful situations.
e. a change in habit patterns	Once new ways of handling stress are identified and tried, successful ones can be developed into new habits.
f. encouragement, reinforcement, or evaluative feedback	Close and honest working relationships with Mr. Nesbit can provide the nursing staff with opportunities to participate in identifying and reinforcing successful ways of handling stress. Reduced acid flow will be reinforcing.

When the discussion was completed, the team decided to work with Mr. Nesbit and teach him a more healthful way to handle stress. The nurse talked extensively with him and discovered that with some help he could identify some recent, very consistent sources of stress. The nurse supplied information about the physiology of duodenal ulcers and the stress—acid—intestinal motility relationship, and together Mr. Nesbit and the nurse worked out several alternative ways of dealing with the stress at the time it occurred. His hospital stay was of sufficient length to allow him several opportunities to cope with stressful situations successfully. The nursing team collaborated to reinforce his changing behavior.

Effective teaching is a learned process. Mastery of teaching requires knowledgeable, careful planning and continuous practice, for it is the teaching, not the teacher that is the key to learning. It is not what teachers are like but what they do that determines the outcome of the instruction and how the learners feel about themselves. Following is a discussion of concepts and predictive principles that are useful to the nurse in the teaching-learning process.

Assessment

Assessment is determining the present status of the individual; goal setting is establishing the changes that are necessary; teaching is facilitating changes; and evaluation is assessing what changes occurred and whether they were the desired changes.

Assessment is the first step in the teaching process and is necessary to establish need, content, and method. Even when incidental teaching occurs, quick assessments are made by the nurse-leader. Often these are so natural that they are engaged in without planning or conscious thought. Some of these easy and obvious assessments are the general health status of the learner, age, general alertness, and any more obvious characteristics.

Planned change requires detailed and methodical assessment of the learner and those things that influence learning. Assessment is not something that ends before teaching begins; it continues throughout the teaching process. Information gathered during all phases of teaching adds to the teacher's total knowledge of what the learner brings to the teaching-learning situation, and this knowledge contributes to better teaching.

The effective teacher gathers information from all available and appropriate sources. The patient, family members, friends, other members of the nursing and health teams, charts, observations, and other agencies contribute to the total data about the learner. The principles elaborated in this section are designed to help the nurse-leader assess the learner so that content and methodology have meaning and are useful.

PREDICTIVE PRINCIPLE: The learner's developmental stage, personal characteristics, and prior experiences influence learning potential and dictate content.

The age and central stage of development of the learner will determine how he interprets what he hears, sees, and experiences.

The age level is an indication of "normal" growth and maturation. The average child grows at a given rate and develops physical and mental skills at certain mean ages. With knowledge of normal growth and maturation the teacher will know at approximately which ages muscular coordination is developed, abstract thinking is developed, and physical decline will begin to occur.

Erikson's stages of development are briefly outlined here. Only the positive senses are listed. The negative senses, which Erikson calls the "dynamic counterpart," are omitted for brevity. The development of these "senses" is a problem or task facing each individual.*

1. Sense of trust (first year)—satisfying experiences or finding biologic and emotional needs taken care of consistently in appropriate ways without pain or harm
2. Sense of autonomy (12 months to 3 or 4 years)—asserting and concluding that the child is an individual with a choice and responsibility
3. Sense of initiative (4 to 6 years)—finding out what the child can do; period of vigorous learning and intrusion into other people's worlds by physical attack, incessant questioning, and locomotion
4. Sense of industry and accomplishment (6 to 12 years)—engagement in real, worthwhile, socially useful tasks that can be completed correctly and well
5. Sense of identity (early adolescence, 12 to 15 years)—clarification of who one is, what one's role in the world will be, and to what group or groups he or she belongs; whether independent or dependent, adult or child
6. Sense of intimacy (middle to late adolescence, 15 to 20 years)—friend-

---

*For a full discussion of the stages of development see Erikson, E.H.: Childhood and society, ed. 2, New York, 1963, W.W. Norton & Co., Inc., pp. 247-273.

ship and companionship; need for warm, close bonds with others, even a need for an inner feeling of fusion with others

7. Sense of generativity (adulthood)—interest in producing and caring for one's own children

8. Sense of integrity (maturity)—healthy integrated personality that accepts life, limitations, people, group, and time period; recognition and acceptance of limitations and potentialities

These categories are presented briefly and incompletely. The ages given are approximate ages of focus for each task. No task is mutually exclusive of other tasks, and most overlap and are repeated at subsequent stages of development.

Glueck, a management consultant, compiled the findings of several psychiatrists and psychologists into developmental stages that concentrate on the adult life more specifically than Erickson did believing this knowledge bears great significance to management.

1. *Leaving the family* (16 to 22 years). Fantasies of life begin to meet reality. The family ceases to be the primary influence and is replaced by peers who have equal standing with the individual, as with age and job. Peers impose group beliefs, and friendships are made and broken easily, usually with feelings of betrayal. Emotions are camouflaged to protect the person's feelings of insecurity. Nurse-managers who have young employees can recognize these behaviors as normal and deal with them accordingly.

2. *Reaching out* (23 to 28 years). During this period the individual becomes more stable, attempting to discover personal identity, which includes trying to understand the meaning of work. More attention is directed to standards of care and quality assurance. Deep relationships are formed, with the person looking to an older, more experienced individual to serve as a role model. This person often becomes the nurse in charge or assistant.

3. *Questioning period* (29 to 34 years). This is the period of crisis when individuals begin to wonder what life is all about and to question their personal and work relationships. Needs such as freedom from restraint versus upward mobility come into conflict. By this time most nurses are married and may have children. At the same time many are trying to be successful in the professional market. Some are feeling a need for educational advancement. During these turbulent years individuals begin to feel that if they do not make the right choices with respect to their lives and careers, they may never become the persons they hope to be. A significant point for the nurse-manager to realize is that if a person does not settle down by age 34, the chances of this individual forming a reasonably satisfying life structure are small. Nurses in this age group may have established goals that are as yet unfulfilled, but they know where they are and in what direction they want to go.

4. *Unstable period* (35 to 43 years). During this period an individual becomes aware that life may be half over or more. These years are sometimes labeled second adolescence. Parents are blamed for unresolved personality problems.

At work the person seeks to become a role model or counselor to someone else. The nurse in this age group is usually intensely interested in achieving or advancing, in proving to be a professional person.

5. *Settling in* (44 to 50 years). Most persons realize that major career decisions are settled and must be lived with. This does not negate their natural thirst for more learning and greater self-development. It usually means that they have attained the highest level of advancement in the work setting they are apt to achieve. (There are many exceptions to this statement, however, particularly with persons in the highest positions). Economic interests become less predominant; the individual looks to family and a few close friends as sources of social fulfillment and support.

6. *Mellowing* (50 years and over). This is the period when a person settles into a quiet pace, giving attention to the satisfactions, irritations, joys, and sometimes sorrows of each day. Parents are no longer blamed for personal problems, and the individual looks for opportunities to nurture others. Little attention is given to the past, but rather to the future. Persons in this age group are very interested in a retirement plan whereby security for life is assured. They are usually dependable and stable workers, unencumbered by the problems of young families. The person over age 50 is intent upon leaving a good record and acquiring as many benefits as possible.

The nurse-leader who can recognize developmental levels and central tasks of learning, whether the learner is a client or staff member, can use this knowledge effectively in teaching. For example, the child who has not developed a concept of time cannot be taught about "tomorrow," for time has no meaning or reference point. Or a 23-year-old new employee who is assigned to work in an unstable staffing environment in which she must be oriented to her role by different nurses almost every day, who themselves may be struggling to become acclimated, cannot identify with a role model. Her developmental need to discover personal identity and to develop deep relationships with peers is denied and personal and professional growth hindered. The repercussions of such an experience can bear great significance to management.

The use of central tasks of development in teaching patients can be seen in the following situation:

Carolyn, a 15-year-old girl, was admitted to the orthopedic ward with a fractured femur and was placed in balanced traction. She was 30 pounds overweight and was placed on a 1000 calorie diet. Maintenance of the diet quickly became a power struggle between Carolyn and the nursing and dietary staffs. The physician ordered dietary teaching for Carolyn, which was given by the hospital dietitian using didactic methods.

High school friends participated in the power struggle by smuggling in favorite candies; parents became caught up in the cross fire between pampering a loved child and cooperating with the prescribed regimen. One day the team leader asked, "Carolyn, does food really mean that much to you?" Carolyn replied, "Not really, but I don't like to be *made* to do anything. I'm old enough to eat what I please."

The nurse assessed Carolyn's present task of development as the need for identity and independence from adult domination. This developmental task was then used by the nurse to foster personal growth. The nurse obtained the physician's cooperation and the diet order was changed to a "regular select." The nurse then acted on the knowledge that the adolescent needs to plan her own life and course of action in collaboration with others but maintaining some degree of independence.

The teacher used Carolyn's additional need for intimacy with the concomitant adolescent preoccupation with appearance and attraction of the opposite sex to interest her in personal hygiene and grooming. Dietary facts and information were supplied in the form of booklets and pamphlets. Carolyn was soon asking for explanations about food values, calories, fats, protein, and carbohydrates. A high school friend brought her a home economics book, and Carolyn requested the dietitian to come back so questions could be answered. By the time Carolyn returned to school, she had lost the 30 pounds and was helping her mother lose weight by planning the family meals. The nurse's skilled use of the central tasks of development of the middle teens enabled the accomplishment of the desired health goal for Carolyn.

Personal characteristics, such as intelligence, curiosity, perseverance, fear, insecurity, ways of handling stress, and adaptability, help to determine the content and method of teaching. Often a learner's inability to speak English or health problems such as blindness or deafness mask intelligence or obscure other personal characteristics. These factors should be carefully considered when assessing the learner.

The nurse-teacher can make some personal characteristic assessments by observing the learner's ability to solve small problems and cope with minor life situations. Entering into ordinary discourse with people can give the nurse further clues about their intelligence and level of curiosity. The nurse can observe (1) the kind of questions that are asked, (2) the frequency with which the same question is repeated, (3) the rapidity with which simple instructions and routines are grasped, and (4) the difficulty or ease with which new ideas and ways are adapted. These observations help the nurse build a picture of the learner's personal characteristics and assist with the adoption of content useful to the learner.

The following are examples in which personal characteristics hinder the teaching-learning process:

Barbara, a baccalaureate graduate, was employed at a general hospital and enrolled in a twelve-week orientation program for new graduates. Although she was graduated with honors, Barbara was hesitant to function independently, even at the end of the training program. She continued to make statements to her preceptor such as "I'd rather you show me again," or "I need to read a little more about that procedure before I try," or "I prefer to restrict my activities to what I am doing for a while until I feel more comfortable."

When these actions were explored, the nurse-leader identified that Barbara was capable but was afraid to move from the student role into a professional arena where she would be required to function independently.

Jan, who spoke no Spanish, was attempting to instruct a woman who spoke no English about how to give herself a vinegar douche. She brought the solution to the bed-side, and through a series of gestures with smiles and nods of affirmation from the client determined the procedure would be accomplished well. Twenty minutes later the nurse found the client vomiting large quantities of fluid. The woman had misunderstood and drunk the liquid. Somewhere assessment and validation had broken down. Clear communication is essential.

Prior experiences influence present responses by providing the conditioning and context for understanding the meaning of educational stimuli. Concepts are learned by building ideas, facts, knowledge, and antecedent concepts, one on the other, pyramiding them into an interrelated whole.

Everyone has antecedent knowledge and concepts on which to build new knowledge. The nurse cannot assess all prior experiences of learners but can evaluate selected prior experiences. Education, family constellation, experiences with teachers and health personnel, hobbies, interest areas, and occupation provide reference points, context, and antecedent knowledge for learning. This information allows the nurse-teacher to start where the learner is and to relate new material to familiar material in meaningful ways.

PREDICTIVE PRINCIPLE: The learner's sociocultural and religious group determines the nature, content, and acceptability of learnings.

The learner's sociocultural and religious group usually determines his or her value system. The value system dictates what is right and wrong, moral and immoral, fair or unfair, honest or dishonest, desirable or detestable. A value system influences ideas and feelings about others and provides guidelines to behaviors.

Teaching and learning objectives consistent with the learner's value system are realistic and achievable; the value system itself can be used as a motivation factor. Objectives in conflict with the learner's values are unrealistic and almost impossible to achieve without first changing the values.

An example of the influence of values derived from cultural groups can be seen in the following:

Alfonso is a 22-year-old Mexican-American with diabetes. Alfonso resisted all health teaching, regardless of methodology, until he saw another diabetic, aged 40, with a below-the-knee amputation as a result of gangrene. The knowledge that a loss of limb could be a consequence of uncontrolled diabetes and inattention to special foot care shocked Alfonso and threatened his "macho" (self-concept of manliness). He became interested in preserving his feet and legs and learned rapidly about all aspects of diabetes.

He also helped the nurse to understand the importance of the "extended family" in the Mexican-American culture so that more valuable and realistic teaching could include reference to the extended family.

Knowledge of and respect for the learner's value system will be a major determinant in the teacher's success or failure and may influence the learner's future relationship with health care personnel. Values govern both the learner's and the teacher's behavior; interpretations of and judgments about other people's behavior are made within the framework of each person's value system. The nurse-teacher must not only be cognizant of the learner's sociocultural or religious values but also must have insight and self-knowledge.

Religious constraints can sometimes create problems as illustrated by the following:

Rosanne, a Jehovah's Witness, asked to be assigned to an acute care medical unit. She stated, however, that she could not "have anything to do with handling blood transfusions" as this treatment was contrary to her beliefs.

The problem was solved by Rosanne agreeing to learn about the hospital's nursing procedure and to monitor the patient during and after the administration of blood. Problems of this kind have more ramifications than teaching and learning, for when one nurse refuses a part of the client's care for whatever reason, another person must assume that responsibility. In this instance, the nursing staff wanted Rosanne as a member of their team, so they worked out a trade of activities when they needed to assume part of her work load. The staff members respected Rosanne's value system and were willing to sacrifice something to preserve it.

PREDICTIVE PRINCIPLE: The learner's prevalent life needs determine what he or she will learn.

The learner, as does any other organism, responds to the strongest stimulus. Adults make most of their own decisions about what they will do, where they will go, what will happen to them, and what they will learn. Adults want to become involved in decision-making that concerns them. A strong need is a strong stimulus, and early in the episode the teacher must identify the most urgent need, for until this need is met little else will be learned. The needs of the learner determine what is seen and heard and the interpretation placed on sensory input. A patient who had just had an electrocardiogram and was anxious over the results was asked by the team leader, who was making patient rounds, if he had been up yet that morning. The patient replied, "Why, what's the matter, is something wrong with my ECG?" Another patient, responding to a different need, might reply, "No, not yet, I wake up slowly, and I haven't had any coffee yet." Each person responded differently to the same stimulus because of different anxieties and needs.

A strong stimulus can create a need and facilitate learning or can interfere or distract the learner so that the stimulus becomes an inhibitor. A patient who is concerned about an errant husband or a sick child may not be able to learn about prenatal diets because of the more pressing worry.

Selective hearing, need, and readiness become problems to the teacher only if the teacher has not assessed the most pressing and current need of the learner collaboratively with the learner. Frequently what the learner wishes and is ready to learn is more important and achievable than what the nurse wishes and is ready to teach. Developing common goals may require a synthesis of teacher and learner goals.

Formulation of objectives

> Oh what, oh what is wrong with my objective?
> Was the affective ineffective?
> Or the cognitive defective?
> For my psychomotor wouldn't start
> And I lost the warranty for it
> Yet I thought I did my part
> Oh, my objective looked so good
> And it sounded very well
> But if any one learned—you couldn't tell!
>
> E.O. Bevis

An objective is a destination, goal, or expected or desired outcome. An objective defines where one wishes to go and what one wishes to accomplish. As someone has said, "If you are not sure of where you are going, you are liable to end up someplace else." An objective tells what the learner will be able to write, recite, construct, identify, differentiate, contrast, solve, compare, discriminate, judge, do, and so on. Objectives tell the teacher what is to be taught and the learner what is to be learned, and they enable both to determine the extent of accomplishment.

Objectives cannot be assumed, for such assumptions lead to conflict of purpose and misunderstandings and defy evaluation. Objectives need to be clearly and concisely stated so that they can be understood, accepted, and used. Vague objectives, couched in erudite but trite jargon, are useless to most teaching-learning participants. Simple, direct, and explicit sentences that spell out in common language the desired outcomes enable the teacher and learner to select content, methods, materials, and activities that are appropriate and can promote goal accomplishment.

PREDICTIVE PRINCIPLE: Participation of the learner in setting learning goals increases the number of learning activities meaningful and useful to the learner.

PREDICTIVE PRINCIPLE: The more congruent and relevant that goals are to life needs of the learner-client, the more likely the goals are to be achieved.

Setting goals with the learner helps to keep them realistic and meaningful. Participation of the learner in goal setting enables goals to be set within the framework and context of the learner's life and needs and ensures that established objectives are goals to which he or she is committed.

Learners have information, insights, and awareness of problems pertaining to their own lives and needs; the teacher has specialized knowledge, skills, experiences, insights, perspectives, and often an objectivity that the learner does not possess. Working together, teacher and learner can set goals best suited for specific needs.

PREDICTIVE PRINCIPLE: Realistic behavioral goal setting enables selection of appropriate and meaningful content.

PREDICTIVE PRINCIPLE: Setting goals that specify the precise degree of attainment required provides the learner with guidelines that can be followed.

When objectives are stated explicitly, it is much easier to find out if the objective has been accomplished. Clearly defined objectives provide the learner with (1) what content is important; (2) the knowledge of what instructional materials are needed, and (3) what method or constraints are to be used. Further, they provide learners with the means to organize their own efforts toward accomplishment of those objectives and give clear guidelines for evaluation of the degree of goal accomplishment. An illustration of construction of such an objective follows:

Objective: The orientee demonstrates the ability to prepare and to set up an additive of antibiotic to a mainline IV solution without assistance and within a time period of ten minutes.

The learner is given clear direction in this objective; it states what content is important (knowledge of the antibiotic), the materials needed (correct additive set, syringe, and solution with which to mix the antibiotic), and the method and constraints expected (according to hospital procedure without assistance, and within a period of ten minutes).

Objectives may cover three domains: affective, cognitive, and psychomotor. An *affective* objective concerns feelings and emotions. For example, an affective objective might be:

In the process of providing morning care to a dying patient, the nurse shows empathy by:
  a. sitting quietly with the client for at least ten minutes, inviting expression of feelings
  b. touching the client gently when communicating with him
  c. validating the client's feelings with such phrases as, "I understand," "Go on," "Tell me more," or "It's OK to cry."

Cognitive objectives include knowledge, understanding, and thinking skills. The following objective illustrates a cognitive objective:

After being given hospital prescribed instruction about the Hickman catheter, the learner states in his or her own words:
  a. where and how the catheter is inserted
  b. the functions of the catheter
  c. how to provide proper care to the catheter

A *psychomotor* objective describes manipulative and motor skills. This type of objective is illustrated below:

In preparation for an eight-hour tour of duty, the nurse:
  a. arrives on duty on time
  b. prepares a worksheet containing the items essential to practice
  c. listens to the off-going shift report; makes notes on worksheet of pertinent information
  d. visits assigned patients
  e. makes assessments of each patient according to the diagnoses.

Psychomotor skills are by far the simplest to prepare since they are task oriented and can be listed, prioritized, written down, and tested; however, danger occurs if psychomotor activity is allowed to become mechanical without cognitive foundations and positive attitudes in the process of implementation.

PREDICTIVE PRINCIPLE: Objectives that describe outcomes in small increments enable successful fulfillment.

Objectives need to be stated in terms the learner can comprehend and follow. If, for example, the objective reads, "At the completion of a guided tour of the unit, the new employee will know where everything is," the learner is left floundering, with no possibility of successful achievement. When the objective is broken down into manageable pieces such as, "At the completion of a guided tour of the unit, the employee will be able to locate the locker room, the medicine room, and the clean and dirty utility rooms," there is clear direction, with criteria established for evaluation of achievement.

Without specific, realistic goals, content selection becomes arbitrary and is frequently motivated more by what the nurse-teacher is comfortable in teaching than by what the learner needs to know. Realistic, specific behavioral goal setting therefore gives structure to learning situations, which decreases the frustration and lowers the anxiety of both teacher and learner by enabling the learner to understand how content will be useful.

Motivation and reinforcement

Theorists differ in basic assumptions about the role of motivation and reinforcement in learning. In this discussion some differences among learning theorists are given with an attempt to choose those theories or aspects of theories that will be most helpful to the staff nurse during everyday teaching responsibilities.

Motivation can be intrinsic or extrinsic. Intrinsic motivation is the impetus, incentive, or driving power within an individual that propels him or her into action. The teacher who can capitalize on an individual's motivation can concentrate on the activities of being mentor, guide, validator, supervisor, enabler, supporter, reinforcer, and evaluator. Extrinsic motivation is provided by the teacher or other external factors that influence the learner's desire to learn. These factors can be identified and manipulated to develop maximally and influence directionally learner motivation.

The nurse-teacher will discover that motivation may be influenced by personal and individual circumstances but that intrinsic motivation is the more important of the two types. Some motivating factors are common to most individuals and groups. This section relates to the common principles of motivation and learning and is primarily concerned with intrinsic motivation.

PREDICTIVE PRINCIPLE: Use of motivation theories enables the development of guidelines for understanding and assessing of behaviors.

Theorists provide excellent clues as to what motivates people to do what they do. Maslow* proposes that humans direct their own actions to satisfy their own needs. He believes that needs can be categorized and compared in their relative importance as they influence a person's actions. When a need at any one level is satisfied, the next level need becomes predominant. McGregor's† theory X assumes that most people are naturally lazy or unreliable, find work inherently distasteful, and want safety above all. Managers therefore plan, decide, and police what everyone is doing. McGregor presents an alternate theory Y, which assumes that people are not naturally lazy or unreliable and that properly motivated workers are capable of directing their own efforts to accomplish goals. McGregor suggests managers push information and responsibility downward, explain to workers the reasons why things should be done, and assume they have an interest in and a willingness to do the job.

Herzberg's‡ theory of satisfaction and dissatisfaction proposes that satisfiers (for example, increase in pay, positive reinforcement for behaviors) are motivators because they have positive effects, thus increasing the individual's output, whereas dissatisfiers on the job (for example, frowns for behaviors, poor environment) have no influence as motivators for high level performance. He concludes that achievement and recognition are the single strongest motivators of work performance.

---

*Maslow, A.: Motivation and personality, ed. 2, New York, 1970, Harper & Row, Publishers, Inc.
†McGregor, D.: The human side of enterprise, New York, 1960, McGraw-Hill Book Co.
‡Herzberg, F.: Work and the nature of man, New York, 1966, World Publishing Co.

Kelly* theorizes that a person's motives cannot be labeled, that saying a person is energetic or lazy, cooperative or uncooperative, happy or unhappy does not make it so. He says that we can only guess at what a person's motive is. Kelly's research led to the scientific theory of behaviorism and behavior modification, based on the premise that all behavior is a function of its consequences. This means that people do the things they do because of the results or consequences to them. This scientific approach to management proposes that not only can people's behavior be changed regardless of what their attitudes might be, but once the behavior has been changed, the attitude change usually follows. Behavior modification deals only with measurable behavior, in contrast to the theoretical, internalized activities of the mind, which are not measurable except by indirect means.

PREDICTIVE PRINCIPLE: An obvious relationship between learning activities and stated goals increases the motivational value of the activity.

The more reasonable and meaningful the activities appear to be to the learner, the more effort he or she will invest in their accomplishment. For example, the patient or aide learning about changing dressings using aseptic techniques may balk at learning the physical principles governing the capillary action of fluids until he sees the influence of those principles on the transportation of microorganisms by moisture. Or the nursing staff may comply half-heartedly with the requirement for mandatory instruction in cardiopulmonary resuscitation or the use of the "crash cart" until there is occasion to use this knowledge and the nurses are found wanting.

The nurse-teacher can demonstrate relationships between necessary knowledge antecedents, content, and objectives by planning overall teaching content with the learner in a graphic way. To the uninitiated learner, knowledge basic or preliminary to goal accomplishment may appear to have little relevance to the goal. Motivation can be stimulated by content and activity plans, either written or carefully described so that relationships between necessary learning activities and accomplishment of goals will be conspicuous to the learner.

PREDICTIVE PRINCIPLE: Accomplishment of beginning objectives reinforces belief in ability and motivates to greater effort for greater accomplishment.

Probably nothing is quite so motivating as success. Success is a lessening of anxiety or tension, because a goal has been achieved. It is a moment of accomplishment when confidence grins a little and takes a deep breath. The next task is then begun with confidence reaffirmed and reinforced. Anxiety about failure is somewhat relieved, and fear of falling short of an established goal is decreased.

Success early in the learning process is necessary even to those who

---

*Kelly, G.: The psychology of person constructs, 2 vols., New York, 1955, W.W. Norton & Co., Inc.

appear most confident. The nurse-teacher who sets a few small but challenging goals that can be met early in the learning process ensures greater motivation and effort for the larger learning tasks. Success can be planned by structuring learning situations with a high probability of success. A case in point is nurse Jan who is being introduced to the unit dosage system by her preceptor:

Preceptor: "I don't have much time to show you, but you are to give meds to all the patients today. Here is the cart. Each patient has his own drawer. The med sheet is here. Be sure you record in all the right places, or you will be called down to the Record Room. You can see what others have done—I'll be around if you need me."

One can easily deduce that Jan will have difficulty in grasping her role in medication administration, and she probably will feel anxious with the threat of accountability for her errors of omission. Her alternatives are to do the best she can by herself, study the procedure manual as she moves along, find her preceptor each time she has a question, or refuse to assume this responsibility until she receives adequate instruction. Had the preceptor introduced Jan to the unit dosage system utilizing clearly defined objectives, Jan could have felt a sense of accomplishment and a motivation to move ahead.

Preceptor: "Today our goal is for you to understand the use of medication administration sheet on which all medications are recorded. To do this, you should observe me as I administer medications and record them. I will explain each step as I go. Please ask questions about any part of the procedure you do not understand. Tomorrow, you will administer the medications and I will observe you, reserving the right to make suggestions as I feel necessary. In the next days, we will cover how to check the meds, order what is necessary, and restock the cart."

This success-oriented approach provides the preceptor with many opportunities to give positive reinforcement and thereby reduce anxiety associated with the task. The reinforcement of having succeeded, even in a small learning task, can be highly stimulating and can motivate the student to greater effort. Success early in learning will promote greater tolerance of failure.

PREDICTIVE PRINCIPLE: Closely monitoring the level and source of anxiety and excitement in the learner enables the teacher to adapt the learning plan to learner needs.

PREDICTIVE PRINCIPLE: Teaching in times of crisis about how to handle the crisis increases the opportunity for reinforcement and retention of learned behaviors.

People learn best when they have a value, need, obstacle, obstruction, puzzle, dilemma, or interruption of some kind. Under ordinary circumstances, this interruption creates a state of mild anxiety, excitement, or anticipation. Resources are mobilized to overcome, solve, or bridge the problem. At this stage learners are highly motivated to learn things that will contribute to their ability to solve the problem or achieve their goal. Statements such as "I function more efficiently under pressure" or "I'm so excited I can't wait to get on this project" refer to the level of anxiety or anticipation described.

When the pressure is increased, anxiety increases and diminishing returns are realized. The learner's activities are no longer goal oriented and tend to function as a pressure release valve without actually contributing to solving the problem. Activities such as telling everyone how overworked one is, making elaborate preparations for work, and making several trips gathering books or equipment when one trip would do, are all clues to the nurse-teacher that learner anxiety has increased.

Mild anxiety is a natural state of the human organism. Dynamic tension is the mechanism by which homeostatic balance is maintained. The healthy state is not a tension-free state; it is a state of tension balance. Anxiety or excitement is energy—energy is a pivotal learning force. Without an increased level of energy, no learning takes place. Anxiety or excitement results from encountering a problem. Sometimes the energy level is so low that it is not readily observable or it may not be within the learner's level of awareness. Encountering a problem or recognizing a goal is always accompanied by an internal "toning up," a sharpening of wits, an increase of alertness that is called excitement or anxiety. McDonald* calls it "anxiety" and labels it "intrapersonal energy change." The energy change then becomes the precursor to motivation. McDonald characterizes motivation as a condition necessary for learning but not sufficient to make learning occur. He defines motivation as having three characteristics: (1) intrapersonal energy change, (2) affective arousal, and (3) anticipatory goal reaction. The *intrapersonal energy change* may be caused by autonomic response mechanisms (as with fear) or basic life support needs. Most of the time the exact nature of the causal sequence of the energy change is unknown. The *affective arousal* is a feeling state or emotion. This state may not be in awareness or it may be a highly charged, intense emotion and well within the level of awareness. The *anticipatory goal reaction* is the purposefulness of motivation. Motivation is goal oriented, for it is through movement toward the goal that anxiety is reduced and satisfaction or pleasure achieved. The consequence is that goal achievement returns the arousal state to normal and reduces the energy change to its prior level.

Generally speaking, the higher the anxiety, the more specific and focused the learner's attention, so that learning goals unrelated to the anxiety are not achieved. Learner attention becomes highly focused on the stimulus causing the anxiety. Teacher activities begin to center around reducing the anxiety, strengthening coping mechanisms, or teaching coping behaviors directly related to the source of the anxiety. Consider the emphysematous patient who has great dif-

---

*McDonald, F.J.: Educational psychology, Belmont, Calif., 1966, Wadsworth Publishing Co., pp. 111-113.

ficulty in breathing. The nurse moves him through a procedure that will ease his dyspnea:

> Close your mouth. That's right.
> Breathe in through your nose. (Nurse inhales with the patient.)
> Purse your lips as I am doing. Good!
> Blow your breath out as though you are slowly blowing on the flame of a candle. Slowly . . . slowly . . . That's very good! Now, let's do this again.

Crisis, a state of very high anxiety and acute problems, provides a fertile field for learning. The person in crisis needs solutions desperately and is very receptive to cues and models, information guidance, and so on. The nurse-leader who takes the person in crisis through the activities necessary to resolve the crisis is capitalizing on prime learning time. The learner uses a real situation to learn behaviors that are immediately useful and have instant reinforcement.

Anxiety is one of the most delicately balanced factors influencing motivation. Perception of anxiety, accurate assessment of the levels of anxiety, and responses designed to control anxiety can mean the success or failure of any teaching endeavor.

PREDICTIVE PRINCIPLE: Rewards consistent with the value system of the learner, such as recognition, praise, peer status, or valued gains, are motivating and reinforcing influences and thus facilitate learning rate, amount of retention, and degree of behavior change.

Reinforcement of desired behaviors is the most influential factor contributing to the retention of learning. Reinforcement takes many forms and assumes many meanings, depending on the reinforcing stimuli and the learner's value system.

Recognition of a successful experience is a prompt reinforcement. Success is probably the greatest reinforcer. The nurse-teacher can promote the reinforcing value of success by preparing the learner to recognize the characteristics of a successful experience, as experienced by the emphysematous patient who realized success as a result of specific behaviors. Behavioral objectives that are spelled out enable the learner to identify what successful behaviors are and to recognize success immediately.

Reward and punishment reinforcement are helpful, depending on the form taken. Reward tends to be more successful than punishment. Rewards can be something tangible received for desired behaviors or positive feedback that causes good feelings. For instance, the relief of anxiety can be an important positive reinforcer.

Recognition by others can be highly reinforcing. Success recognized and appreciated by a meaningful individual or group and mentioned to other people important to the learner acts as a strong reinforcer in the learning experience.

For employees, rewards may take the form of statements in efficiency reports, letters to the employer or supervisor, commendations made to committees on promotions, and written memos to people in a position to give employment rewards such as salary raises, promotions, bonuses, and educational leaves. Copies of all such commendations should be sent to the employee.

Reinforcement therapy in the form of behavior modification is being conducted currently for both selected psychiatric and pediatric patients. This method uses rewards of valued objects, tokens that can be exchanged for privileges, favored foods, candy, or other desired objects as tangible rewards that can reinforce desired behaviors effectively. There must be careful selection of candidates for the controlled use of this teaching technique; if used inappropriately, it can become a way to obtain a desired object rather than a way to learn successfully.

Status rewards can be very important to learners. "Face," family pride, superior achievement, special mention, or public acclaim can fit into a value system and fulfill a need that can be more reinforcing than any tangible form of reward.

Punishment is an often-used negative reinforcer, but it has limited effectiveness in the teaching-learning process. Punishment of patients usually takes the form of reprimands, deprivation of privileges, exhibition of angry behavior by authority figures, ridicule, or sarcasm. Punitive statements such as "I'm not speaking to you today; I heard how bad you were last night" or "That was a stupid thing to do; what in the world made you do that?" do not contribute to the motivation of the learner and probably only serve some ego need of the nurse-teacher. Punitive measures may cause the learner to avoid the teacher and withdraw from learning situations. Fear of punishment or failure can cause learners not to try. This does not imply that failure should be ignored, nor can the teacher positively reinforce *nonlearning*, for that would negate *positive* reinforcement of *learning*. The teacher can recognize degrees of less failure as achievement. The nurse-teacher can compliment progress when the learner is trying and gives evidence of potential success, even though it is less than satisfactory. The wise teacher thanks the learner for achieving more, rather than punishing with sarcastic or embarrassing remarks. An evaluative statement can be made about whether the objective has been accomplished and can help learners to evaluate their own progress.

The optimal use of reinforcements most meaningful to each individual requires the nurse-teacher to utilize the reinforcement judged effective for each person or group in each separate learning experience. The closer the reinforcement follows the successful learning experience, the more valuable the reinforcement for both motivation and retention. Continued reinforcement at later times also provides increasingly greater reinforcement and greater motivation and retention. The reinforcement that takes place at a later time can take the form of additional comments from the nurse-teacher or opportunities for repetition of the successful experience.

PREDICTIVE PRINCIPLE: Practice of learned activities in a variety of ways reinforces learned behaviors and promotes the ability to generalize and discriminate.

Repetition of the same material over and over again has little value for learning beyond habit fixation. Repetition, to be valuable, must have an improvement aspect. When repetition contains an improvement aspect, it becomes practice. Accompaniment of each repetition of the behavior by using feedback for correction enables the learner to improve each time he performs the behavior.

Repetition and overlearning are necessary for the purpose of achieving skill. Beyond achieving the required skill, repetition of learned behaviors in the same manner or in a similar situation is unnecessary and adds nothing to the learner's knowledge or skill.

Learning experiences spaced to allow the time lapses necessary for maturation are most effective for promoting retention. Rapid repetition of activities within a short period of time increases skill in narrow or single applications but contributes little to the learner's ability to generalize and discriminate.

Providing the learner with situations that require extraction of central principles and application of these principles to several problems or learning situations does three things: (1) it requires the learner to recognize and extract the central and uniting themes of situations (conceptualization); (2) it requires the application of principles to like situations (generalization); and (3) it requires the learner to perceive variables and make decisions and judgments about the selection of principles to apply to a given situation (evaluation and discrimination). An example of this type of reinforcement can be seen in the nurse's aide who learned that microorganisms can move rapidly through moisture, which was an important consideration when sterile dressings were changed. Opportunities to work in other situations where sterile fields were important enabled the aide to extract selected central uniting concepts and principles of asepsis. The preparation of injections and emptying and changing urethral catheter drainage bags required that aide select and apply the applicable aseptic principles.

Practice, either spaced or continuing, and application to similar situations require periodic review, supervision, and evaluation by the learner and the teacher to ensure continued quality behaviors.

Establishing the learning environment

The learning environment is not so much a matter of architecture as a matter of atmosphere. The building, patient units, classrooms, conference and office spaces, lighting, temperature, air circulation, paint color, piped-in music, and intercommunication systems affect the teaching-learning process to some degree. Physical environment can facilitate teaching and learning through technologic aids, convenience, and comfort. However, the teacher with something to teach and the imagination, enthusiasm, and will to teach and the student with the need, ability, and determination to learn will create an environment where teaching and learning can take place regardless of the surroundings.

Authority figures in the teaching-learning situation in health agencies set the tone and atmosphere for learning. However, learners are equally important contributors to the learning environment. The learner who brings negativism into the learning situation as a predominant characteristic can negate efforts of the teacher to establish an environment conducive to learning. Mutual contributions and consistent effort to create and maintain a positive learning environment are required of all participants. The nurse-teacher sets the pattern for learning interactions by implementing principles of teaching and learning that elicit positive responses from the patients, co-workers, and ancillary workers who are the learners.

PREDICTIVE PRINCIPLE: A reciprocal relationship of trust and security facilitates teacher-learner communication and allows accurate assessment, learner participation in goal setting, and better utilization of resources.

The optimal learning environment is basically one in which freedom is fostered by mutual trust. This allows the learner (1) the freedom to question without feeling foolish or stupid, (2) the freedom to participate in decisions, (3) the freedom of choice when there is a choice, (4) the freedom to learn as much as possible, and (5) the freedom to establish one's own goals and obtain help in reaching them. These are important freedoms in learning, and either the teacher or learner can alter the learning climate and decrease learning potential by tampering with the trust on which the learning freedoms exist.

Accurate assessment, learner participation in goal setting, and full utilization of resources are possible only if the teacher has self-trust. If the knowledge of self as a competent, adequate nurse depends on knowing all answers and solutions to nursing problems, then the nurse-leader will not have the ability to participate freely in the teaching-learning process. Lack of self-trust can cause the teacher to guide learners only into content areas in which the teacher feels secure. This lack of self-trust places a rigid restriction on both content and method.

PREDICTIVE PRINCIPLE: Recognition of the effect environment has on learning enables the nurse-teacher to mobilize environmental factors for the reinforcement of content.

The physical environment and the climate in which learning takes place have a major effect on all phases of learning, and the inclusion of environmental considerations in teaching plans will help determine what is learned. Nurse-teachers often comment, "He knows better; why doesn't he do it?" The factors causing a discrepancy between what an individual "knows to do" and what he "does" are not specifically known. It is known that all behavior is meaningful, although not always understandable, and all behaviors are in response to some internal or external stimulus. The most usual approach to solving this problem is for the nurse-teacher to attack the overt behavior when some simple alteration in the forces that cause the behavior might enable real learning to take place.

Teacher behavior frequently exerts more influence on learning environment than does the material being taught. Following is an example of behavioral influence on the learning environment:

A nurse-leader was orienting two new ancillary workers. After describing their duties, the leader assigned them to care for two clients and told them, "If you have any questions or are in doubt at all, just come and ask me." Later, when they did ask for information the nurse answered the questions, but by her behavior communicated impatience at being interrupted, and the ancillary workers felt stupid for asking questions. The verbal message was clear and simple; it was the behavior that communicated negatively. The ancillary workers sought no more help from the nurse-leader because her behavior created an environment that taught them not to ask when in doubt.

Contradictions between content and climate and lack of congruity between words and behavior cause confusion. Learners will respond to the clearest or least threatening message.

PREDICTIVE PRINCIPLE: Accountability for learning that rests with the learner enables him to meet his own learning needs and goals and enables the teacher to act as resource person, facilitator, validator, conferee, and consultant.

PREDICTIVE PRINCIPLE: Verbal or written contracts with client-learners for attainment of specific learner needs enable the nurse-leader to enact the teaching role more precisely.

The nurse is in the peculiar position of being employed (usually) by an agency, yet being the servant of the client. As in any profession, the professional loyalty of the nurse belongs to the client. Seldom do the nurse's allegiances to the client and to the employing agency conflict, because in health-related fields the objectives of all are geared to attaining and maintaining or retaining the highest possible health level. Teaching needs of clients do sometimes cause some conflicts, since hospitalization of a client may not be timed for the best possible teaching, and teaching needs may span the involvement of several agencies. There are several ways around this problem, but none is entirely satisfactory and none gets at the problem created by the nurse being agency based rather than client based. Some of these ways are discussed here.

1. *Involvement of the learner.* The nurse-teacher involves learners to such a great extent that they assume the responsibility for their own learning program. Continuity then rests with them. The client collaborates with the nurse, who makes the placement of responsibility explicit and helps him establish what he needs and wants to learn to solve his health problems (for example, increase his exercise tolerance). Together they attempt to establish alternative ways he might go about learning (physical therapist, local gym, assistance at home) and establishing checkpoints or criteria for measuring progress (monthly tests by physical therapist, public health nurse, or physician).

2. *Use of learning contracts.* A second alternative for solving this problem is use of learning contracts. Once the learning program is established, the nurse and client enter into a learning contract that incorporates both content and time so that mastery of specific content is completed within certain time constraints. Converting the goal of increased tolerance into a contractual agreement, the nurse and the patient record that for the first week, the patient will:
   a. Do breathing exercises for ten minutes, four times a day.
   b. Walk fifty feet each morning and afternoon.
   c. Climb up and down three stairs two times a day, between walks.
   Mastery of content is recognized by the attainment of specific criteria. Mastery means the ability to perform up to some established standard considered to be within the parameters of safety or desirability by both nurses and client.

3. *Continuity of care on a contractual basis.* Some agency-based nurses have a third alternative. With agency support they can incorporate, enabling them to follow patients at their homes on a fee-for-service basis to ensure continuity of nursing care. This makes them available for helping the family and the patient and makes teaching continuity possible.

4. *Continuum of care on a donated basis.* Nurses on their own time often follow patients at their homes or other agencies. If a patient is discharged from an agency before completion of the learning episode, the nurse may use time off to conclude the contract. Care-oriented nurses find it satisfying, yet this activity can overextend them. Nurses should not make a practice of this; there are other agencies to carry out this responsibility.

PREDICTIVE PRINCIPLE: Structure, limits, and feedback provide an environment that promotes security and trust.

Structure means guidelines and road maps. Structure in learning situations means the provision of directions, limits, specific goals, specific outcomes, time constraints, and other formats that enable the learners to know where they are going; it provides a means for getting there and signposts useful for determining when they have arrived. Structure does not mean control or restriction on the independence of the learner; quite the contrary, structure is often a mechanism for providing for learning independence. One can provide a little structure and therefore a lot of independence, or a lot of structure and less independence. Often all the learner wants or needs is for someone to validate learning or perceptions and to help detect misconceptions. Establishing a mechanism for validation is a form of structure. The balance between structure and nonstructure is delicate and difficult to maintain. However, it is essential to the learner's independence, creativity, and own need system to provide him or her with some sense of the parameters of environment, for example, time constraints and the types of learning aids available, and the parameters of learning needs, that is, the value of knowing certain things or behaviors.

Structure in the form of specific learning objectives, limits, available learning experiences, expected relationships, and requirements for success provides a secure environment that promotes learning. Comments such as "I never really knew where I was with that nurse; I did not know what I was supposed to do or what was expected of me" indicate distrust caused by a lack of the structure necessary for optimal learning.

PREDICTIVE PRINCIPLE: Awareness of legal aspects of client education provides the nurse-teacher with the scope and limitations of content to be taught.

Patient education activities are often conducted without legal descriptions of their parameters and restrictions. Who should teach, what should be taught, and the rights clients have to information about their care and treatment are major issues that must be addressed.

Physicians, functioning under the state medical practice act, have control of the client's medical treatment plan, including diagnosis, prescription of medication and treatment, and determination of the prognosis. Physicians therefore are legally responsible for communicating information about diagnosis, treatment, and prognosis to their clients. The nurse, on the other hand, practices under the state nurse practice act, which usually speaks in general terms and does not describe everything a nurse can do. Many nurses interpret the act to mean that they may teach clients about anything that is of concern to the patient and may do so without a physician's written order. However, unless there are policies or standardized procedures written to this effect, the nurse may not infringe upon medical practice legally without a written order. Fortunately, with the advent of primary nursing and the collaborative relationship that has been established with physicians in some areas, nurses are becoming more and more accountable for assessment and need for implementation of the teaching role.

All hospitals require that clients sign a form at the time of their admission indicating willingness to be treated by the physicians and hospital personnel. The implication is that the client may ask questions and receive answers. Informed consent given by the client at the time of admission to the hospital or at the time of treatment is a common approach for protection of the client, physician, and nurse. Informed consent is often medical in nature with the client giving written permission to the physician and hospital (or other health facility) to do a specific procedure. It is the physician's legal responsibility to teach the client about the procedure, but it is frequently the nurse's responsibility to witness the client's signature on the consent form. By witnessing, the nurse is confirming that the client signed of his or her own free will and understands the meaning of the document. It is advisable therefore for the nurse to refuse to witness if in her assessment she believes the client lacks sufficient information for proper decision making.

The nurse is responsible for teaching the client about nursing care that is being provided. Each time the nurse performs a client-centered task, it is the nurse's duty to inform the individual about what is to be done, not only to gain the client's cooperation but also to gain informed consent. For example, before administering medications, the nurse should be sure the client understands what is being given and why. If this step is overlooked, the nurse may be open to charges of negligent conduct.

Nurses should consider keeping the client informed about what is happening by including teaching as a necessary part of the care plan. Since the physician and nurse are partners, this leaves the issue even more ambiguous. The physician will also need to be informed about what is being taught to the client, and the teaching should be documented in the nursing record.

Learning activities

All nurse-teachers utilize activities in teaching, whether by accident or by intention. Activities are all those things that will make learning take place. Activities can involve people, agencies, books, charts, or any source of content; they can be projects, audiovisual aids, or any teaching tool. Thus learning activities enable the acquisition of knowledge and recall; they reinforce, promote, transfer, and foster generalizations and discrimination. The planning of learning activities for the maximum benefit of the learner will ensure efficient accomplishment of behavioral objectives.

PREDICTIVE PRINCIPLE: Ability to use a varied number of learning theories increases the probability that varied strategies will be used in the nurse-teacher's teaching repertoire.

There are many theories of learning. This book presents only two—behaviorism and cognitivism. These two theories are at opposite ends of the learning spectrum. *Behaviorism* is sometimes called stimulus-response associationism, behavior modification, or instrumental or operant conditioning. Whereas classical conditioning (Pavlov's dog) deals with inevitable, or reflex, responses, operant conditioning deals with voluntary behavior. When the desired response occurs, whether accidental or guided, a reward in behavior meaningful to the learner is provided so that the probability of the desired response recurring is increased. The basic thesis of operant conditioning is that *the frequency with which any act occurs may be altered by the consequence of the act.*

Gestalt field theory or *cognitivism* has as its salient feature that a person *in the environment is a unit participating in what is called a simultaneous mutual interaction.* This theory of learning conceives of perception as all the different ways one becomes familiar with the environment and not mere consciousness of the environment. Things and people are perceived differently by different individuals because perception depends on the sum total of life experiences and the way other things in the person's life space are perceived concomitantly. (Whereas stimulus-response associationism emphasizes single units—one organism [human being], one stimulus, and one response—and an effective reinforcer, cognitive field theory deals with the concept of person [meaning the individual] within his whole field.) Cognitive field theory proposes that hypotheses that help to determine causal interrelationships and organize facts to provide direction and predictability are the heart of a science. Reality for the cognitivist is what each individual perceives and experiences it to be. Nothing exists in and of itself to people; things exist in relationship to a person's total experience. The cognitivist theory has the following characteristics:

1. Insight (realize the meaning)
2. Putting things together to make a pattern (seeing consistency, category, size)
3. Seeing things in relationship to each other, or relativity (for example, sickness can only be viewed in relation to health; passive can only be viewed in relation to active; happiness can only be viewed in relation to sadness)
4. Always developing

Other theoretical frames of reference for learning can be derived from learning theory source books. Since the nurse-leader has a teaching role, one of the tasks essential to role development is an exploration of learning theories. From this base the nurse can develop a useful eclectic approach to teaching-learning situations. For example, the nurse teaching a ten-year-old child may choose behavior modification to help the child learn to use an atrophied arm and cognitivism to help her learn to avoid foods to which she is allergic.

PREDICTIVE PRINCIPLE: Learning episodes that contain input, operations, and feedback increase retention and utility of learning.

Learning is a change in behavior that is acquired as a result of practice and can be repeated when needed. Learning has three identifiable aspects that exist regardless of the learning theory adopted:

1. An input aspect
2. An operation aspect
3. A feedback aspect

These aspects are sometimes called sequences or phases, but since both sequence and phase imply a serial order in time, "aspects" is used here, since aspects can occur simultaneously. Graphically, learning is like a pyramid with three sides, one each for input, operation, and feedback.

1. *Input* is the acquisition of information and the organization of the information into action hypotheses (predictive principles). These activities may be assessments, content information, instructions, recognition that a response is appropriate, or any of the *cognitive* activities associated with acquiring input.

2. *Operation* is the *activity phase;* it is directly observable behavior, responses to the input and interactions. It is practice (prescriptive theory). In memorization, it is repetition (either oral or written). In discovery learning it is testing out ideas, either by putting them into action or interacting with another person. The operation aspect is *response.*

3. *Feedback* is the result of the operational test or the result of evaluation—verbal, nonverbal, or written.

In order for feedback to be useful to someone, the person must understand the feedback, accept it, and be able to do something with it. Guidelines for giving feedback effectively include: (1) avoid generalizations and use specific, recent examples of behavior, (2) provide privacy when giving feedback, (3) validate the data or information with the person in question, and (4) speak only in descriptive terms of what the teacher has seen and its effect. For example, "When I observed you emptying the Hemovac, I noted you used good aseptic technique throughout the entire procedure." In order for the feedback to be useful, the person receiving the communication must be able to change or confirm the behavior involved.

The three aspects of a learning episode frequently occur with such speed that clear delineation among aspects is not always possible. For instance, the operational phase is in effect a test or trial or acting out of the input. The very act of doing generates immediate feedback that becomes input for corrections. The most useful element about familiarity with the three phases is that the presence of all three phases in any learning episode increases the likelihood of the learner actually having a change of behavior.

PREDICTIVE PRINCIPLE: Varied teaching strategies and operations available to and usable by the nurse-teacher increase the nurse-teacher's selection of a strategy based on learner and situational needs.

Choosing a teaching strategy depends on several variables. Most of these options are simple logical ways of looking at the factors governing the means by which the learner and the teacher can find a common learning medium. If the learner is a client in the hospital or home, consideration must be given to mobility, energy level, the availability of resources (books, pamphlets, audiovisual materials), the content to be taught, the amount of anxiety surrounding the teaching subject, and the number of other stimuli being received by the client and family. Families and other people significant to the client have a part in choosing the learning strategies if they are going to participate in the learning episode.

Most teaching strategies are passive in nature. The learner reads, watches, and listens. These teaching strategies provide the major modality for cognitive input. They will probably continue to remain a central learning modality because early in a person's life reading, listening, and watching play prominent roles in gathering information. People seldom experiment and rediscover information each time it is needed—that method is too inefficient. Many advances in modern technology assist learning—television, super 8 mm film, video and tape cassettes, telephone dialing information systems, film strips, slides, programmed books, transparencies, and the whole gamut of audiovisual materials that bring information to learners in a wide variety of formats. These informational packages can be put together in learning modules tailor-made for learner and situational idiosyncrasies. The bibliography for this chapter contains references to resources helpful to the nurse who wishes to make multimedia learning modules for clients or other health caregivers.

The nurse-leader who teaches the same or similar content repeatedly to clients may wish to make (or work with the agency to purchase) learning modules using several media as the input mode for selected clients. Examples of excellent programs available to the public include the subjects of exercise, diet, hypertension, cardiac recovery, administration of medications, primary care, teaching, and management. Some clients depending on their cognitive style, may wish to participate in the development of an individualized program of study, to complete a programmed text designed to meet their needs, or simply to read or listen to the nurse talk with them about the content.

The operation sequence of learning demands that the learner *do* something with the information. This activity may involve solving a simulated problem, practicing a procedure, recalling, building, creating, making, using, or any other active operationalization of the input (information). The act of *doing* provides a basis for the feedback sequence. Feedback arises not only from the formal evaluative material available on tests but also from the act itself. As learners practice or get involved in some utilization of information, the information begins to correct itself, to make further sense, to fit into patterns, and to make generalization insights possible.

Each phase of the learning process—input, operation, and feedback—

needs to be devised in collaboration with the learner and chosen for its ability to meet the client's specific needs and the needs of the situation in which learning will take place.

Simulation teaching techniques offer the nurse-teacher an opportunity to develop teaching skills with exciting dimensions. Usually health teaching involves information giving, demonstration, and return demonstration. Creative teaching strategies provide the learner the opportunity to experience behaviors that are the objectives of the learning episode. For instance, the caregiver who is teaching the child diabetic to give insulin often uses a syringe, a bottle of water, and a lemon, orange, or sponge for this purpose. This technique is a form of simulation. Role playing a patient interview with a colleague provides the nurse with alternative approaches and interviewing behaviors that are difficult to learn in the real situation. Children learning balanced dietary habits are sometimes given models of food to put on a plate to illustrate a balanced meal. These forms of simulation provide practice when the "real thing" cannot be studied directly because it is too expensive, not available, or too dangerous.

Children and adults enjoy playing games, and games lend themselves well to learning. Games are contests requiring skill or luck. Skill or good memory retention can provide the nurse with the structure for a game. Bingo provides a model for a game to aid memorization, as is needed for classification of foodstuffs or vitamin content. Guessing games such as "my ship comes in sailing" and "20 questions" are models for information games. Problem games also make good learning exercises. For good simulations, structure in the form of specific behavioral objectives and directions will make the difference between success and failure.

PREDICTIVE PRINCIPLE: Utilization of problem-solving processes promotes continuity and ease of learning.

The ability to use the problem-solving process is a skill that promotes a systematic use of appropriate resources. Problem solving takes place in many ways; however, the more systematic the problem solving, the more reliable the result. The neophyte in systematic problem solving will find that a logical format or model contributes to skill. The following is a suggested guideline for problem solving in tasks or stages.

Stage I, problem identification or establishment of objectives, is the initial task and the keystone of problem solving. Stage II is the gathering of appropriate data or the selection of appropriate principles. This stage requires (1) a survey of all the learner or problem solver knows about the problem, (2) a collection of the antecedent knowledge patterned into concepts, and (3) formulation of the concepts into predictive principles. These predictive principles enable the learner to list possible alternatives of action (stage III). Stage IV, a listing of the risks inherent in each alternative, helps the learner to make a logical choice of alternatives, choosing the one that has the greatest chance of solving the problem with the least chance of damaging the patient or the situation. An additional stage (stage V), in which all possible applications of the theories, facts, concepts, and principles used in the problem are listed, will be useful as an aid to further generalizations. The additional stage will also help the learner or problem solver to reinforce learning. Utilizing problem-solving processes in a tangible form can make content logical and sensible to the learner. Use of such methodology will provide an overview of all elements of the content.

Since much of nursing and health maintenance is applied science, health teachers frequently draw facts, concepts, and principles from the basic sciences of anatomy, physiology, chemistry, bacteriology, physics, and the social sciences. Often the learner has difficulty in seeing the relationship between these antecedents and the goal. The nurse-teacher who begins the teaching process with the basic science concepts may lose the learner because the antecedent-goal relationship is not apparent. Conversely, teachers who initiate the process with the application or "nursing action" phase may lose the learners because they do not understand the antecedent information that supplies the "why."

Objectives can be realized when the teacher and learner participate together in the problem-solving process using a simple graphic model so that individual parts of knowledge can be patterned into a meaningful whole. The table on pp. 150-155 is an example of a problem-solving tool in which the hygiene activity of mouth care is the subject. The topic chosen is simple to enable emphasis to be placed on the process and not the content. The example can be used as a model and can be successfully employed for any content regardless of complexity. The goal may be stated as a behavioral objective or as a problem, depending on which is appropriate to the situation. Both a behavioral objective and a stated problem are given here for clarity and to demonstrate the flexibility of the tool.

Problem-solving sample

Both the problem and the behavioral objective require the learner to have knowledge of facts, theories, concepts, principles, and risks involved so that he may generalize, discriminate, and perform to accomplish the objective or solve the problem.

The process enables the nurse-teacher to identify all the knowledge relevant to the development of a module or small unit of teaching. Once the necessary components of the sample model are identified, the nurse-teacher can share the overall pattern with the learner and through learner participation can select knowledge that (1) does not need to be covered, (2) needs to be reviewed, and (3) needs to be learned. In this way the teacher can start where the learner is and utilize what the learner brings into the learning situation. Once the content is selected, the methods, teaching tools, and other resources to be used can be chosen or devised. Use of the tool itself as a single method rather than as an overall guide stereotypes teaching and develops rigidity, which can decrease the creative enthusiasm in teaching and learning.

PREDICTIVE PRINCIPLE: Increasing the difficulty of learning material in small increments promotes learning success.

Difficulty is measured by complexity. Complexity in learning material is a function of five things:

1. The number of variables with which the learner must deal at one time
2. The degree or amount of structure provided by the setting, the teacher, and the learning activities
3. The level of theory with which the content deals
4. The degree of familiarity of the content to the learner
5. The intensity of the situation

When the nurse-teacher attempts to teach material that has a high number of variables, has very little structure, has a high level of theory, and is highly unfamiliar to the learner, successful achievement is jeopardized. When approaching new subject matter, it is easier to learn one thing at a time than to try to cope with something with several aspects. The number of aspects or variables with which the learner must deal is directly related to the complexity of the material. Simplification can be achieved by decreasing the number of aspects of the material to be presented at one time and allowing one small part of the total learning package to be dealt with before proceeding to the next part. The second problem is to select and provide the amount of structure. Sometimes the structure is provided by the setting. Nurses who are learning new procedures have access, within health agency settings, to policy and procedure manuals that provide structure. Nurses in acute care agencies are aided by and receive guidance from nurse colleagues, ancillary personnel, other health provider departments, as well as supervisory level management. This not only provides structure but also promotes the security of the learner. The teacher's role, then, is to provide structure by formulating clear, concise, attainable behavioral objectives and by giving clear directions, instruction, or other relevant information.

The level of theory involved is an important aspect of difficulty. Low level theories (see Chapter 1) are easier to learn than high level theories; in other words, it is easier to learn to identify, name, describe, and list things than it is to predict or develop causal connections and prescriptions. Creative, or inventive learning, that is, at level IV, is the most difficult level of theory with which to deal. Nurse-teachers must be sure before teaching level III and IV theories that the learner is well acquainted with level I and II theories which are fundamental and basic to these higher levels. For example, identifying, naming, listing, and de-

Problem-solving sample*

Statement of problem and objective	Necessary facts or concepts	Principles†
Problem: How to get the nurse to use appropriate mouth care with two critically ill patients who are given nothing orally (NPO) and are mouth breathers	1. Mouth is the portal of entry for food.	A. A well-cared-for mouth during critical illness increases the patient's ability to return to normal eating habits on recovery (1).
	2. Digestion is started in the mouth, where food is thoroughly chewed and mixed with saliva, which contains the digestive enzyme ptyalin.	B. A sensitive or infected mouth produces discomfort (2). (Food is often swallowed before it is thoroughly chewed and mixed with saliva or food may not be eaten at all.)
Objective: The nurse is (1) able to select the correct type of mouth care for each patient and (2) able to give adequately the correct type of mouth care to meet the individual needs of each patient	3. If the jaws are not used for mastication and if there is no acid or alkaline intake, there is little or no stimulation of parotid secretion.	C. NPO causes the parotid glands to become inactive (3). D. Meticulous mouth care prevents the massive invasion of microorganisms from the mouth through the parotid duct to the inactive gland(s) (3, 11).
	4. Salivary flow is decreased in severe illness.	E. Decreased salivary flow creates the need for frequent and special mouth care (4).
	5. Salivary flow has a constant cleansing action.	F. Local treatment of dry mouth with fluid and emollients promotes temporary relief (5).
	6. Anaerobic organisms do not ordinarily grow in the mouth.	G. The use of lemon juice for special mouth care causes an increased secretion of saliva (5, 7, 8, 9).

*This problem is the work of Honor B. Dufour and is used with her permission.
†Numbers after principles refer to number of facts or concepts used to compose them.
‡Letters after statements refer to principles used to devise action.

Prescriptions ‡	Possible risks involved	Generalizations
Frequent examination of the mouth to ascertain its condition. Observe for dryness, collection of undesirable excretions, redness, and odor. If patient is responsive, question him concerning subjective condition of his mouth—discomfort, pain, difficulty swallowing, foul taste (A, B, C). Use tongue blade and light when necessary to improve visualization of oral cavity (A, B, C).	Examination may be incomplete because of poor visibility. A tongue blade may be necessary to hold tongue down during examination, but care must be taken *not* to damage delicate tissues. Patient may not give dependable answers to questions. Aspirating agent used for oral care.	This procedure for special mouth care would be applicable to any patient in whom the salivary flow is decreased. Some common examples would be: Patient who is comatose Patient suffering from severe dehydration Patient unable to swallow Patient receiving oxygen therapy Patient with collection of foul debris in the mouth Patient who is NPO Patient receiving chemical therapy that has drying effect on the mouth *Discrimination:* This procedure would *not* be applicable in any situation where blood clots were necessary for healing (oral surgery).

Problem-solving sample—cont'd

Statement of problem and objective	Necessary facts or concepts	Principles†
	7. The accumulation of dried secretions in the mouth provides an environment conducive to the growth of anaerobic organisms.	H. The use of hydrogen peroxide, an oxidizing agent, for mouth care inhibits the growth of anaerobic organisms in the mouth (7).
	8. When the mouth is dry, local treatment with fluids and emollients gives temporary relief.	I. The use of hydrogen peroxide for mouth care results in a bubbling action that facilitates the removal of undesirable excretions in the mouth (8).
	9. Application of lemon juice and glycerine to the tongue and gums is a classic treatment for dry mouth.	J. The use of concentrated glycerine alone (which is hydroscopic) for special mouth care predisposes to dehydration and irritation of mouth tissues (9, 12, 13).
	10. State of hydration of the patient does not depend on the moisture of the mucous membranes of the mouth.	K. Small amounts of glycerine promote softening and protect mucous membranes (9, 12, 13).
	11. Antiseptic rinses stimulate saliva flow and decrease microorganism population.	L. Use of an antiseptic mouth wash results in lessening of halitosis (11, 13, 14, 15).
	12. Glycerine (concentrated) is hydroscopic and is a drying agent.	
	13. Small amounts of glycerine can protect and soften.	

Prescriptions ‡	Possible risks involved	Generalizations
Give mouth care with lemon juice and glycerine if there is danger of the patient swallowing the substances (E, F, G, J, K).	Glycerine must not be too concentrated, since it can be dehydrating and irritating. The nurse must obtain help to position the patient if she cannot do it alone.	
Careful positioning of patient with head to one side to prevent aspiration; suction machine should be available if patient is not responsive or cooperative (O).	If suctioning is required, care must be taken *not* to damage delicate tissues.	

Problem-solving sample—cont'd

Statement of problem and objective	Necessary facts or concepts	Principles†
	14. Excretions such as dried blood, mucus, and sputum in the mouth may be removed by the use of hydrogen peroxide, which is an oxidizing agent.	
	15. Saliva putrefies rapidly, giving rise to objectionable odors.	
	16. Water is not effective in removing odors.	
	17. Substances such as petroleum jelly and cocoa butter applied to the lips and tongue have a protective action.	M. Petroleum jelly applied to the lips and tongue after special mouth care results in a slower drying of these tissues (17).
	18. Mechanical action and friction remove dried and putrefied materials and stimulate salivation.	N. Careful use of mechanics and scrubbing promotes removal of dried blood, mucus, and sputum (18).
	19. Cleaning patient's mouth while he is positioned on back makes it easy for patient to aspirate.	O. Positioning of patient on side during mouth care promotes drainage of secretions outward and prevents aspiration (19).

scribing the anatomy and physiology of the skin and subcutaneous and muscular tissues is prerequisite to predicting absorption time of insulin based on whether or not it is injected into the muscle or subcutaneous tissue.

The next aspect of difficulty, familiarity, is a factor that enables the learner to be the nurse-teacher's greatest resource. The teacher who assesses what the learner knows, not only about the subject in question but also about other areas of interest, can relate this familiar knowledge to the unknown. For example, a maintenance worker in a factory that used steam boilers suffered a heart attack. Arteriosclerotic heart disease was diagnosed. The community health nurse used the client's knowledge of the precipitation of mineral content of water in boilers and pipes and the resultant dangers of clogging and pressure

Prescriptions ‡	Possible risks involved	Generalizations
If the mouth is foul with dried blood, mucus, and sputum, use hydrogen peroxide to remove crusts, followed with antiseptic mouth wash and then apply petroleum jelly to lips and the tongue (unless the patient complains of the taste) (E, H, I, L, M).	Hydrogen peroxide can injure the gums if used improperly, may cause gingival hypertrophy if used over a long period of time. Hydrogen peroxide not diluted to a strength of about 1% can injure tissues. Oils, such as mineral oil, are contraindicated because of the danger of aspiration and the development of lipoid pneumonia or lung abscess. All special mouth care performed with inappropriate tools can injure tissues or be ineffective in accomplishing goals. Applicators are rarely effective.	
Special mouth care is best carried out with a toothbrush; however, in some instances a protected forceps and soft gauze sponges may be substituted (N).	If protected forceps are used, care must be taken not to injure the buccal tissues or disturb oral injury, surgery, or dental work.	

in the boiler system to teach the patient about arteriosclerosis, blood pressure, and myocardial infarcts.

It is not always possible to teach material from the "simple" to the "complex" because "simple" and "complex" are relative terms to the learner and actually depend on the related knowledge and experience the learner brings to the learning situation.

Intensity is a factor that can be measured by the following guides: (1) does the job depend upon the speed, skill, or manner in which the job is done? (2) is the time factor critical? and (3) is life endangered or at stake? Situations that are highly structured, have few variables, and are fairly familiar may still produce problems because of their intensity.

Evaluation

Evaluation is the bugaboo of all those engaged in the teaching-learning process. Evaluation is the process through which the teacher and the learner determine progress toward the learning objective.

Evaluation for the purpose of establishing a "grade" may only tell the learners their achievement as rated on some established scale and usually compares them to other learners attempting to master the same content. Evaluation provides the learner with a guide that will enable him or her to determine progress toward accomplishing a desired goal. It helps the learner ascertain goal achievement. In health teaching and problem solving, evaluation means assessing behavioral changes in relationship to the goal or defined problem.

Evaluation for better learning enables the nurse-teacher and the learner to determine (1) that a desired behavior has or has not been learned and (2) how well a desired behavior has been learned.

Quantitative evaluation is of little use to the nurse-leader. Quantitative evaluations are characterized by words such as *always, frequently, sometimes, rarely,* and *never. Qualitative* evaluations are characterized by descriptions of behaviors that indicate the stage the learner has reached in the theory-building or problem-solving process and how skilled he or she has become in that stage. Qualitative evaluations tell the character and nature of success or failure.

An example of the differences in quantitative and qualitative evaluations may be drawn from the situation in which the nurse-leader was teaching an elderly man to administer injections to his wife, who had pernicious anemia. The man had extreme difficulty in manipulating the syringe and vial without contamination. The nurse's evaluative note, which states, "Very rarely draws up solution correctly" and "Frequently contaminates the syringe," does not convey to either the teacher or the learner what has or has not been accomplished. A qualitative evaluative statement would read, "Has identified the components of aseptic technique but has difficulty with the coordination necessary to master the handling of the vial and syringe without contamination. He is aware of breaks in techniques and is developing manipulative skills slowly." This statement conveys specifically and clearly the stages of learning achieved in behavioral terms.

PREDICTIVE PRINCIPLE: Objectives expressed as learner behaviors enable the teacher and learner to know the limits of expected outcomes and to evaluate in meaningful, specific terms.

PREDICTIVE PRINCIPLE: Criteria by which to measure success, established through collaboration between teacher and learner, provide motivation, reinforcement, and guides for determining achievement.

The time required to write detailed behavioral objectives is compensated for by the efficiency with which one can plan the content necessary to accomplish the objective and the ease with which behavioral objectives can be evaluated. Behavioral objectives definitely describe the precise activities necessary to demonstrate that the desired learnings have occurred. For example, the practical nurse who was learning aseptic technique would not know what was expected of her if she were trying to achieve the objective "to become increasingly knowledgeable about aseptic technique." "Knowledgeable" does not indicate what behaviors result from the knowledge. However, "to recognize when aseptic technique is required" and "to perform tasks requiring aseptic technique in any situation" are two objectives that tell the learner and teacher exactly what behaviors must be achieved to accomplish the objective. They spell out criteria for both teacher and learner to use in judging accomplishment.

The foregoing principles indicate that evaluation in meaningful and specific terms is an activity of both teacher and learner. Evaluation carried out by either, exclusive of the other, reduces the effectiveness of the evaluation by making it impossible for one half of the teaching-learning team to use the evaluation in activities designed for further goal accomplishment. For successful evaluation, both teacher and learner profit by having the data necessary to assess the present situation and to structure additional experiences for achievement of the desired behavioral changes.

Staff development: use of predictive principles of teaching and learning in in-service or nursing education departments

Education programs for the provision of staff development have three distinct purposes:
1. To increase the health worker's ability to be congruent with and supportive of the health agency's philosophy and/or statement of mission and goals as provided in its charter, organization plan, or appropriate documents
2. To meet the specific learning needs of the individual nursing care given in order to facilitate the employee's optimal development

Both of these purposes synthesize to form a third purpose:
3. To enable each employee to provide the most effective and efficient client care possible in the setting where employed

In-service programs are organized to meet these purposes by responding to the following three basic in-service needs:
1. The need for orientation to the health care agency, its policies, procedures, physical environments, culture, goals, organization, communication flow, and people
2. The need for mastery of health care—oriented content; learning nursing behaviors necessary to:

a. care for clients (general or specialty content)
b. use physical plant and equipment better
c. work with nursing group
d. work with health care team
3. The need for promotional mobility, which involves expertise needed:
   a. for vertical promotions and merit raises in salary
   b. in leadership and management group work and clinical knowledge and skill for vertical promotion up the organizational ladder

Therefore all instructional designs for in-service education programs are devised to respond to one or more of these three areas of need:

1. Orientation
2. Client care improvement
3. Promotion

PREDICTIVE PRINCIPLE: In-service education programs structured to separate orientation, clinical experience, and management aspects promote clarity of content and staff growth.

In-service education is one of the biggest problems managers face. Nursing attrition (turnover) is a constant problem for nursing managers. Nurses and ancillary help tend to go from agency to agency looking for better pay, fringe benefits, better working conditions, and greater job satisfaction.

Good in-service educational programs alone will not alter attrition rates but will provide one positive factor for staff stability. "Good" in-service education is in-service education that is:

1. Planned to separate the three aspects of in-service education: orientation, client care, and promotion
2. Planned congruence with the conceptual framework of the agency
3. Slanted toward active rather than passive teaching strategies
4. A total curriculum package
5. Tied into merit raises, promotion, retention, and other concrete reinforcements
6. A mechanism for self-improvement and for increased job satisfaction

PREDICTIVE PRINCIPLE: Effective orientation programs contribute to retention of personnel and promote job satisfaction.

Orientation is the simplest, most routine, and most repetitious of the three areas. It is also the area most likely to lose the interest of the learner. Orientation is uninteresting to the learner if it lacks relationship to a real or felt need. Learning in the abstract is more difficult than learning in the concrete. The time frame for orientation depends on such factors as (1) provision for employment of the individual while in the process of induction, (2) experience and competency of the employee, and (3) needs of the job to be filled. Some practical guidelines for making orientation programs more concrete, usable, attractive to the learner, and efficient are:

1. Conduct all the tours of the physical plant, grounds, offices, etc., as taped guided tours. The in-service education director can carry a mobile tape recorder with a map around the agency and conduct a guided tour as if for one individual. Some hints for this are:
   a. Speak as if speaking to one person on a tour.
   b. Make it personal, interesting, and relaxed.
   c. Speak in the first person singular.
   d. Walk the employee around the facility using a map with numerically designated spots.
   e. Instruct the employees how to use the tape recorder, ear jack, and map to tour themselves around the agency.
   f. Allow the employee to keep the map at the end of the tour.
2. Meet important people in the situation through slides and taped voices. Take several slides of each important person doing his or her job in the agency. Have voice on the tape: "Hello, I'm Miss Important. This is my office. It's marked on your map as '10.' My job is . . ." You might ask the person to tell something about responsibilities, lines of authority, communications, and committees. Ask the person to tell something about his or her professional life, previous work experiences, biographic data, work history, values, hobbies, religious affiliations, or anything else of interest or use to the employee.
3. Devise active learning experiences to teach new employees about policies and procedures. This can be done by assigning problems that must be solved correctly by using the policy/procedure manuals, for example, instead of telling a nurse what to do with diet orders, give her a "simulated" chart of diet orders and allow the problem to be solved using the policy/procedure manuals. (This format will also point out areas in the manuals that need clarifying in order to be useful.)

   EXAMPLE 1: Mr. Jones has been on a regular diet. His doctor just ordered a low-fat diet. It is ten minutes before the trays are due to be served. Use your policy and procedure manual and list the steps you would take to ensure that Mr. Jones receives the proper tray. Now fill in the correct forms and state where you would send each form.

   EXAMPLE 2: Mr. Jones is admitted with orders for complete isolation. Do all the appropriate things to ensure that isolation is established for him and all appropriate departments are notified.

4. Give simulated experiences (problems) to teach the use of the computer and all routine desk work. For example, use of tickler files; all chart work; admitting and discharging clients; handling orders such as medications, x-rays, laboratory work, activities, physical therapy, and social services; and giving public health referrals.

One orientation program is suggested as a sample:* Thirteen days of full-time orientation are provided the new experienced nurse employee. (If inexperienced, the nurse is scheduled to take a six-week preceptor program.) The first day includes (1) introduction to the health agency's purposes, goals, and organizational structure, (2) tour of the facility, (3) brief presentations given by representatives from key support areas such as pharmacy, laboratory, chaplain's office, and personnel, and (4) distribution to each new nurse of a manual containing general information about the hospital and the nursing department, a nursing skills inventory, and printed objectives and content for a review of major systems and nursing procedures relevant for practice in the hospital. An additional manual is provided each nurse assigned to specialty areas (such as ICU/CCU, neonatal, or open heart surgery), addressing more specific information pertinent to these areas. The second and third days are given to (1) presentations by hospital nurse-educators relating to nursing process, documentation, computer system, code policies, and quality control, (2) validation of recent CPR certification, or instruction and validation, and (3) an introduction to the new employee's charge nurse and nurse preceptor assigned for the orientation period.

The remaining ten days are spent in reviewing basic nursing knowledge and in assessment and validation of nursing skills, utilizing the nursing skills inventory provided (for example, respiratory and cardiac assessment, oxygen therapy and chest tubes, abdominal assessment, neurologic assessment, fluid and electrolytes, TPN and CVP, and specific drugs and equipment). Fig. 4-1 provides a sample of skills expected of the nurse, showing how the new nurse is required to assess levels of achievement based upon the hospital's policy and procedure and to have the procedure validated by the preceptor. The "remarks" column can be used by either person. The new worker also keeps a diary, reflecting satisfactions, needs, and concerns; this is gone over with the nurse-educator in charge of orientation. This log helps offset issues that might become problem areas. For example, the new employee might record, "I am having difficulty in finding enough patients to validate my nursing skill in chest tubes." The nurse-educator can then arrange for this nurse to go to another unit where the experience is available. Or the orientee might log, "I cannot relate to my preceptor. She makes me feel stupid." The nurse-educator and nurse-preceptor can discuss this problem with the orientee and identify what precipitates the feeling. If the problem cannot be resolved satisfactorily, a new preceptor is assigned, since the primary goal of the program is to achieve a smooth transition into the job. If the new employee continues to have similar reactions, then the agency personnel take serious note before assigning this person to permanent status.

---

*Provided at The Good Samaritan Hospital of Santa Clara Valley, San Jose, California.

Skill	Self-assessment				Hospital policy and procedure	Validated by preceptor	Remarks
	A	B	C	D			
Ostomy care (irrigation, changing, patient teaching)							
a. Colostomy							
b. Iliostomy							

Fig. 4-1. Example of a nursing skills inventory format.

PREDICTIVE PRINCIPLE: Establishment of preceptor training programs for new nurses bridges the gap between education and service and reduces turnover rate.

One method proved successful in hospitals throughout the country is the establishment of nurse preceptor programs. A preceptor is an experienced nurse specially selected by the head nurse or counterpart. The preceptor is a full-time employee who has demonstrated proficiency in technical, nursing process, intellectual, and interpersonal skills. To be selected the preceptor must indicate an interest in teaching and in helping a new employee in a one-to-one relationship. She or he serves as a role model and a resource person to ease the novice into the work assignment.

Nurses who meet the selection criteria and have no experience may consider a preceptor training workshop. The workshop usually runs for one or two days with content developed by in-service educators, with input from nursing staff. Following is an example of content selected for a two-day preceptor workshop in a general hospital.*

1. Nursing process as a basis for practice:
   a. *Assessment and planning:* Collection of data, definition of problems, establishment of nursing objectives. Accomplished through general and complex orientations, post-tests, skills inventory, and process evaluation. The preceptor monitors the new orientee in these activities using the tools provided.
   b. *Intervention or implementation:* Accomplished through independent nursing actions (assessment skills, patient teaching, safety, nursing procedures, etc.), and interdependent nursing action (standardized procedures), and dependent nursing actions, or those dependent on medical instructions and orders. The preceptor's actions are intended to meet those objectives established in the assessment and planning stage.
   c. *Evaluation:* The orientees' response is compared to objectives and parameters established by clinical instructor, head nurse, preceptor, or orientee.

*The Good Samaritan Hospital of Santa Clara Valley, San Jose, California.

Evaluation tools are process evaluation, validation of skills inventory, and an individual record. The preceptor is guided through the use of each of these increments.

2. Concepts of the adult learner and group membership:
   a. Theories of adult learning are presented, including self-concept, experience, readiness to learn, and orientation to learning. Group membership strategies include theories of bonding, competition, compromise, cooperation, and collaboration. The preceptor's responsibility is to help the orientee to assess herself in relationship to learning and adaptation to the new work environment, and then to apply these concepts to nursing practice.

3. Definition of role, responsibilities, and precepting and mentoring: Guidelines for the roles of assessment, planning, implementation, and evaluating are defined for the department manager, preceptor, nurse-educator, and orientee. (See Chapter 6 under accountability for learning new behavior.) The preceptor accepts her role as it describes and follows the progress of the orientee.

4. The art of coaching: Concepts are introduced regarding motivation, teaching skills, and support systems. The preceptor role-plays situations given in the workshop with her peers.

5. Evaluation methods and process: Discussion of how tools are used such as the skills inventory, individual record, and clinical orientation evaluation. The preceptor demonstrates understanding of these tools by verbal feedback and a practice session.

6. A "mini-teach": Each preceptor teaches the participants in the workshop for ten minutes as if they were new orientees. The preceptor selects a nursing skill that is commonly practiced in her clinical area, develops behavioral objectives for the mini-teach, and names the criteria she will use in evaluating the learner's progress. The audience of fellow preceptors evaluate the presentation verbally and in writing using a checklist with space for comments.

Nursing preceptors are selected to attend the workshop from every area of the hospital, since the basic concepts of precepting apply to all. In addition to learning the art of precepting, the participants have two days in which to become better acquainted with disciplines other than their own. While precepting, assistance with problems is obtained from the head nurse or clinical instructors. After about one year of precepting, nurses attend a follow-up workshop entitled "Preceptor Enrichment." Experienced preceptors gather to share their experiences of the year through a structured framework of the preceptor as helper, counselor, facilitator, and evaluator. They discuss such items as problem identification and conflict resolution.

The degree of success in overcoming excessive nurse turnover depends on recognition of the problem, identification of the causitive factors, and implementation of programs that will promote congruence among personal, professional, and organizational goals. Each agency requires a program unique to its institution, but the predictive principles offered here can be applied in all settings.

Maintaining currency in the field. The educational process for nurses employed in an agency is a significant factor leading to effective and efficient staffing and satisfaction of the employee. Even with excellent orientation, nurses can anticipate that jobs will change. With highly sophisticated professions such as medicine and nursing, there is a need for periodic updating of knowledge and skills. Many times both nurse-managers and staff are lulled into a false sense of security by the gradualness of change and are brought face to face with reality when confronted with a situation for which they lack coping skills. It is far better to anticipate the need for continued learning and to make the necessary provisions before a crisis develops.

There are three ways in which nurses maintain currency in their field. One is through on-the-job training, where each nurse is responsible for teaching part of her job. At this decentralized level the nurse-manager teaches staff, and staff help teach one another. A second approach is through a formal training department, usually called a "nursing education" or "in-service education," conducted at a centralized level. Depending on the size and purposes of the institution, one or more individuals are responsible for ascertaining educational needs and offering short-term programs to supply those needs. The focus of in-service education is specifically job related. Keeping current with new concepts, knowledge, and techniques that relate to health care and nursing activities is called continuing education (CE). Many states have legislated that a nurse must complete a specific number of hours of continuing education before each license renewal. This provides some impetus for nurses to avail themselves of ongoing education. Careful documentation of each educational experience assists in determining the extent of educational exposure needed for updating knowledge and skills.

The final phase of the staffing process is that of employee appraisal.* An employee appraisal is conducted for the purposes of assessing performance on the job and determining potential for development. The issue is discussed in relationship to the staffing process, because retention, compensation, and promotion directly correlate with performance evaluation. Both formal and informal methods, ranging from verbal assessments to ranking methods, checklists, or rating scales, are used to determine proficiency. Performance, experience, and qualities of employees are reviewed and compared with the job description. Whatever approach is taken, it is important that the employee be apprised in advance of the procedure concerning methods used and frequency of evaluation. A planned evaluation system helps the employee and nurse-manager consider all factors carefully and reduces the chances of personal biases. The employee appraisal allows the nurse-manager to scrutinize the work of employ-

---

*Chapter 8 is devoted to evaluation of personnel, giving predictive principles for the management of ongoing evaluation and scheduled periods of summative review.

ees in terms of how well they are performing their jobs and also from the standpoint of what can be done to improve performance. The nurse-managers may detect inadequacies in supervising and can improve their own performance.

Client care improvement. Many nurses speak of wanting to improve client care. It is often difficult to plan a curriculum individually tailored for each nursing caregiver and yet common enough to be practical. If one refers to the needs of the setting, the client, and the knowledge base of the conceptual framework of the agency, cues can be found that are helpful in designing a curriculum responsive to the nurse and the agency and beneficial to the client. The nursing or in-service department may work with a coordinating committee comprised of nurse-educators, head nurses, and staff nurse representatives to make decisions as to what offerings are most useful. Some ideas are as follows:

1. Keep a frequency count of the types of nursing care problems that occur in a two- or three-month period.
2. Keep a list of admitting and discharge diagnoses.
3. Keep a running list of the incident reports or notification forms.
4. Ask the pharmacy for a list of the ten drugs used in largest volume in the agency.
5. Ask the dietary department for a list of the five most common diets issued, except regular and soft.
6. Ask housekeeping what constitutes its three most commonly recurring problems.
7. Find out from clients (through interviews) what kinds of things they find most and least helpful.
8. Ask employees what course they would enroll in if offered any course they wanted in nursing.
9. Ask each employee what his or her professional goals and ambitions are.
10. Ask supervisors, head nurse, and clinical specialists what recurring problems are attributable to human ignorance or carelessness.

Regardless of the content of the in-service educational programs, there are guidelines helpful to managers that will enable the education program to be responsive to the needs of the agency, the nurses, the clients, and the community. Some of these guidelines are as follows:

1. Plan as few single-topic, one-shot programs as possible. Instead, plan courses consisting of five to fifteen hours, or the equivalent of a course of study, so that the learner can become involved in the course.
2. Build in some assignments and requirements for the learner that take into consideration the learner's individual problems, needs, areas of interest, and life goals.
3. Use clients of the agency as a resource for learning activities so that there is a practice component required for the completion of the courses.

4. Provide some rewards for work accomplished, for example, time and a half for attending, compensatory days off, letters of commendation, efficiency reports for permanent files, merit raises, mastery certificates, or credit for continuing education.
5. Allow the learners to help structure the course, its objectives, learning activities, etc., through preplanning sessions and postevaluation.
6. Buy, make, beg, or borrow some individualized learning materials, multimedia learning materials, books, and films on the subject under study.
7. Always have topics that are immediately applicable to the "real world" work situation.
8. Tailor all interactive learning (learning where nurses interact with teacher, other nurses, or patients) to the personal needs and characteristics of the learner.

Promotion. Many agencies promote nurses who have shown promise or expertise in nursing up the managerial hierarchy into positions of greater and greater responsibility as openings occur. More and more agencies are establishing requirements for skills in organizational leadership and management for these promotions. Civil service-type examinations and interviews often are used to test for skills. Sometimes it is presumed that nurses have managerial skills because they have previous work experiences. All these methods for selecting persons for promotion have assets and liabilities. Agencies are increasingly adding another dimension to the prerequisites for promotions—a requirement that employees have completed an in-service course in leadership and management especially tailored for the setting of employment. Staff development directors design courses that teach the philosophy and content of leadership and management as practiced or desired at the agency. In order to qualify for promotion up the administrative line the employee must complete a specified series of courses. Each promotional slot requires additional courses of study and preparation. Sometimes several agencies in a locale combine to offer the courses for greater cost effectiveness. Completion of a course of study does not ensure promotion; it only satisfies one qualification for a promotion.

Some topical examples are as follows:

Team leadership
Primary nursing
Principles of management
Budgeting and cost accounting
Evaluating personnel and peer review
Philosophy and goals of health care
How to critique a procedure
Working with people—a communications course
Assessing patient care—a supervisional function

Patient teaching—a basic nursing leadership activity
Teaching ancillary personnel
Quality assurance
The nursing audit

Application of predictive principles of teaching and learning

Mr. Scarborough, a 34-year-old alert man, has acute thrombophlebitis of the right leg. He is on complete bed rest with his legs wrapped with elastic bandages to midthigh (rewrapped every four hours) and taking anticoagulant therapy. The nurse observed Mr. Scarborough twisting a towel tightly around his right thigh. When asked why, Mr. Scarborough stated, "It eases the pain."

Problem	*Predictive principles*	*Course of action*
How to teach Mr. Scarborough healthful ways of alleviating the pain of thrombophlebitis	The learner's developmental stage, personal characteristics, and prior experiences influence learning potential and dictate content.	Assess prior experiences, previous knowledge, and personal characteristics.
	The learner's prevalent life needs determine what he or she will learn.	Use learner need to decrease pain as starting point.
	A reciprocal relationship of trust and security facilitates teacher-learner communication and allows accurate assessment, learner participation in goal setting, and better utilization of resources.	Establish open and trustful communication using appropriate activities.
	Participation of the learner in setting learning goals increases the number of learning activities meaningful and useful to the learner.	Collaborate (his need and nurse's specialized knowledge and skill) in establishing learning goals in behavioral terms, that is, identify a variety of methods for reducing the pain without jeopardizing his health; choose the appropriate method for each situation; perform the activities necessary to the implementation of the chosen alternative.
	An obvious relationship between learning activities and stated goals increases the motivational value of the activity.	Develop a brief overview of necessary content in collaboration with patient.

Problem	Predictive principles	Course of action
	Rewards consistent with the value system of the learner, such as recognition, praise, peer status, or valued gains, are motivating and reinforcing influences and thus facilitate learning rate, amount of retention, and degree of behavior change.	Determine appropriate rewards and use as reinforcers.
	Utilization of problem-solving processes promotes continuity and ease of learning.	Use flexible approach building toward a useful body of predictive principles based on valid antecedents.
	Increasing the difficulty of learning material in small increments promotes learning success.	Use meaningful similes (based on prior experiences), such as that a clogged drain causes drainage backup and overflow and collection of solids at point of obstruction, causing further clogging.
	Objectives expressed as learner behaviors enable the teacher and learner to know the limits of expected outcomes and to evaluate in meaningful, specific terms.	Evaluate patient's ability to behave in the manner specified and thereby gain relief from the pain. If possible, reinforce behavior. If not possible, determine with patient what would be necessary steps for achievement of success.

BIBLIOGRAPHY
Books

Berni, R., and Fordyce, W.: Behavior modification and the nursing process, ed. 2, St. Louis, 1977, The C.V. Mosby Co.

Bower, F.: The process of planning nursing care, a model for practice, ed. 2, St. Louis, 1977, The C.V. Mosby Co.

Buck, R.: Human motivation and emotion, New York, 1976, John Wiley & Sons, Inc.

Cazalas, M.: Nursing and the law, ed. 3, Germantown, Md., 1978, Aspen Systems Corp.

Creighton, H.: Law every nurse should know, ed. 3, Philadelphia, 1975, W.B. Saunders Co.

De Tornyay, R.: Strategies for teaching nursing, New York, 1971, John Wiley & Sons, Inc.

Douglass, L.: The effective nurse: leader and manager, St. Louis, 1980, The C.V. Mosby Co.

Drucker, P.: Managing for results, New York, 1964, Harper & Row, Publishers, Inc.

Erickson, E.: Childhood and society, ed. 2, New York, 1963, W.W. Norton & Co., Inc.

Foley, R., and Smilansky, J.: Teaching techniques: a handbook for health professionals, New York, 1980, McGraw-Hill Book Co.

Gagne, R.: The conditions of learning, New York, 1970, Holt, Rinehart & Winston, Inc.

Gardner, J.: Excellence, New York, 1961, Harper Colophon Books.

Ganong, W., and Ganong, J.: Help with innovative teaching techniques, Chapel Hill, N.C., 1976, W. Ganong Co.

Herzberg, F.: Work and the nature of man, New York, 1966, World Publishing Co.

Houle, C.: Continuing learning in the professions, San Francisco, 1980, Jossey-Bass, Inc., Publishers.

Huckabay, L., and Dadenian, M.: Conditions of learning and instruction in nursing, St. Louis, 1980, The C.V. Mosby Co.

Kelly, G.: The psychology of personal constructs, 2 vols., New York, 1955, W.W. Norton & Co., Inc.

Mager, R.: Preparing instructional objectives, Palo Alto, Calif., 1962, Fearon Publishers, Inc.

Maslow, A.: Motivation and personality, ed. 2, New York, 1970, Harper & Row, Publishers, Inc.

McGregor, D.: The human side of enterprise, New York, 1960, McGraw-Hill Book Co.

McKeachie, W.: Teaching tips: a guide for the beginning college teacher, ed. 7, Lexington, Mass., 1978, D.C. Heath & Co.

Practical Management Associates: how to teach grown-ups, Charleston, Ill., 1980, The Association.

Rogers, C.: Freedom to learn, Columbus, Ohio, 1969, Charles E. Merrill Publishing Co.

Shaffer, S., Indorato, K., and Deneselya, J.: Teaching in schools of nursing, St. Louis, 1972, The C.V. Mosby Co.

Sheehy, G.: Passages: predictable crises of adult life, New York, 1976, E.P. Dutton & Co., Inc.

Williams, J.: Human behavior in organizations, Palo Alto, Calif., 1978, South-Western Publishing Co.

Zander, K., and others: A practical manual for patient-teaching, St. Louis, 1978, The C.V. Mosby Co.

Periodicals

Bavaro, J.: Questioning the key to learning, Superv. Nurse 11(6):26-31, 1980.

Bennett, A.: Education and training need to be brought up to date, Hospitals, Dec. 16, 1978, pp. 75-76.

Benner, P.: Characteristics of novice and expert performance: implications for teaching the experienced nurse, Proceedings of Second Annual Conference, National Second Step Project, Sonoma State University, 1981.

Bowman, M.: Specifically objective . . . the need for educational aims and objectives in nursing, Nurs. Mirror, Sept. 1979, pp. 28-29.

Clark, M.: Staff nurses as clinical teachers, Amer. J. Nurs. 81(2):314-319, 1981.

Crisham, P.: Measuring moral judgment in nursing dilemmas, Nurs. Res. 30(2):104-110, 1981.

Flanagan, J.: The critical incident technique, Psycholog. Bull. 51(4):327-358, 1954.

Glatt, C.: How your hospital library can help you keep up in nursing, Amer. J. Nurs. 78(4):642-644, 1978.

Hartsborn, J.: The role of nursing education in critical care, Superv. Nurse 12(6):64-65, 1981.

Katefian, S.: Critical thinking, educational preparation, and development of moral judgment among selected groups of practicing nurses, Nurs. Res. 30(2):98-103, 1981.

Kirkis, J.: Teaching and evaluating nursing management, Nurs. Mgmt. 13(6):14-51, 1982.

Knowles, R.: Dealing with feelings: handling depression through positive reinforcement, Am. J. Nurs. 81(7):1353, 1981.

Mauksch, I.: Nurse-physician collaboration: a changing relationship, J. Nurs. Admin. 1(6):35-38, 1981.

McCaffrey, C.: Performance check-lists: an effective method of teaching, learning, and evaluating, Nurs. Educ., Jan.-Feb. 1978, pp. 11-13.

Meisenhelder, J.: A first-hand view of the unit teacher role, J. Nurs. Admin. 12(1):35-39, 1982.

O'Shea, H., and Parsons, M.: Clinical instruction: effective and ineffective teacher behaviors, Nurs. Outlook 79(6):411-415, 1979.

Perry, J.: Effectiveness of teaching in the rehabilitation of patients with chronic bronchitis and emphysema, Nurs. Res. 30(5):219-221, 1981.

Smith, C.: Planning, implementing and evaluating learning experiences for adults, Nurs. Educ., Nov.-Dec. 1978, pp. 31-36.

Sossong, A.: Motivating others, Nurs. Mgmt. 13(6):26-28, 1982.

Stafford, L., and Graves, C., Jr.: Some problems in evaluating teaching effectiveness, Nurs. Outlook 26(8):494-497, 1978.

Villeneuve, M.: The patient compliance puzzle, Nurs. Mgmt. 13(5):54-56, 1982.

Zonca, B.: The role of the patient education coordinator, Superv. Nurse 11(12):21-28, 1980.

chapter five

Predictive principles
of effective communication:
interpersonal and group

The communication process

Understanding the communication process facilitates effective communication
in interpersonal relationships.
The process of group communication enables collaboration in finding
solutions to problems and meeting needs.
Effective communication leads to influence and power.

Perception of self and others

The leader's self-perception directly influences the development of positive
perceptions in each group member.
The value systems of the leader and group influence the establishment
of goals and priorities as well as govern the amount of effort given to goal
attainment.
Continuity of competent leadership and management facilitates the efficiency
of the communication process.
Characteristics of client and leader/manager determine the types of
communications that will evolve.

Reinforcement and feedback

Integrative positive reinforcement increases individual identification with
group goals and the participation level of the individual.
Perceiving negative feedback enables group members to become aware of
others' responses and to modify behavior accordingly.
The dependent, interdependent, and/or independent natures of relationships
affect the structure of the communication process.
The interdependent collaborating group facilitates accomplishment of its
goals.
Continuing reference to and clarification of goals enhance the ability to attain
those goals.

Communication strategies

The type of communication at work in a group dictates member perception
and consequent action.

Congruent behavioral and verbal messages promote clear communication.
Recognition and use of informal communication channels by the leader can
lead to enhancement of organizational goals.
Threat and resulting anxiety, unless resolved, can inhibit individual and group
communication.
Questions and discussion geared to second- and third-level theories promote
cognition that is more useful in nursing activities than questions and
discussion geared to first- and second-level theories.
Use of simulation facilitates decision making and provides efficient means
for learning problem-solving methods in a nonthreatening and safe
environment.

Goal setting, achievement, and evaluation

Preassessment of individual and group knowledge, skills, and expectations
establishes baseline data for measuring progress or change.
Mutual understanding and agreement on goals appropriate to the client or
agency ensure support for goal achievement.
Circumstance and member capability determine the type of directions to be
communicated.
Opportunity to express expectations of the individual or group, when
translated into meaningful terms to members, determines individual
identification and invites commitment of members to goal achievement.
Realistic and valid goals promote achievement.
The extent of involvement of each group member determines the group's
proficiency.
Group involvement in goal setting requires the endorsement of the agency
and commitment of membership to participate in the outcome.

Effective conferences

Adequate preparation by the leader for all conferences expedites fulfillment
of expectations for the conference.
Relieving caregivers of responsibility while the conference is in session allows
members to proceed without interruption.
Prior announcement of time, place, purpose, and duration of conferences
to all concerned promotes assembly of a group well prepared and ready
to focus attention on the purpose of the conference.

Direction-giving conferences

Obtaining the most recent data available prior to conference ensures the
leader that imparted information is pertinent, inclusive, and accurate.
Information that is paced, systematic, and inclusive allows participants time
to assimilate the content and provides them with information necessary to
function.

Client-centered conferences

Interaction of conference members on an equal basis encourages active
participation and leads to usable solutions to the problem.
Identification of the nursing problem to be considered expedites the
formulation of nursing intervention.
Analyzing nursing care given in the light of established goals enables members
to validate their behavior and to devise ways to improve nursing care.

Formation of written nursing orders or care plans from client-centered conferences provides a central, continuous source of information.

Content conferences

Member participation in problem-solving processes during content conference results in more meaningful learning.

Nursing care conferences

Conferences held between nurse and client as well as with significant others contribute to reciprocal development of care plans and lead to optimal health service for the client and satisfaction for the nurse.

Periodic care review conferences held with colleagues provide a mechanism for the nurse to validate care plans and maintain quality control.

Reporting conferences

Directions given to conferees before report reveal expectations the leader has for the members.

General problems conferences

Sharing feelings through conferences unifies and integrates the membership and allows work to progress.

Understanding and managing group behavior require ability to predict the processes through which feelings and meanings are transmitted among group members.

Involvement in group process results in specific gains or losses for the individual member.

The communication process

Effective communication is extremely important for leaders and managers for two reasons. First, communication is the necessary process by which the management functions of planning, organizing, directing, and controlling are accomplished. Second, communication is the activity to which managers devote an overwhelming proportion of their time. The process of communication makes it possible for managers to carry out their task responsibilities. Information must be communicated to nurses so that they will have a basis for planning; the plans must be communicated to others in order to be carried out. Organizing requires communicating with members of the health team about their job assignments. Directing requires nurses to communicate with members so that the group goals can be achieved. Written or verbal communication is an essential part of controlling. In the final analysis, nurses do not function in isolation; they carry out their management responsibilities only by interacting and communicating with others. The communication process is the foundation upon which the management function depends.

Nurses are involved in two kinds of communication: interpersonal and organizational. *Interpersonal communication* is the process of exchanging information and meaning from one person to another or in small groups of people. *Organizational communication* is the process by which managers use the established system to receive and relay information to people within the organization as well as to relevant individuals and groups outside it. A nurse-manager works toward creating an environment that promotes ease in communication among individuals and groups, within the formal communication system defined by the authority structure in the agency. This chapter considers the importance of the communication process in organizations and the nurse-manager's role within the system.

PREDICTIVE PRINCIPLE: Understanding the communication process facilitates effective communication in interpersonal relationships.

An effective communication model consists of six steps: (1) the message, (2) encoding, (3) transmitting, (4) decoding, (5) action, and (6) continuous feedback (Fig. 5-1).

The message. Senders must have something to say before they send a message. The first step is to choose a fact, concept, idea, or feeling to communicate. This is the content of communication; it is the basis of a message. In an organization the nurse is a person with needs, feelings, information, and a purpose for communicating them. A nurse-leader wishes to communicate information about clients for the purpose of motivating other members of the nursing team. Without a reason or goal, the sender has no need to begin the communication process.

Encoding. Encoding means translating the message into words, gestures, facial expression, and other symbols that will communicate the intended

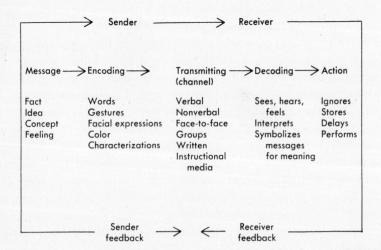

Fig. 5-1. The communication process. (From Douglass, L.M.: The effective nurse: leader and manager, St. Louis, 1980, The C.V. Mosby Co.)

meaning to the receivers. Words have many meanings. It has been pointed out that each of the five hundred most often used words in the English language has an average of twenty-eight different meanings. The meanings of words are determined by dictionary definitions, by the way they are used in a sentence, and by the context and setting in which they are used. All communication employs symbols to represent persons or things, and only symbols are transmitted. The meaning received depends upon the receiver's interpretation of those symbols. For example, the cross has meaning to the Christian just as the Star of David has to the Jewish person. There are symbols depicting male and female, and a host of symbols used in medicine to convey messages (e.g., $\bar{c}$, $\bar{p}$, tlc). Words, gestures, facial expressions, and all other symbols are learned through the influence of parents, school, religious affiliation, friends, and employment. To the extent that all symbols used in communication do not have universal meanings, there is communication difficulty.

Encoding the message requires decisions not only about what will be said, but how, when, and where it will be said. Encoding may also involve decisions about expressing or concealing emotion. Effective communication depends on the right degree of intensity for the message. The nurse may, for example, decide not to show fear or frustration and to communicate in a matter-of-fact, unemotional manner while working with an emergency or crisis situation. The nurse may ultimately decide to talk with clients and nursing personnel later, tailoring the message to the unique circumstances of each, communicating with them informally or formally as the appropriate occasion arises. Visual materials can help the human mind comprehend information. Media most commonly used to transmit messages are records, charts, computer printouts, slides, overhead projectors, and movies.

These four ideas affect encoding:

1. Words mean different things to different people.
2. Words that are supplemented with nonverbal cues are clearer than when used alone.
3. Complex messages are better if expressed in several ways.
4. The language of the message reflects the personality, culture, and values of the sender.

Encoding may occur within a few seconds, as when one person greets another with a "Hi" rather than with a more formal greeting. Regardless of the time required and the degree of conscious planning, the transmission of a message depends upon proper encoding.

Transmitting. Transmitting is the channel used to communicate a message. The message may be in any form that can be experienced and understood by one or more of the receiver's senses—speech may be heard, written words may be read, and gestures or facial expression may be seen or felt. A touch of the hand may communicate messages ranging from love and comfort to anger and hate. A wave of the hand can communicate widely diverse messages depending on the position ("Come here!" or "Get lost!"). Nonverbal messages are often more honest or meaningful than verbal or written exchanges. The client who smiles and laughs while saying "I have an unbearable headache" and the team member who frowns and is uncooperative while saying "Everything is fine" are transmitting nonverbal messages different from the spoken word. Odors can communicate a great deal to the receiver. The astute nurse soon learns to use olfactory senses in perceiving such things as infection, postpartum signs, and need for dressing changes.

Decoding. In the fourth step of the communication process the initiative transfers from the sender to the receiver who perceives and interprets or decodes the sender's message into information that has meaning. Ideally, the information communicated consists of what the sender believes the receiver should know and what the receiver wants to know. Understanding is the key to the decoding process. Words and other symbols have multiple meanings, and there is no assurance that the intended meanings of the sender have been encoded to mean the same thing to the receiver who decodes or interprets them.

The decoding process is affected by the receiver's experiences, personal interpretations of the symbols used, expectations, and mutuality of meaning with the sender. Normally, receivers make a genuine attempt to understand the intended message. Even with the best of intentions, however, a receiver may not understand the intended message because perceptions of the two people are different. As shown in Fig. 5-2, the more experiences the sender and receiver have in common, the more likely it is the sender's intended meaning will be communicated. In order for people with different experiences to communicate, at least one must speak the language of the other. Nurses who aspire to communicate with members of the nursing team with varied fields of preparation and experience must learn how they think, feel, and characteristically respond in a variety of nursing situations. By applying such knowledge, nurses are usually able to predict with acceptable accuracy how a given message will be decoded.

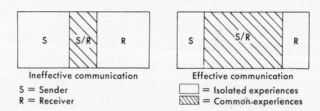

Fig. 5-2. Effectiveness of communication depends on commonality of experiences. (From Douglass, L.M.: The effective nurse: leader and manager, St. Louis, 1980, The C.V. Mosby Co.)

Action. Action in the communication process is the behavior taken by the receiver as a result of the message sent, received, and perceived. Action is the process of doing or performing something; it is behaving or functioning in a certain way. The sender of a message has no guarantee that what has been heard and decoded will be put into the action intended. The receiver chooses whether to act on the message. Many nurse-leaders overlook this important fact when giving instructions or explanations. They assume that merely giving a staff member a message ensures that the intended action will take place, but communication is not successful until the message received has been understood and acted upon appropriately.

Several options are available to the receiver once a message has been received: (1) ignore the information and fail to act, (2) store it as reference material until choosing to respond, (3) respond by saying one thing and doing another (credibility gap), or (4) respond to the message according to the receiver's interpretation.

Feedback. The communication process is not complete until feedback occurs. Feedback is an integral part of the communication process whereby senders and receivers exchange information and clarify the meanings of the message sent. Two-way rather than one-way communication allows both sender and receiver to search for verbal and nonverbal cues. Effective two-way communication occurs when a receiver acknowledges a message and then sends meaningful feedback to the sender. The more complex the information the nurse is trying to communicate, the more essential it is to encourage receivers to ask questions and to indicate areas of confusion throughout the entire communication process.

Feedback may be in direct and indirect forms, both verbal and nonverbal. Behaviors such as recording information in a direction-giving conference, nods of acknowledgement, smiles, and movements to accomplish the task given offer one kind of feedback. On the other hand, actions such as a blank stare, lack of motion to respond, or a frown provide quite different feedback. For nurse-leaders feedback serves as a control measure. In most organizational communications the greater the feedback, the more effective the communication is likely to be. For example, early feedback will enable a team leader to know if the instructions given team members have been understood and accepted. Without such feedback the leader might not know until it is too late whether the instructions given were accurately received and carried out.

Accurate feedback is more nearly achieved with face-to-face communication, use of simple and direct language, and sensitivity to individuals' values, attitudes, and expectations. Much can be learned in the feedback process if the communicator (1) expects to gain some information, (2) tests the information for accuracy by asking pertinent questions and repeating information, (3) determines the relevance of the information to the work situation, and (5) listens for meanings that may not be communicated verbally.

PREDICTIVE PRINCIPLE: The process of group communication enables collaboration in finding solutions to problems and meeting needs.

The purpose of group communication, like individual communication, is to enable collaboration in finding solutions to problems and meeting needs. This differs markedly from making statements and giving directions or providing information. These are one-way messages not geared to collaboration.

Communication breaks down for several reasons:

1. *Overloading the system.* Human communication shares a characteristic with animal and machine communication, that is, overloading causes it to break down. A computer will click out on overload; an animal under excessive stress will show signs of purposeless or erratic behavior, motor neuron synaptic failure, or other signs of "nervous breakdown." A human being will replace normal modes of communication with private modes (jabber) or will restrict communication to the intrapersonal system (talk to himself) or use some other protective device. Reduction of the communication load and other stimuli is necessary for intervention and reestablishment of successful communicating patterns.

2. *Malfunction of the communication apparatus.* This can be from disease or from poor or insufficient mastery of the communication apparatus (eyes, ears, touch, smell, and vocal ability).

3. *Incorrect information.* This is erroneous perception or interpretation of data or faulty data. Anytime the input is faulty, the response will probably be inappropriate.

4. *Misuse of or use of too few communication strategies and tactics.* Strategies and tactics provide for the sending of messages and the obtaining and utilization of feedback. In addition to the clarifying and validating tactics discussed earlier, communication modalities are included here.

5. *Crossed ego states.* According to Berne,* each person has three ego states: Parent, Adult, and Child. Communication proceeds from one of these states. When the person with whom communication is occurring responds from a parallel ego state, breakdown does not occur. Breakdown does occur when communication lines cross (Fig. 5-3).

6. *Perceptual differences.* Perceptual differences among people exist because of differences in experiences, expectations, levels of education, and ethnic, cultural, and religious backgrounds. Two people hearing

---

*Berne, E.: The structure and dynamics of organizations and groups, New York, 1966, Grove Press, Inc.

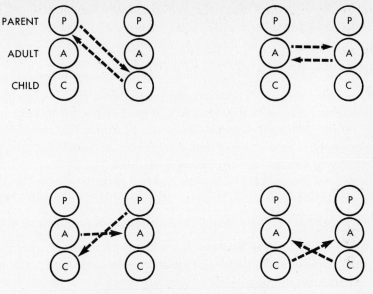

Fig. 5-3. Crossed communication.

the same message will interpret it differently, based on perceptual "programming." These perceptual differences often cause breakdown in communication.

7. *Cognitive style differences.* Several types of cognitive styles have been mapped, and differences in cognitive style account for communication problems. Some people reason by comparing and contrasting. Others synthesize what they hear into categories meaningful to them and responsive to individual needs. Some people are highly theoretical and perhaps esoteric in their cognitive styles, while others are quite concrete and prefer examples and explanatory material. Differences in cognitive styles can lead to communication breakdown.

8. *Private fantasies.* Private fantasies occur because people's imaginations provide them with the structure they deem necessary to operate in ordinary life. When private fantasies become very real, people operate on their fantasies rather than checking out the landmarks of reality. For instance, an employee may imagine that the manager will not like a particular event in the day's work. Operating on that fantasy the employee may begin to defend himself or to dissemble. The manager in such an instance may not know why the employee is defensive or how to respond. Communication breaks down.

Group work extends throughout all health services. Nurses are called on routinely to work with groups of personnel who have a diversity of experience and preparation. The nurse-leader learns to use effective communication in any structural care pattern (for example, case, functional, team, or primary) or within varied organizational systems established for provision of care.

In this context, *group* refers to a number of people, small or large, who work under a leader for a common purpose: that of providing quality nursing care to a specific client or number of clients in any setting. *Process* refers to the goal-oriented operations of the group and the forces at work within operational procedures. For many years the dynamics of group behavior have been studied intensely by psychologists, sociologists, and educators. The scientific study of group process is relatively new; hence there are no absolutes, but there are sufficient data to indicate the processes most useful to leaders and managers. Efforts to classify groups and to identify internal processes reveal that the general laws concerning group life apply to all groups, large or small.

PREDICTIVE PRINCIPLE: Effective communication leads to influence and power.

When nurse-leaders and managers share information with individuals and groups, communicating that information effectively and with legitimate power derived from the organization, they are more apt to be viewed by other persons involved in the process as the ones who exert influence. Claus and Bailey* report several studies showing that leaders depend upon many different channels of communication as power bases. These include nurse-patient/client, nurse-nurse, nurse-physician, nurse-supervisor/administrator, nurse-support service personnel, and so on. Interrelationships occur face to face, by telephone, written memorandums, and in groups, both formal and informal, as discussed previously.

Nurse-managers are central in the communication network, enabling them to acquire vast amounts of information, to use that information to achieve organizational goals and objectives, and to provide opportunity for individuals to grow personally and professionally. There is a direct relationship between power and position with high status in the communication system as those who hold power and position can receive and give more messages and exert more influence than can people with lower status. For example, the director of nursing services can use influence with the board of directors to open a new wing of the hospital or to achieve an across-the-board increase in nurses' salaries, while the lower or first-level nurse can exert influence to institute a treatment or to change the entire direction of nursing care. Through effective communication the nurse-manager can influence nursing supervisors to adopt a different system for delivery of care or to add another member to the nursing staff.

Communication of power can result in a chain reaction. The nurse-

---

*Claus, K., and Bailey, J.: Power and influence in health care: a new approach to leadership, St. Louis, 1977, The C.V. Mosby Co.

manager who feels secure in personal skills and abilities will be likely to release power to others, creating an atmosphere in which staff members feel secure and capable of assuming responsibility for their work. As a result productivity will rise and more goals will be accomplished.

Perception of self and others

Perceptions, like beauty, are in the eye of the beholder. The nurse's perceptions are affected by the total self-system. Value systems, ideals, life goals, experiences, preconceptions, expectations of self and others, and context all affect perception. What a person sees and hears and how he or she interprets this information are regulated by the self-system. Perception is more than seeing and hearing; it also includes interpreting these data. Interpretations are functions of values, social conditioning, and life experiences and expectations. The leader's perception of self affects his view of others. Individuals who expect to receive affirmative responses from people elicit positive responses through their approach. The converse is also true, as people who expect negative reactions usually communicate such expectations behaviorally and elicit similar negative responses.

Perceptions of others also affect communications. The leader's perceptions of an individual or group are usually only parts of reality; the same is true of the group's or individual's perception of the leader. The invalidity or lack of authenticity in perception greatly influences interpretation of behavior and communication. Sharing insight about perceptions and self within the group will aid the efficiency of communication. No attempt is made to deal specifically with therapeutic communication; however, the predictive principles discussed have relevance to all phases of nursing.

PREDICTIVE PRINCIPLE: The leader's self-perception directly influences the development of positive perception in each group member.

Since much of leadership and management is individual and personal, these roles demand involvement of oneself as a person. It is essential that the leader have both the ability to share and the capacity for self-discipline. Perceptual psychologists have indicated that the deeply deprived self cannot afford to give itself away. The self must possess a satisfactory degree of adequacy before it can venture commitment and encounter with individuals or groups. Leadership depends on entering into an interaction relationship with others, and effective leaders possess sufficient self-esteem to make sharing and supporting relationships posible. The nurse-leader needs to feel personally adequate to deal effectively with others.

Effective leaders believe themselves fundamentally adequate, which facilitates the giving of adequate attention to the needs of both client and care-giver. Those who feel inadequate and deprived cannot afford the time and effort required to lead and assist others. In the University of Florida studies* of the helping professions, a number of perceptual psychologists studied the nature of self-fulfillment and personal adequacy in professional leaders and directors. It was found that effective leaders felt themselves being (1) identified with rather than apart from others, (2) basically adequate rather than inadequate, (3) trust-worthy rather than untrustworthy, (4) wanted rather than unwanted or ignored, and (5) worthy rather than overlooked or discounted.

The nurse-leader with a positive self-perception is able to provide the necessary positive support to clients and members of the health team. This posi-tive perception is communicated to others, thereby increasing the self-esteem of individuals and group members. With the self-concept strengthened, partici-pants can often develop in turn into support agents for other relationships, as for example with clients.

Another element in positive supportive relationships is the ability to care. Persons with successful caring experiences find it easier to care about others successfully. Caring managers and leaders learn names, obtain vital statis-tics, and personal and professional information, and use these data in positive, supportive, and growth-provoking ways.

PREDICTIVE PRINCIPLE: The value systems of the leader and group influence the establishment of goals and priorities, as well as govern the amount of effort given to goal attainment.

Value systems are those ethics, ideas, objects, behaviors, or philosophies important to an individual. As the outgrowths of life experiences, life goals, ambi-tions, and ethnic background, values dictate the moral, ethical, material, and religious "set" of individuals. The leader and every member bring a value system to their group. This pooling of values creates an amorphous group personality. Because of the makeup of a group and its climate, leadership, and task, its value system becomes evident in what is important to it, that is, in what receives its attention and efforts. Changes perceived by the leader and the group as having great worth will receive high priorities and much effort, whereas changes or goals viewed by the group as unimportant or of little value will receive slight effort and be of low priority. Priority setting is a direct function of individual and group values.

If the goals established are not valued by the group, the personnel will usually not work toward them. However, extraneous factors may enter in. If re-wards for goal achievement become important enough, the group will strive for the established goal to achieve the reward.

PREDICTIVE PRINCIPLE: Continuity of competent leadership and management facilitates the efficiency of the communication process.

Continuity with reference to nursing care means provision for daily, uninterrupted service for a prescribed period of time. To ensure continuity there is an unbroken chain of related communications, events, and responsibilities. When a link in this chain becomes weak or severed, the probability of discontinuity increases in proportion to the number of persons involved. There is a return to the concept of primary care where those persons most concerned and involved in health care services are in contact.

Continuity necessitates adequate coverage for days off, illness, vacations, and leaves in order for communications to be maintained at the desired level of operation. The manager attempts to select replacements who are skilled in nursing, are familiar with client or agency policies and procedures, have the ability to work well with others, and have the potential to guide the client or group members in achieving their purposes.

Staffing formulas can become inadequate when prolonged absences occur. Provision for vacations, illnesses, attendance at workshops, and leaves for other purposes requires the addition of personnel. It is well for new nurses to become familiar with the overall plan of nursing care, to assess potential client needs, and then to be assigned for individual orientation into group processes within the work setting.

The importance of having a second person qualified to assume a managerial role is determined by the length of absence of the regular manager and the role the manager plays in the agency. Leadership does not always depend on the physical presence of the leader. If the individual or group understands its direction and if its behaviors are established, basic functions can take place under minimal direction. When absences are extensive, it is important that a prepared person be available. The opportunity to experience group process in operation helps the alternate or associate leader carry on the pattern of activity established by the primary leader. It also provides a basis for joint evaluation of the process by both leaders.

Having someone ready to take over during absences is important, but there are other benefits of having an associate manager. The process of teaching and preparing others for leadership helps the manager to learn. The manager gains a clearer picture of the job in the process of explaining it, learns more about the abilities of the client or caregivers, and gains increased insight into the group processes.

The sense of cohesiveness built up in the members when management is shared results in a more reliable process. Each person clarifies his or her role and relationship to others. There is a reinforcement of the rationale for care and a sense of accomplishment in seeing that plans run smoothly.

PREDICTIVE PRINCIPLE: Characteristics of client and leader/manager determine the types of communications that will evolve.

The practice of nursing is gradually shifting its focus from being essentially curative and restorative and practiced in hospitals or client facilities to the promotion of health and prevention of disease. This latter practice is increasingly becoming a part of community or emergent institutional programs. Consumers of nursing services are being looked on not as "patients" but as "clients" who may initiate and participate in their own health care. This procedural shift from a passive to an active role by clients influences attitudes and behaviors concerned with communication.

The average consumer has increasing geographic and economic access to health care. Hospitals and similar agencies are often overcrowded and unable to provide for all clients who seek admission. There is also the economic problem faced by those who are unable to finance the higher cost of institutionalized service. Subsequently, there is a shift in the role of the nurse-leader from hospitals and other institutions to outpatient health care. This requires a varied technique of communications, for the nurse must be acquainted with many types of facilities that offer health treatment in various locales. These range from national, state, and regional facilities to those provided by local communities, churches, and other groups interested in fostering health improvement among all strata of society. These health programs incorporate maintenance, curative, restorative, and rehabilitative services for the various types of health needs such as physical health, mental health, family planning, mother-child relationships, health supervision, teaching, and counseling.

Despite how or where client and nurse begin their relationship or contractual agreement, the nursing process involves partnership between nurse and client in planning and implementing problem-oriented care. As mentioned earlier, Berne proposes that every individual has three basic ego states—parent, adult, and child. The parent ego state governs an individual's values, conscience, and moral and ethical behaviors. Parent messages given to self and others contain words such as "should," "ought," and "must." Parent ego states are derived from early injunctions learned in the primary family and are part of the "scripting" of early childhood. They are necessary in the socialization of an individual and enable people to conform to the mores and folkways of their cultural environments. Parent ego states can be nurturing (loving, protective, supporting, caring) or critical (cross, criticizing, discounting).

The adult ego state is the logical state that looks at consequences, weighs risks, and makes decisions on a strictly rational level. It is mathematical in its precision, objectivity, and freedom from emotional overlay.

The child ego state is an emotional, "little kid" state. It has two facets:

1. Adaptive, which can be sweet, loving, dependent, seductive, and eager to please; or rebellious, which can be easily angered, contrary, negative, and not wanting to be bossed or managed

2. Free child, which can be playful, mischievous, enthusiastic, caring, and insightful, or a "little professor" who figures out how to get what he wants

Nursing, because of social set and traditional role enaction, proceeds primarily from the parent and child ego states. Communication patterns with clients usually place the nurse in the "parent" position, "telling" the client (child) what he or she should or should not do. Clients get "hooked" into playing the child ego state, whether adaptive, rebellious, free child, or little professor.

Nurses' relationships with physicians are also child-parent oriented, with the physician playing the parent role and the nurse playing the child role. The physician is nurturing and critical by turns, and the nurse adaptive, rebellious, free child, or little professor in response.

Communication flows well as long as each participant plays out prescribed roles, but when any participant attempts to establish another ego state from which to communicate, communication can break down.

Nurse-managers usually set the stage for communication. Managers who communicate with staff as "the boss" are in the parent ego state and, through role modeling, set a climate of "parenting" for their subordinates. Clients, last in the chain of command, are then treated like children and are placed in the "one-down" position. This decreases the decision-making powers of clients and strips them of individuality, rights, and responsibility for their own care and destiny.

Fig. 5-4 illustrates the traditional communication flow in nursing, just discussed. Fig. 5-5 illustrates the communication pattern adult-to-adult, that is, the desirable flow of communications among physician, manager, staff, and client. This is not to say that participants in the health care setting need never proceed from any but the adult ego state. This would indeed be a coolly logical,

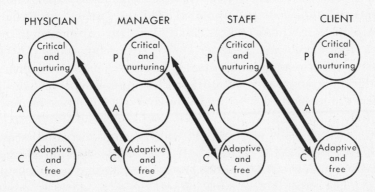

Fig. 5-4. Traditional ego state communication patterns in health agencies.

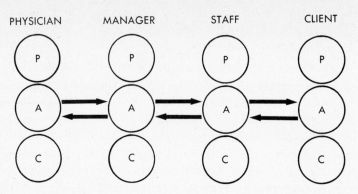

Fig. 5-5. Desirable ego state communication patterns in health agencies.

and not necessarily desirable, communication flow. There are times when every individual needs and requests nurturing, and it is productive for a manager to play that role when requested. It is helpful when one gets into the child ego state to have another willing to also enter that state and "play." Indeed, this section is not intended to convey that because the adult ego state is the most reality oriented the other ego states are undesirable and should never be used. What is desirable is that each individual recognize the ego state from which communications are derived at any given time and be aware of the ego states of those with whom he is communicating, so that adjustments can be made that keep communication flowing.

Managers who are willing to relate to staff on an adult level and reinforce adult communication among staff succeed in raising the level of productivity, accountability, and shared responsiveness to clients' rights and privileges. When communication is (1) uncrossed, (2) clear, and (3) proceeding from the adult ego state, the client is the beneficiary. As a result, clients make verbal contracts and agreements about the care they want and need and thereby participate in their own care; families can make choices about their own involvement in the family member's health problems. In general, when communications proceed from managers on adult-to-adult levels, there is a better climate for healing.

The successful leader will work to keep interpersonal relationships at a level where group efforts will be productive and will encourage members to be cooperatively interdependent. With this type of leadership and management, it is probable that a process will evolve in which there is increased member participation, increased client participation, more rapid decision making, more achievement within the group, and more progress toward accomplishing purposes and goals. Effective communication increases productivity, group cohesion, and quality of client care.

Reinforcement and feedback

In human relationships, some form of reinforcement, positive or negative, is communicated. The effective leader will use reinforcement as a means to increase each participant's identification with and effort toward individual or group goals. According to Professor B.F. Skinner of Harvard, reward, not punishment, is the most effective force for shaping human behavior. Positive reinforcement may be food, money, praise, a kiss, a smile, a nod of approval. More significant, however, is that positive feedback may consist of eliciting a right answer and knowing it is correct, working out a problem to one's satisfaction, mastering a skill, or finding new beauty and order in words, music, and art. Every culture and subculture, all institutions such as hospitals and health agencies, and every home has its own methodology, acknowledged or unacknowledged, of employing rewards and punishments. Studies have shown, however, that in many cases the direction of various group processes has relied on punishment or the threat of punishment to control subordinates and other members of the group. Ineffective forms of positive reinforcement are used, forms that are not in keeping with the value system for participating. These practices ignore the most effective forms of positive reinforcement.

Steiner* has done much work in stroking patterns. Steiner defines strokes as reinforcements. They can be (1) positive-conditional, (2) negative-conditional, (3) positive-unconditional, or (4) negative-unconditional.

Positive-conditional strokes are strokes given for things well done—pleasing and acceptable behaviors. An example is "You certainly took good care of Mrs. Jones while she was in such a panic state during that procedure."

Negative-conditional strokes are those that are critical, providing negative feedback. They are given for things incorrectly and poorly done or things omitted that were displeasing to someone. An example is "You really blew that! Now we'll never get Dr. Morris to cooperate in our new drug plan."

The best strokes are *positive-unconditional* strokes. These are positive compliments given a person for just being—just existing. Comments such as "I really do like you," "I really like being around you," and "You're such a fine person" are positive-unconditional strokes.

The worst strokes are the *negative-unconditional* strokes. These punish one for just being—not for anything that has been done or not done—but for just existing. Battered children and battered managers and staff are often the products of negative-unconditional stroking. For example, "I just don't like you" is a negative-unconditional stroke. Character assassinations that evolve during arguments or reprimands are common negative-unconditional strokes. These

---

*Steiner, C.: Scripts people live, New York, 1974, Grove Press, Inc.

are such remarks as "You are such a turkey!" or "You dumb broad!"

According to Steiner, there are five stroke injunctions. These injunctions have been taught to people in the United States as a part of their socialization process. Much of our inability to provide reinforcements can be attributed to these injunctions:

1. Don't ask for strokes—even if you want them.
2. Don't give strokes—even if they are deserved.
3. Don't reject strokes—even if they are given for something you don't want them for.
4. Don't stroke yourself—even if you think you deserve it.
5. Don't accept strokes given to you—even if you want to.

One can see by looking at these injunctions why strokes are so difficult to give and receive, for the messages are mixed. A person who asks for strokes is often perceived as conceited or having excessive ego needs. A person who gives strokes often perceives himself as giving away too much or somehow detracting from his own worth and value. People are taught that if someone gives a stroke, positive or negative, one must accept it whether or not it is wanted. It somehow is not legitimate to say, "Please don't compliment me on that thing—I'm not very proud of it," or "Don't criticize me for that—I'm very pleased with myself about that," or simply "No, thank you, I don't think I'll take that compliment." People who stroke themselves say, "Gee, didn't I do a great job!" or "I really like the way I handled that situation," or "I wish I had done such and such; it would have produced a better job" and may be seen as either too prideful or too critical of themselves. As a result of the injunctions listed, it is extremely difficult to enter into a healthy, even-keeled, balanced stroking system that reinforces positive growth, promotes feelings of self-worth, provides adequate feedback, and enables continued clear communications. Leaders and managers who are conscious of stroke injunctions and individual workers' stroking needs and patterns can help workers ask for and receive the strokes they need to alter behaviors, grow, and be more productive.

Positive and negative stroking patterns (or positive and negative reinforcements) form the basis for all growth patterns and communication patterns and affect the goals that are set; how one manages time, energy, resources, and materials to achieve those goals; and how one evaluates whether or not the goals have been reached.

PREDICTIVE PRINCIPLE: Integrative positive reinforcement increases individual identification with group goals and the participation level of the individual.

Since the mid-1950s Flanders, Amidon, Hough, and others have been experimenting with a system to measure verbal and nonverbal group interaction styles called *interaction analysis*. A significant aspect of this analysis scheme is to measure the group leader's or instructor's ability to reinforce verbally the participants' behavior in order to induce the members to initiate positive action toward group goals and to increase retention level of the participants. *Integrative behavior influences* of the instructor or group leader are (1) accepting feelings of participants, (2) praising or encouraging participation, (3) accepting or using ideas of participants, and (4) asking questions of participants. These are positive-conditional and positive-unconditional strokes from the adult ego state. *Directive behavior influences* are (1) lecturing to the group, (2) giving directions to individuals or the group, (3) criticizing, and (4) justifying authority. These are communications from the parent ego state and include negative-conditional and negative-unconditional strokes.

The integrative leader is one who accepts, clarifies, and supports participants' ideas and feelings and who praises, encourages, and stimulates participation in the decision-making process. Directive or dominative leaders, on the other hand, tend to focus on introspective ideas and knowledge, giving many directions and orders, criticizing participants, and being concerned with justification of their own position and authority. Other studies have replicated the described analysis system, indicating that the more integrative the leader (or the more he or she uses positive reinforcement), the higher the identification by group participants in achieving group goals. Instruments have been devised to measure group participants' retention of substance in group sessions, and again it was discovered that the greater the positive reinforcement, the greater the retention.

A direct positive relationship exists between the group leader's ability to reinforce the members' supportive interaction and individual initiative in achieving group goals. There is a statistically significant positive relationship between a leader's ability to reinforce group participants and the frequency of group members' support and reinforcement of one another. This is especially true in cases where the leader uses more integrative positive reinforcement of group participants. The more a nurse-leader accepts, clarifies, or uses the ideas of a member, the more that member will tend to participate in the group process and positively support other members by recognizing, clarifying, and accepting their ideas and input. The behavior of nonparticipating members in a group may be changed from passive to active if the nurse-leader provides sufficient positive reinforcement to the group. The more active participants will in turn desire to support these less active group members through questions, encouragement, or praise or, in general, will communicate a feeling of acceptance.

PREDICTIVE PRINCIPLE: Perceiving negative feedback enables group members to become aware of others' responses and to modify behavior accordingly.

Negative feedback or negative strokes are reinforcing in that they provide individuals with important information about what is not occurring that should be or what is happening that should not be. It enables individuals to know how they affect others in displeasing or unacceptable ways. Negative feedback is the counterpart of positive feedback, and both are important reinforcing factors. If a member is not contributing to group goals, not participating in collaborative efforts, or is exhibiting undesirable behaviors, it is more important for that individual to know what those noncontributory behaviors are than to proceed in ignorance.

Negative feedback is difficult for most people to give or receive. People like to be liked; therefore criticism is hard to give. People want to behave appropriately, to contribute to group effort, and to be working, interdependent members. Negative feedback is often interpreted as not fulfilling to a positive self-image. The pain of receiving negative input is partially offset by the knowledge of the "caring" behind the critique. Negative feedback is uncomfortable for most people and is therefore avoided. Inherent in any feedback, negative or positive, is the message of "I care about you and your contribution to this group." Negative strokes can be very effective if they are given in supportive ways. Brutal negative-unconditional strokes are counterproductive. The person who is given only negative strokes will not grow.

PREDICTIVE PRINCIPLE: The dependent, interdependent, and/or independent natures of relationships affect the structure of the communication process.

Dependence in relationships takes three forms: (1) dependence of one member on another for guidelines and support; (2) interdependence, where members share decision making and responsibility; and (3) independence, where members engage in an activity on their own.

Group members seek to achieve some balance of dependence, interdependence, and independence within group structure according to group climate. Successful exercise of authority requires not only a recognized dependence on the part of the members or the leader, but also a reciprocal and acknowledged recognition of the leader's dependence on the members. This interdependence results in greater mutual confidence between leader and members.

Some people find comfort in maintaining close dependent relationships. These individuals usually seek constant direction and reassurance from others and may become attached to another person or persons. They operate primarily from the adaptive child ego state and "hook" others into communicating with them from the parent ego state. Often dependency is shown by what people do not do; it makes them unwilling to take chances, to exert extra effort, to use their imagination, or to display initiative. They achieve a degree of security without risk by getting others to take care of them. It is unwise to attempt to move the insecure individual beyond what he or she is capable of accomplishing without a clear agreement or contract concerning goals and growth.

Interdependence is a reciprocal reliance between group leader and participants. In a cooperative environment, whenever one member performs a beneficial act all others benefit simultaneously.

An example of interdependence in action can be illustrated by the following:

A vocational nurse observed that Mr. Cable, a 68-year-old man hospitalized for treatment of a fractured femur, was developing a reddened area on his coccyx. He resisted lying on his side and disliked massage. In checking his record the licensed vocational nurse (LVN) noted that no reference was made to this problem. After discussing the matter with the nurse-manager and Mr. Cable and involving them in the decision-making process, the LVN obtained an air mattress for Mr. Cable and then began to make plans with him for exercises he could do to increase his circulation. She followed through by recording the care plan on the nurse's notes.

This worker initiated preventive measures that would prove beneficial to the client (possibly saving him a long hospitalization) and would help other caregivers by affording them the satisfaction of knowing they had participated in problem-oriented care and had possibly avoided many hours of unnecessary nursing care. This communication pattern proceeded from the adult ego state, avoided "preaching" parent messages (of what Mr. Cable should or ought to do), and involved all concerned persons in making the decision.

A state of dependence among members can foster characteristics detrimental to group goals. The nurse who asks the leader or manager for directions or specific instructions for every move, refuses to make decisions, blames others when things go wrong, and gets others to "rescue" her or do her work is dependent and operates from the child ego state. Each person in this relationship expects the others to keep the status quo, and there is resentment if moves are made to alter the nature of procedures designed to keep the dependency going. The alert group membership will know when conditions warrant group decision to solve the problem. The leader who can create conditions of interdependence and adult communication patterns will have facilitated productive communication processes.

PREDICTIVE PRINCIPLE: The interdependent collaborating group facilitates accomplishment of its goals.

Group participation in coordinating activities is a natural by-product of a democratic managerial philosophy. If nursing groups can facilitate coordination at the unit or team level, the entire organization is benefited.

Ingredients for group success in devising plans for cooperative effort include (1) a willingness on the part of all members to participate in the planning, (2) a sharing of common purposes, (3) careful communication, and (4) adherence to the authority of the employing person or organization. Responsibility for group action is often invested in the leader by bureaucracies, but this does not imply that authority must be given to a single individual. In an interdependent group, each member shares equally in the responsibility for group decisions and actions. Within guidelines, members are free to explore processes through which care can be administered to a number of clients.

Interdependent activity operates on the basic premise that groups have the power to produce changes in individual behavior so that more work will be accomplished collectively than would be individually.

Cooperation depends on routine relationships developed and practiced over a long period of time. It relies on codes of behavior whereby people work together in a group without conscious choice of whether or not they will cooperate. Cooperation demands a certain stability in the ways of the group. In nursing, this stability is often in jeopardy because of fluctuating staffing patterns. In agencies where round-the-clock coverage is necessary, membership is relatively unstable and ways must be found to overcome this problem.

Group consensus presents an element of danger. The pressure of conformity, the urge to become like every other member, and the fear of the consequences if group norms are not adhered to may make a member function in a manner contrary to the group expectations:

The new nurse's aide is told by her peer, "I know they told you in in-service to bathe everybody every day, but let's face it!—we don't have that kind of time. You do up the worst ones and take care of the rest the best way you can. I give patients assigned to me a bath about two times a week. I do the best I can and report 'bath given' when we sign off."

The new aide is in a dilemma. She needs the job and wants to give good nursing care but feels pressure from all sides. She is caught in a power struggle between the stated authority figures who set the standards and one member who digresses from the rules. The solution rests in the leader's and individual's ability to recognize that a power struggle exists and to deal with the situation openly. The leader can help the members face the problem by stating directly, "I notice there is a conflict between policy and practice. I need to know more about the situation. What is really going on? What caused this to happen? How do you feel about the situation?"

In all probability, group process will lead to the formation of a work structure that will resolve the conflict. The leader can ask the group how they believe priorities can best be established to ensure the administration of good care without rigidity. Possible alternatives are as follows:

1. Provide personal hygiene for every patient daily.
2. Every day bathe those patients having fevers, diaphoresis, or incontinence.
3. Bathe geriatric patients every other day (unless in category 2).
4. Establish round-the-clock activities (bathe some patients in the evening, unresponsive patients at night).

Through interdependent action the leader has helped turn a negative situation into one that can prove highly beneficial to all concerned.

Positive relationships facilitate cohesiveness and achievement of goals with speed and efficiency. Independent activity has a definite place in group activities. When members experience feelings of security in their ability and in relationships with others, they will begin to seek ways of utilizing their capabilities and skills more fully. This active search is constructive and should be nurtured. The process of allowing independence among membership is a delicate one. A willingness to assume authority for special tasks does not ensure success. Self-development must have reached a level where the individual can move into the desired role with ability to achieve. Independence can be fostered by giving additional tasks gradually, so that workers are not suddenly made insecure by too great a load but can exercise authority with discretion.

Independent action within nursing takes several routes, ranging from physical activity to mental exercise. The nurse might have sanction to manage and complete a complex assignment (for example, primary care), to take responsibility for reorganizing the medicine or treatment room, or to devise a new way to administer a treatment. The individual expresses ideas and contributes suggestions on matters that involve the client, himself, and group operation. Participation of this kind leads to member satisfaction in knowing that individual efforts have been recognized and that options and ideas are given consideration in a search for increased effectiveness and efficiency and solutions to problem-oriented nursing care.

PREDICTIVE PRINCIPLE: Continuing reference to and clarification of goals enhance the ability to attain those goals.

Goals will seem more attainable to the participant if the nurse-leader provides opportunity for membership input. Often the group leader will assume that the preestablished goals are clear, relevant, adequate, and interesting to the extent that mere exposure will motivate the participant to achieve the goals. Empirical data suggest that increased group participation in clarifying individual and group goals is important to continued goal-directed effort; tangential activities are fewer and group effort more consistent.

Management by objectives (MBO) is a system in which management and labor at all levels participate through organizational strategies in the identification of worthy goals for the whole division as well as individual units and individual workers. Joint participation in goal-setting enables common or agreed on goals to be established. Once this is done, each person within the structure has a responsibility for meeting the defined goals. Each person knows what is expected in the effort to achieve the goals. These goals are then used to generate criteria by which individual, unit, and division efforts can be evaluated. MBO is a science in itself, with strategies for implementing, working with, and evaluating the system. Research findings generally indicate it to be highly effective.*

Goal-setting is the key to any successful management program, whether that management is the care of one client, a team, a nursing unit, several nursing units, or a whole nursing division. Goal-setting may or may not lead to MBO, but it always leads to more effective and efficient coordination and collaboration. The goals are clear and accomplishment easily evaluated. MBO is not designed to create major changes in organization but rather to assume the smooth, daily operation of an organization.

There are several methods the nurse-leader may use to determine whether the participant has perceived the relevancy of a purpose and accepts its value. The group leader can provide various types of incentives or positive reinforcement to encourage discussion of goals, values, and motivation. For example, when a client is motivated to learn or participate in isolation technique, rewards may be in achieving self-protection and in demonstrating to himself and the nurse that a complex skill has been mastered. At times the reward may be so far removed from the goal that the participant does not see the relationship. For instance, the client may see no relationship between hand-washing and contamination and thus may fail to become interested in the subject.

Communication strategies

Strategies are heuristic devices or tools useful for accomplishing goals. A mechanic is equipped with a huge number of tools, each of which is designed to achieve a specific purpose and has a definite use. Some tools are helpful for a wider number of "jobs" than others. For instance, a spark plug wrench is singularly designed for removing and replacing spark plugs and is not applicable to many other functions, whereas screwdrivers, pliers, and other more nonspecific tools can be used for a variety of mechanical problems. Strategies are similar. The direct question, as a strategy, is useful for eliciting specific answers and definite information but may not be helpful in eliciting discussions about problems important to the group but not included in the question. Nondirective techniques may enable clients to follow their own needs and lines of thought but may not provide the nurse with information vital to a nursing diagnosis and prescription.

There are literally thousands of communication heuristics—communication group laboratory experiences, books, and courses—each filled with devices that enable individuals and groups to communicate more advantageously. This discussion does not attempt to cover even a representative number. A few devices are chosen as examples.

---

*From McLemore, M., and Bevis, E.O.: Planned change. In Marriner, A., editor: Current perspectives in nursing management, St. Louis, 1979, The C.V. Mosby Co., chap. 9.

PREDICTIVE PRINCIPLE: The type of communication at work in a group dictates member perception and consequent action.

PREDICTIVE PRINCIPLE: Congruent behavioral and verbal messages promote clear communication.

As discussed previously, methods of communication employed by participants are important, for receiving and sending ideas clearly are essential to accomplishing purposes. Improvement in communication depends on daily work among all participants.

People who know what is expected of them, who learn about changes before they take place, who feel free to clarify vague messages, and who check out unknown factors will perceive their roles in the best light and will work with heightened interest and enthusiasm.

Careful use of verbal delivery, written messages, and physical behavior is an effective means of increasing communication with others. Effective communication depends on all participants understanding the meaning of the encounter. Without effective communication a group becomes merely a collection of individuals working in close proximity and engaged in ill-defined tasks.

PREDICTIVE PRINCIPLE: Recognition and use of informal communication channels by the leader can lead to enhancement of organizational goals.

Formal communication uses established organizational channels and standard media such as conferences, telephone messages, memorandums, and policies and procedure manuals. Informal communication exists because of personal and group interests of people. In health care organizations much of the coordination that occurs among units in the organization comes about through the informal give-and-take of information exchanges.

Informal or casual groups emerge whenever people come together and interact regularly. This type of communication is commonly called the "grapevine," a term that was coined during the Civil War when intelligence telegraph lines were strung loosely from tree to tree. The messages were often garbled. Grapevines occur when one group member appears to be more informed than others in the group about what is going on in the formal organization. Through this means false as well as accurate information can easily spread. The grapevine is direct, fast, and flexible; yet it does not have access to official information sources.

Keith Davis,* one of the foremost authorities on informal communication, has said some pertinent things about the informal process:

1. The grapevine is a social interaction, fulfilling people's needs for

---

*Davis, K.: Human behavior at work: organizational behavior, ed. 5, New York, 1977, McGraw-Hill Book Co.

communication and recognition. Therefore it is as varied as the people who communicate.

2. The grapevine is based on a natural motivation to exchange information—so much so that if members of a work team do not talk about their work and the people involved informally, they are probably maladjusted.

3. The grapevine occurs at all levels in an organization in horizontal, vertical, and diagonal patterns.

4. The grapevine is extremely influential, shaping persons' attitudes and having the capacity to carry information both helpful and harmful to the organization.

5. The grapevine has an unusual ability to find out even the tightest organizational secrets.

6. Employees become active on the grapevine when they have news that is fresh and "hot."

7. The grapevine can become active when information is of high interest to the individual and the messages regarding that interest are vague or unclear. If a subject has no interest to a person, then that person has no cause to spread a rumor about it. And if enough facts are known to satisfy the individual, there is no need to set rumor into motion.

8. The source of information directly affects the strength and duration of the grapevine, as does the believability of the information passed along. The greater the believability, the more legitimate the grapevine becomes.

9. In organizations the grapevine is more a product of a situation rather than of a personality. The grapevine flourishes wherever anticipation or fear becomes dominant within an organization, for example, when a major change in the agency's management causes fear of transfer or dismissal or uncertainty regarding wages and benefits. The grapevine can and does thrive when an individual member becomes known for some achievement, good or bad.

Davis identifies four channels used in the grapevine: (1) single-strand chain, (2) gossip chain, (3) probability chain, and (4) cluster chain (Fig. 5-6).

Single-strand chain. The single-strand chain is very like the game of telephone, where A tells B, who tells C, who then tells D, and so on until the final person gets the message very incorrectly.

Gossip chain. In the second channel the gossip chain is used, where one person seeks out and tells everyone who will listen the information obtained. This channel is used most often when information of an interesting but nonwork-related nature is being passed on (marriage, separation, divorce, family activities or problems, etc.).

Probability chain. In the probability chain individuals are indifferent

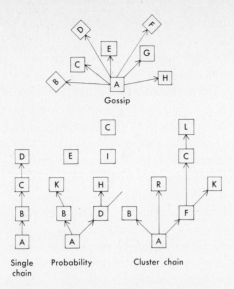

Fig. 5-6. Grapevine patterns of communication. (From Douglass, L.M.: The effective nurse: leader and manager, St. Louis, 1980, The C.V. Mosby Co.; adapted from Davis, K.: Human behavior at work: organizational behavior, ed. 5, New York, 1977, McGraw-Hill Book Co.)

about whom they inform; they tell people at random, and those people tell others at random. This chain is likely to be used when the information is mildly interesting but insignificant, and by people who are not as interested as the gossiper in receiving or sharing other people's affairs.

Cluster chain. The pattern by far the most commonly used is called a cluster chain. Davis believes that most people who learn information do not spread it. They do so only when there is enough interest in the subject. There is selectivity of information in the process. Generally persons choose details that fit their particular interest. In the cluster chain, A tells three or four others, such as B, R, and F. Only one or two of these receivers are interested enough to pass on the information, and they will usually tell more than one person. Then as the information becomes older and the proportion of those knowing it gets larger, it gradually dies out because those who receive it do not care enough about the information to repeat it. The details transmitted in the cluster chain may be true or false.

According to Davis, the accuracy of the grapevine in normal situations tends to be about 75%. Serious problems may arise with inaccurate information transmitted. Often the whole story is not shared. Managers sometimes hope the grapevine in an agency will go away, but it will not. Informal communication channels will emerge whether or not managers encourage them. If suppressed, the grapevine will emerge in another place or in another form. The best approach for nurse-leaders is to use the grapevine to help the organization as much as possible to offset negative impact. Following are methods a nurse-manager can utilize:

1. Keep staff as well informed as possible concerning work-related issues that have relevance to them.
2. Maintain an open communication system that encourages feedback.
3. Listen and learn from the grapevine. Learn who the leaders are, how the grapevine operates, and what information it carries. The object is to determine what is important to nursing staff members. Omissions in information or false messages can be identified; then strategies can be developed to heighten areas of satisfaction and reduce anxiety, conflict, and misunderstanding.
4. Try to influence the grapevine by giving relevant information to liaison or key people. This is especially necessary when the grapevine has been spreading incomplete or inaccurate information such as possible lay-offs, transfers, or mandatory rotation of shifts.

In management the nurse-leader will discourage the development and use of grapevines for work-related matters and will promote the use of formal communication channels. The effective nurse-manager will recognize the need for informal communication by the staff and use the grapevine to enhance organizational goals.

PREDICTIVE PRINCIPLE: Threat and resulting anxiety, unless resolved, can inhibit individual and group communication.

Threat is a device that usually results in anxiety and can have detrimental effects on individuals and groups. Anxiety can appear when there is uncertainty regarding some event or series of happenings. The tension may be expressed internally, or the feeling may be communicated to all those who have contact with the disturbed person. Anxiety can be relieved constructively through exploration of the cause, with appropriate follow-up by the manager.

The effect that anxiety can have on a staff member is illustrated through the following incident:

John, an aide, was evidencing anxiety that was affecting his ability to function adequately. It was nearly time for his six-month evaluation, when he would be informed whether he would be placed on permanent status or asked to leave. He was a medical student and depended on the job for his income. In addition, he liked the work and all the members of the group. When the nurse-manager had given him his three-month evaluation, he had been told that his work was "OK" but that he needed to improve. Nothing specific was mentioned. Since that time, he found himself increasingly anxious.

The leader talked with John. Discussion revealed that he was "worried sick," and because he had not heard any positive feedback except for an occasional noncommittal remark from his group leader, he knew no positive ways to improve. Together they devised a plan of improvement, established evaluation and feedback schedules, and planned a program for John to ask for and receive positive strokes. He was soon clearly asking for feedback by such things as "Mr. Cox sure looked better today after I finished with him, don't you think?" "I categorized all the traction equipment this afternoon. It should be easier for everybody to find what they need from now on, right?"

The two members worked through the problem by analyzing the specific incidents and recognizing when feelings of anxiety were generated. The leader recognized the lack of specificity in the three-month evaluation and failure to provide structure for follow-up. John sought more direct ways for ascertaining his progress from the leader.

Another manifestation of problems with the communication process is the introduction of threatening stimuli. Threat occurs when impending danger is made known by word or action. The term is applied to both important and trivial matters. When the member becomes aware of the threat, he or she concentrates on ways to handle the problem. In interrelationships, threats are conveyed both through conscious and subconscious means. If, for example, two members of a group distrust each other, threatening actions that express their feelings may be manifested in both overt and covert ways. Innuendos, verbal exchanges, and failure to assist one another are examples. These actions have a deleterious impact on group efforts. Threats can also exert a positive influence by serving as strong motivators to action. The group that is presented with a challenge for which it feels ill-prepared can offset the threat of failure by mobilizing forces to obtain the tools that will enable its members to accomplish the charge. Overt threats are usually more counterproductive than productive.

Resistive behavior is another negative force that can deter the communication process. The apprehension of not wanting certain things to take place can evoke resistive responses in clients or group members. The inspection process may create feelings of resentment. The client or caregiver may ask, "Why should I be checked on? I'm capable of completing an assignment." Opposition may also take the form of reluctance or failure to accept assignment, hostility, rigidity of action, regression, absence, or nonresponsiveness.

PREDICTIVE PRINCIPLE: Questions and discussion geared to second and third level theories promote cognition that is more useful in nursing activities than questions and discussion geared to first and second level theories.

Alert observers will attest that more than 80% of the verbal exchanges in group process are initiated with a question. Traditionally, questions are used to determine what has been learned or the status of one's thinking. Most questions posed by group leaders or instructors are asked so that the response and thinking of the respondent are at the first two levels of theory and require only memory or recall. There is, then, a wide range in the quality of quesitions. The effective leader will use questions geared to levels III and IV of theory (discussed in Chapter 1), which call for prediction or prescription. Responses to these levels of inquiry require synthesis, imagination, and creativity and encourage varying forms of problem-oriented thinking.

In developing a questioning strategy the leader will realize that (1) raising questions and issues helps to increase group interaction and establish feedback, (2) questions are used to assist participants in sharing, (3) questions are employed to lead the participant step by step to think about experiences, and (4) questions are a means of sampling respondents' understanding of or ability to make application of concepts.

The skilled leader tends to have other techniques available to accomplish the goals itemized. Statements that elicit remarks are one way; examples of these "eliciting remarks" are "Please tell me about . . ." or "Help me to understand. . . ."

Gallagher and Aschner* developed a system that classifies questions into four categories:

1. *Recall-descriptive*—narrow questions calling for specific facts, information, or descriptions to be presented by rote. Participants are asked only to give a response, not to do anything with it. Answers to these questions require only the lowest intellectual level (first and second level theories).

2. *Convergent-explanation*—calling for the analysis and integration of given or remembered data. Problem solving and reasoning are often involved in this category. The answers may be predictable, but the task requires application of two or more recall items (third level theories).

3. *Divergent-expansion*—calling for answers that are creative and imaginative and not empirically provable. Many different answers may be correct and acceptable (third level theory).

4. *Value-evaluative*—dealing with judgment, value, and choice. The participant states a preference based on individual values and standards (fourth level theory).

Productive groups soon learn the value of third level discussions and concentrate remarks on that level. The payoff for the group is more efficient and valid problem solving.

PREDICTIVE PRINCIPLE: Use of simulation facilitates decision making and provides efficient means for learning problem-solving methods in a nonthreatening and safe environment.

Simulation, as used in this discussion, affords the participant opportunity to elicit various response patterns to a set of circumstances, the content of

---

*Gallagher, J., and Aschner, M.: A preliminary report on an analysis of classroom interaction, The Merrill Palmer Quarterly of Behavior and Development **9:**3, 1963.

which is comparable to that found in a real-life situation. Thus members attain particular knowledge, understandings, or skills while being confronted with lifelike situations; also they are required to apply this learnings in constructing a response. The manner in which they respond becomes a measure of the participants' grasp of the original learnings and an indicator of their abilities in real situations.

Simulation is useful to develop decision-making skills (see Chapter 1). Since it is a structured method, feedback can be built into the format, which enables the participant to benefit from the experience in one of two ways: (1) The learner may observe if the course of action embarked on resulted in a desired payoff, which improved understanding of the problem-solving process. If so, then wise action is reinforced by the simulation. (2) Conversely, if the feedback shows the procedure resulted in ineffective decision making, the learner will then resort to alternative steps that lead to desirable results. One advantage of simulation is that an individual can alternatively be participant and observer and can see the whole situation in a nonthreatening and safe environment.

Participation builds a high degree of motivation and gives purpose to activity. A major benefit of using the simulation process is that more members of a group are immediately and actively involved in problem solving or decision making. Because of increased insight, changes in behavior are more rapidly facilitated. Simulation also supplies a number of contingencies that may often be encountered in the nursing arena and may not be experienced in the clinical work setting.

A further advantage of the simulation strategy is the acquisition of particular skills and knowledge. In life, normally a time lag occurs between making a decision and receiving information about the effects of the decision; there is also the possibility of making costly mistakes. Simulation provides a laboratory where experience can be gained and mistakes made. It also accelerates training and shows the effects of decisions quickly.

If properly structured, simulation will make it necessary for the participants to envision the whole of the problem: to be certain of their observations and facts; to collect, evaluate, and analyze the available information; and to develop prescriptions for nursing action. Another advantage is that alternative actions for a given circumstance can be identified and explored. During the post-simulation stage, reflection, interpretation, and discussion are often needed for final synthesizing and evaluating. Role playing is a simulation technique often used in nursing to learn to handle difficult situations.

Goal setting, achievement, and evaluation

Goal setting, prescribing nursing actions, and evaluating progress are key nursing responsibilities requiring a network of communications. Determining effective goals for nursing leadership and management depends on an accurate assessment of what comprises effectual management for the work situation. The individual or group setting goals must know professional standards for nursing care, be aware of policies and expectations for the nurse-leader set by the client or employer, be familiar with the work environment (physical setting, design for administration of nursing services, personnel, lines of authority), and be alert to needs and wishes of the clients who are served. Since democratic groups are facilitated by leaders to set their own goals, this task is a shared one.

Furthermore, the nurse-leader helps goals to be communicated in meaningful terms, recognizing that (1) behavior implies active participation, (2) the learning procedure consists of acts that require a change in behavior, (3) people respond more quickly if they assist in establishing their own goals for learning, and (4) the committed individual is motivated to achieve optimal levels of performance.

The effective leader develops skills in awareness of problems, formulation of goals, appropriate activities, methods of evaluation, and sharing this process with involved participants to establish aims and devise activities for their accomplishment. With this leadership, efforts are more effective, quality of care is improved, job satisfaction is increased, and costs are reduced.

PREDICTIVE PRINCIPLE: Preassessment of individual and group knowledge, skills, and expectations establishes baseline data for measuring progress or change.

The primary purpose of the preassessment process is to determine what the individual or group brings to the nursing arena in terms of prerequisite knowledge for nursing activity. Planning nursing prescriptions without first making an assessment of participant characteristics is akin to prescribing medicine without first diagnosing the patient. If individuals from the least to the most skilled are to be given adequate opportunity to progress and achieve, the nurse-leader needs to assist members in determining their status and the procedural methods. As the leader gains information regarding each caregiver, strategies can be developed and plans made for reducing the discrepancy between what the participant is able to achieve at the point of preassessment and what he or she can be expected to accomplish within a prescribed period of time.

It is vital to ascertain what the participants have learned, what skill levels they have achieved, and what characteristics they possess in order to avoid problems and facilitate growth. Through the preassessment process the leader can develop baseline data for the measurement of progress or change that results from the members' experiences and instruction in nursing practice. An example would be a leader's preassessment determination that a nurse is unable to take a maternal-child health history. If at the end of the designated learning period the member is able to make a complete nursing assessment, success has been attained. Without preassessment it would be difficult, if not impossible, for the leader to ascertain how or when learning and change in behavior occurred.

Although it would seem impossible for the leader to be totally aware of the interests, concerns, and expectations of each new group member, goals are achieved with greater efficiency when the leader communicates closely with the members by preassessing, accepting, and clarifying the expectations, interests, and concerns of each member. Often a client or worker enters the nursing scene expecting a certain experience only to be disappointed, confused, and frustrated because the direction and focus are not what he expected or perceived himself as needing. The effective leader will preassess expectations of each participant and align these expectations with related activities to the extent that the care plan and environment permit.

PREDICTIVE PRINCIPLE: Mutual understanding and agreement on goals appropriate to the client or agency ensure support for goal achievement.

Agencies are established for specific and defined purposes. These purposes are dictated by social and community health needs and are written into charters and agency objectives. When an individual becomes an agency employee, he or she is committed to the agency's established purposes. An agency supports activities designed to accomplish goals in keeping with its defined purposes. Support for activities outside the defined purposes is not economically feasible and dissipates the manpower necessary to accomplish established agency purposes. Such purposes change when social, health, or community needs dictate alteration, either by evolution or through responses to emergency situations (civil, natural, or national disasters). Agency purposes seldom change simply because nursing care groups adopt goals not in keeping with established ends. Therefore it behooves nursing groups to select goals appropriate to the institution to ensure its support. The following example illustrates this principle:

Jimmie Bigalow, an 8-year-old boy, had been in Sundown Children's Convalescent Hospital for 18 months for convalescence from rheumatic fever with several complications when he became acutely ill with pneumonia, laryngeal edema, high fever, and severely compromised respiration. The hospital management wanted Jimmie transferred to an acute care hospital immediately. The nurses had become extremely attached to Jimmie and were very concerned about his care. The nursing group volunteered to "special" Jimmie and to devote their days off to his care. They requested that the hospital secure the necessary equipment through rental or purchase and give permission to the unit to keep and care for Jimmie. The request was denied for the following reasons:

1. The hospital plant and equipment were designed for convalescing children.
2. Other patients on the unit would feel the impact of a critically ill patient through the nurses' preoccupation with Jimmie and the necessity of maintaining a quiet atmosphere.
3. Time off should be spent away from the job to enable full devotion to the job during scheduled work time.

An astute nurse-leader would have determined if group purposes were consistent with the agency goals and would have attempted to lead the membership to adoption of objectives compatible with the agency. Examples of appropriate objectives for the nursing group and goals that would have secured the support of the agency would have been (1) to prepare Jimmie for smooth transfer to another hospital and (2) to adopt measures that would decrease the separation anxiety of both client and nursing staff.

To ensure successful cooperation of and support from the client in primary nursing or independent care systems, it is vital that communication lines exist in the operation. Goals, implementation, and evaluative measures must be defined by the nurse in conjunction with the client or representative and the group or agency, where appropriate. Of equal significance in establishing a procedural health measure are the nurse and the client. In all independent negotiations, care will be exercised that the legal rights of both the consumer of health care services and the rendering person or agency be protected.

PREDICTIVE PRINCIPLE: Circumstance and member capability determine the type of directions to be communicated.

The types of directions most nurse-leaders are likely to give are (1) the command, (2) the request, (3) the suggestion, and (4) the call for volunteers.

A *command* is an authoritative direction or order; it is an exercise of direct authority. Commands imply set directives and structure and require little discussion. Some directions are communicated as commands because the implementation of the directives is important to safety, subsequent activities, cooperation with other departments, or the implementation of physicians' orders.

Most times the *request* can be used to better advantage and, as far as the worker is concerned, can carry almost the same weight as a direct command. Usually the request is given in situations where the time schedule is flexible and the worker is capable of exercising judgment. An example would be "Mrs. Blanton, when you have a chance would you investigate other ways of arranging Mrs. Sampson's personal effects so she can use them more easily? Her right arm is becoming less useful to her each day. She has indicated a desire to use her left arm more." Another form of request could be "Would you be willing to spend some time with Mr. Berra? He feels lonely because his son and family have moved from this area." The request indicates that compliance is expected but that freedom of choice exists.

In the *suggestion* category, decisions are left to the worker as to whether or not something will be done. Suggestions offer alternatives or choices. "If Mrs. Hill is having difficulty swallowing liquids, you might try semisolids," and "You could call the welfare department and find out what they think" are examples of suggestions. Suggestions are offered only when requested; those offered when not requested are usually not used. Suggestions can do much to stimulate initiative and cooperation in the members, because they provide opportunities for the use of independent judgment.

The *call for volunteers* is a form used occasionally in soliciting people for assignments that are difficult, unpleasant, or beyond usual duties. Assisting in another area, serving on a special committee, or assuming responsibility for reorganizing the utility room are examples of situations in which all members have a choice. Again, the leader must exercise caution not to assume the awkward position of having to refuse a volunteer for a job for which the leader feels the worker is not qualified or of having no one volunteer for a job that must be done. If the possible candidates are limited, the call should go out only to those who are qualified to accept. For example, "I would like John, June, or Mary to take care of this; will one of you volunteer?"

There is dual responsibility (leader and member) for preventing continuous delegation of extra tasks to the same few individuals. In every group, certain workers are more cooperative than others and, unless protected, may be exploited.

Conversely, there is a reciprocal relationship in which clients may at times be the communicators of directions. They may determine in collaboration with caregivers the manner in which they desire the care or health plan to be implemented. The client may outline specific times, places, procedures, resources, and persons to fulfill the care plan.

Several rules of thumb hold firm in giving directions or suggestions:

1. *Do not give a choice if there is no choice.* "Would you like to help Mrs. Jones?" implies that a "no" response is acceptable. If "Please help Mrs. Jones" is meant, say so. A better alternative for giving choice yet eliciting a positive response is the question, for example, "Would you be willing to help Mrs. Jones?" Many people who do not "especially" want to would be willing to.

2. *When offering suggestions, make certain they are viewed as suggestions and not dictums.* After offering a suggestion, recommend that the person get ideas from others so that there will be a wider choice of options.

3. *When issuing a command or order, make it clear it is an expectation.* "Mrs. Jones' tray is here now" is a simple statement of fact and does not even imply what you want done with that tray. If the expectation is that Mrs. Jones is to have her tray while it is hot, say so: "Mrs. Jones' tray just arrived from the kitchen; please take it to her while it is still hot."

4. *Provide choices when choices are possible.* Even a limited amount of freedom of choice is better than no choice at all: "I'm sorry, Mrs. Lucie, you cannot save your break until this afternoon and take off early because there is a meeting that Mrs. Copty and Mrs. Gill must attend

at that time and you and I will be alone for thirty minutes. However, you can alter your schedule either Thursday or Friday—both those days are clear."

PREDICTIVE PRINCIPLE: Opportunity to express expectations of the individual or group, when translated into meaningful terms to members, determines individual identification and invites commitment of members to goal achievement.

Goal setting and evaluation are the lifeblood of nursing effort. Goal setting gives nursing activities meaning; evaluation allows the group to measure fulfillment; success whets the appetite for more achievement and motivates the individual or group to further meaningful activity.

Whether an individual or group goal or process is sufficiently important to exert an effect on a participant's behavior depends on the relationship of the goal to the person. The possibilities of what might be expected are many. Confronted with a goal or process, participants will be uncertain about what to expect but will seek that which has meaning for them. Perceptions and expectations are a selective process and are based on past experiences and present awareness. The participant will attend to those matters and anticipate goals and processes that have a relationship to self or to an extension of the self. Information will affect behavior only to the degree to which the individual has discovered its personal meaning.

It is important, therefore, that the nurse-leader provide opportunity for the client, individual, or group member to express and clarify initial expectations. An individual who has opportunity to participate in setting goals is more willing to accept the goals. The more responsive the leader is to the participant's expectations, the less will be the participant's resistance to the group's intended goals or processes. The effective group leader will structure the situation so that the client or member will express and clarify individual expectations.

To achieve group commitment and resultant behavior a goal must have value and meaning. The goal must be something the members can define, put into their own experience, and accept into their own value system. The following is an example:

Miss Swanson, a young graduate, was attempting to interest a group composed primarily of new nursing assistants in foot care for a middle-aged diabetic man. She discussed, at great length, improving circulation, proper shoes, the care of toenails and corns, and bathing and powdering the feet. The group was completely passive until an experienced aide said: "Miss Swanson, are you trying to tell us that if we don't do something, Mr. Taylor's sore toe could turn black and he could lose his foot?"

The aide's translation of the objective into something that had meaning for the group and was familiar to them aroused interest and achieved commitment to the goal.

PREDICTIVE PRINCIPLE: Realistic and valid goals promote achievement.

Setting goals the group can achieve motivates the individual or group to success. Goal setting and record keeping produce gratifying results. With these tools, delegation becomes less difficult and the role of the nurse expands to an amazing degree. The old saying "Goals just beyond reach keep one striving" is false. Goals beyond reach are self-defeating and lead to discouragement and apathy. Realistic means achievable; valid as used here means relevant to the problem. Use of the following three simple, precautionary steps enables the nurse-leader to guide the group in the selection of realistic, valid, attainable goals:

1. *Identify problems.* Descriptions are essential to problem identification. Full, detailed descriptions of the situation and feelings about the situation help the group to identify the problem accurately.
2. *Set goals.* Accurately identified problems make it possible for the group to foresee termination, or at least an alteration, of the problem that would make the situation more tolerable. This imagined absence or alteration of the problem becomes the goal.

   EXAMPLE: The goal for a patient who has trouble with contractures is free movement with full range of motion.

Problem	*Goal*
Contractures	Free movement with full range of motion

3. *Determine ability to accomplish goals.* Determining the group's ability to accomplish the goal establishes whether the goal is realistic. Qualities necessary to accomplish a stated goal would include such things as the following:
   a. *Resources*—either have or can acquire the collective or individual talent, knowledge, and skill appropriate and effective to accomplish the goal. When each desired behavior is defined behaviorally in terms of outcome, the learner knows what is specifically expected and can then determine capability or resources for the tasks.
   b. *Time and energy*—consideration must be given to other tasks facing the group concomitantly.
   c. *Commitment and will of the group.*

PREDICTIVE PRINCIPLE: The extent of involvement of each group member determines the group's proficiency.

Membership in a group necessitates some degree of personal involvement. Behavior as a group member is guided mainly by the individual's perception of his or her needs and interests. A member who receives satisfaction from the work experience will be motivated to join inextricably with the group.

Consideration of variables that influence member involvement is essential to understanding the working of groups.

All individuals are members of several groups, any one of which may exert much more influence on the member's life than does the work situation. Family, social clubs, religious and political affiliations, and community projects are examples of group associations that involve the individual.

Membership in a group does not necessarily engage the entire person, but group proficiency requires that each member be involved fully toward the achievement of group purposes while present with the group. A few dedicated persons virtually live and breathe nursing and evidence little interest in outside activities. These members have much to contribute, but unless they are carefully controlled they can dominate the group and destroy its effectiveness. The overly zealous member becomes wearisome to others and eventually creates a backlash of negative reaction that takes its toll in group productivity.

The leader can utilize the devoted member's zeal constructively by channeling some of the worker's energy into activities that can be performed on an individual basis. Keeping the unit library up to date is one way of providing helpful diversion. The interested member could search nursing literature and bring pertinent materials to the station for members of all teams. Another avenue for the individual deeply engrossed in the profession is to serve on nursing procedure committees, policy boards, and so on. Care must be taken to ensure broad representation, but usually all who wish to do so have the opportunity to participate in these kinds of activities.

A problem of equal significance is the member who works eight hours a day, five days a week for a paycheck and evidences little or no interest in the endeavors of the nursing group to which he or she is assigned. This person must be assisted to progress from the dormant or even inhibitory stage to one of productivity or his position as a group member will become untenable.

Possible reasons for the lack of involvement may be that conditions in the work setting are not contributing to member satisfaction. Perhaps the staff member suffers from burnout or does not feel accepted as a necessary part of the group process or rarely has the opportunity to complete assigned tasks without interruption. Perhaps the member does not feel secure in the ability to perform assigned tasks. Tests in management reveal a close relationship between ability and interest. On the other hand, the member may not experience sufficient outlet for individual abilities. It is up to group participants to discover conditions that will promote and maintain interest in their work situation to foster member involvement and pave the way for group proficiency.

Another factor that influences the extent of an individual's involvement is the degree to which the beliefs, values, and attitudes of the group conflict or agree with those of other groups to which that individual belongs. Conformity pressures may be exerted from both sides, thus forcing the individual to make a choice between the two, as shown in the example below:

A community health nurse was assigned to head a team in a district predominantly populated by Mexican-Americans. The first three-month report revealed very little progress with the families to which she was assigned. On consultation with the nurse the supervisor learned that the leader had been indoctrinated since childhood by family and social groups to believe that "Mexicans are stupid and lazy, do not wish to work, and have as many children as possible in order to collect welfare."

The manager felt assured that the nurse could become a competent and contributing member of the staff. Accordingly, a learning contract was devised and the nurse was assigned to work with a Mexican-American nurse in the district with the provision that a study of Mexican-American culture be undertaken through a planned program. The supervisor reasoned that families could not receive help from a biased nurse; therefore a change was necessary. The assignment to attend classes and seminars and to read was based on the assumption that, with increased understanding of Mexican-American culture, increased exposure to Mexican-American people, and close work with a Mexican-American colleague, the nurse would have an opportunity to examine her preconceptions and would become able to work on the assignment.

One primary aim of the leader is to bring a functioning relationship to all members of the group having different norms or values. Possible means include providing the group members with a role model through exemplary leadership, group discussions, individual conferences, and workshops to provide them with continuous exposure to a democratic point of view.

Actions in the interest of the client are to be fostered. If the decision is reached that a member cannot resolve conflict and become involved in the achievement of the group's purposes, the leader may recommend that member's removal from the work group.

PREDICTIVE PRINCIPLE: Group involvement in goal setting requires the endorsement of the agency and commitment of membership to participate in the outcome.

Group decisions in formulating goals can have a place in employee relations but must be limited to issues that are reasonable and obtainable through the conscientious efforts of all personnel.

Like most business and industrial organizations, health agencies follow established patterns of operation. A governing board gives direction and overall guidance, the administrators furnish the physical environment and services that support the medical and nursing staff, and formulated and stated policies provide guidelines for all administrative action. Ideally, leaders of nursing groups have a part in the formulation of overall policy, but in any case the leader is governed by the stipulations of the employing agency.

In nursing teams formation of group goals usually means selecting subgoals that are consistent with objectives outlined for all nursing services. Overall goals for the agency are usually stated in general terms, such as "to provide nursing care commensurate with the standards established by the American Nurses' Association" or "to treat all patients equally." Although these goals may be desirable and members of the group may wish to become involved in their implementation, it is important to recognize that they are too vague for specific operation. Examples of goals that imply member involvement are (1) complete a course in cardiac resuscitation, (2) develop a plan to facilitate interaction among members, and (3) increase caregiver skill in the operation of cardiac monitors. Each of these aims can be worked through operationally and can be successfully accomplished according to the extent of member involvement.

With that kind of objective, participants can work cooperatively to design a plan that will lead to realization. The latter objective could be operationally defined by the group in the following way:

Goal: To increase caregiver skill in the operation of cardiac monitors.
Operation:
1. Provide each member with a copy of a manual containing necessary background information.
2. Allow two weeks for individual study.
3. Set up a series of five one-hour seminars with in-service director and staff in charge of the cardiac unit.
4. Arrange for practice sessions with equipment. Arrange schedule so that each member has adequate time to attend seminars and practice sessions. (Equal time does not necessarily have to be given to each member.)
5. Have each member take test on theory and practice.
6. Plan additional seminars and practice sessions according to individual need.
7. Allow time for review periods at least once per month.

As the members become involved in planning steps to reach their goal, they will designate the persons to assume responsibility for implementation. Total involvement takes place throughout the process, thus committing members to the outcome.

A managerial error is made when a group is allowed to participate in decisions for which there can be no subsequent fulfillment. The following is an example:

Mrs. Beaux, leader of a nursing team, attended a seminar on group dynamics and was particularly impressed with a series of lectures about employees who were setting their own goals for job fulfillment. The speaker emphasized that co-workers, if given the opportunity, could meet together to consider intelligently and then formulate goals appropriate to the situation.

At her nursing station Mrs. Beaux decided to practice some of these principles. She called together the five members of her team and told them that, in her opinion, the team members would be more satisfied if they decided just how much work they could accomplish in one day. She then gave the team members the opportunity to discuss and decide among themselves as a group what their work loads should be. Mrs. Beaux left the room, believing the group would doubtlessly assess their jobs and establish much higher goals for themselves than she herself would have dared propose.

After the discussion period was over, the group informed Mrs. Beaux that they believed they were overworked. Since they had been given the authority to establish their own work loads, they would reduce the patient census on their team by two and would relinquish their responsibility for distributing fresh linens to all teams.

The weakness in the original proposal belatedly became clear to Mrs. Beaux. She had allowed individuals to participate in a decision that could not be realized, for she did not have the power to implement the proposal. She had failed to equate her naive assumption with reality and was left with a difficult situation.

The fiasco could have been avoided had the leader consulted with the head nurse first to see if the plan was feasible and workable. Mrs. Beaux must now use the situation as a bad start toward something better. She can tell the group where the idea originated, what she thought would happen, and the situation in which she finds herself now. She can discuss with the group the matter of feelings of overload in work assignment and attempt to work out a solution with them and the head nurse that will be mutually satisfactory. By this method the leader's ideas, the group's wishes, and the guidelines and policies of the institution can be blended into a constructive approach.

Effective conferences

Conferences are necessary to the practice of nursing to give and receive information. Grouping persons involved in accomplishing common goals for the purpose of interchange of ideas and solving problems provides a useful tool for building and maintaining mutual understanding.

Nursing conferences are not limited to providers of health services. It is now generally recognized that to attain and maintain optimal mental and physical health, all significant persons must be included in each phase of client care, if possible. Thus, in addition to members of the health team, the client, family, and others who have an interest in the purpose of the conference are included.

A nursing conference is usually called for the purpose of finding out or deciding something. This means there is a reciprocal relationship for the exchange of information. Nurses convene conferences for a variety of purposes, including (1) direction-giving conferences, in which the leader gives information and directions specific to the assignment; (2) client-centered conferences, in which members identify problems and attempt to arrive at solutions and decide on courses of action; (3) content conferences, in which participants assemble to acquire knowledge about a specific subject; (4) reporting conferences, in which participants give progress reports; (5) general problems conferences, in which individuals express their impressions about the work situation and try to resolve work or personnel problems; and (6) nursing care conferences, in which participants collaborate for problem-oriented nursing care.

Effective communication necessitates a systematic plan for providing and maintaining contact between the leader and group and for person-to-person exchanges. Gathering groups together at specific times for clearly defined purposes will help to realize this goal.

The time for nursing conferences is usually relatively short; therefore the participants must work for brevity and exactness. Conference style is most often informal and more conversational than formal meetings; the group that is cognizant of the need to be purposeful and well organized therefore accomplishes more.

The conference situation is not a "natural" one for nurse-leaders, and many are tempted to find reasons for not meeting with the entire group at one time. The leader who feels ill at ease in conducting group sessions may look for reasons to cancel meetings. The excuse may be offered: "There never seems to be a right time to get the group together—when I'm ready, they're not. I would like to have them meet all at one time, but there are just so many hours in a day!" The alternative action is to "catch them on the run" or, worse yet, to trust that the members will discover for themselves what is expected of them.

Time is an important factor, as most caregivers spend the greater share of their work period attempting to meet the numerous demands placed on them. It is true, however, that most people find time for activities they deem important and in which they feel comfortable. If one accepts the principle that effort to arrive at group consensus for nursing action cultivates positive outcomes, time must be given to meetings where the process can take place.

The nurse-manager can become adept in the role of conference leader if effort is channeled into acquiring and applying principles of conference technique that will contribute to the realization of effective amalgamation of ideas and feelings.

All conferences have certain commonalities. Accomplishment of purpose is enhanced when members have the opportunity to meet without interruption and come prepared to participate and when behaviors enhance goal accomplishment. Another contributing factor to successful conference sessions is understanding of behaviors each individual uses to impart ideas or feelings to others and recognition of the effect specific actions have on the group.

PREDICTIVE PRINCIPLE: Adequate preparation by the leader for all conferences expedites fulfillment of expectations for the conference.

Realities of life are such that adequate preparation for all situations and at all times is impossible. Nursing is particularly susceptible to disruptions. New patients are admitted just prior to conference time; substitute staff members are assigned; new procedures are introduced; emergencies occur; and friction occasionally arises among personnel. In addition to these disruptive elements, the nurse-leader will not necessarily have acquired competency in all phases of nursing. Deviations from the ideal, however, need not deter the leader from proceeding with preparation as current conditions allow.

Preparation for a conference will depend on the purpose of the meeting. Instructional conferences call for imparting information to members to facilitate completion of assignments. Content and client-centered conferences require acquisition of knowledge specific to a particular client or subject. Reporting conferences demand that the reporter know what needs reporting; the content and shared feelings conferences depend on group needs coupled with judicious use of interpersonal relationship skills.

PREDICTIVE PRINCIPLE: Relieving caregivers of responsibility while the conference is in session allows members to proceed without interruption.

In most clinical settings, more than one nurse or group are assigned to care for the total client population. Leaders will want to coordinate their schedules to allow time for necessary meetings and to arrange for the care of clients assigned to them while each group is in session.

Clients cannot be left unattended by nursing staff. This is especially true in acute nursing care units where lack of supervision can have serious consequences. For example, intravenous fluids can accelerate or reduce in rate within seconds; clients may require assistance with bodily functions; and there is the ever-present possibility of crises such as hemorrhage, shock, myocardial infarction, or cardiac arrest.

In structured settings a conference time schedule that considers the needs and desires of all personnel equally will prove to be the most successful. Most leaders consider the ideal time for a direction-giving conference to be as soon after the workday has started as possible. The leader will then have the opportunity to give directions to members before the group becomes involved in a multiplicity of tasks. The preferred time for the reporting conference is usually about forty-five minutes before the end of the shift. This arrangement gives members the opportunity to sum up the day's progress before completing last-minute details. Scheduling of content and client-centered conferences does not usually become an issue other than to find time when members can get together.

Nursing functions cover myriad activities. Each member has a job to do that usually must be done within a certain time limit. Some tasks demand strict compliance to a schedule, for example, giving preoperative medications or collecting specimens. Other assignments, such as the administration of hygienic care, allow for a degree of flexibility. Agency and client routines must be taken into consideration. Serving of meals and provision for treatments given by those other than the nursing personnel further complicate planning care. Community health agencies work around appointments, clinic-school visits, and other problems. Regardless of setting, all conferences require careful programming.

PREDICTIVE PRINCIPLE: Prior announcement of time, place, purpose, and duration of conferences to all concerned promotes assembly of a group well prepared and ready to focus attention on the purposes of the conference.

The importance of holding conferences for the purpose of giving direction, coordinating activities, and evaluating progress is patent. It is equally evident that each member must know in advance when, where, how long, and for what purpose the conferences will be held.

A written schedule of meeting times is helpful. A printed format may be devised to fit any situation. Information concerning specific conferences can then be filled in easily and posted for all staff members to note. The following is a model of scheduling for an area that has three groups.

Conference	Group I	Group II	Group III
Direction-giving	7:30-7:50 (daily)	8:00-8:20 (daily)	7:30-7:50 (daily)
Patient-centered	1:00-1:30 (Monday)	11:00-11:30 (Tuesday)	1:00-1:30 (Wednesday)
Content	1:00-1:30 (Tuesday)	11:00-11:30 (Wednesday)	1:00-1:30 (Thursday)
Report	2:15-2:35 (daily)	1:40-2:10 (daily)	2:15-2:35 (daily)

When there are three groups, two can meet at one time with careful planning. The head nurse and unit secretary assist the third group in alerting the attending staff to the clients' needs. Leaders in conferences will have informed the covering nurse-leader of any specific needs that require attention during the time of the conference. When there are only two groups, scheduling is simplified. It becomes a matter of one covering for the other while they are in conference and alternating times of meetings from week to week. When only one group is involved, times for meeting together should still be scheduled although flexibility in timing is more easily managed. In this event, coverage will be arranged on an individual basis.

All members realize there will be occasions when it is impossible to hold to the conference schedule. At such times the situation is usually stressful, often causing members to forget the times of meetings. If at all possible, however, the leader involved in the disruption should alert another leader to arrange for a trade in times for meetings. If the cause for the delay does not permit this step, the coordinator of nursing services must be alerted to proceed with alteration or trade in the conference schedule with the detained leader. Keeping one group waiting for a conference that will not be held is a waste of time; where more than one group is involved, the time lost is proportionately increased.

In addition to timing, clear purpose and agenda contribute much to successful conferences. People who understand the purpose and agenda can prepare for the meeting and contribute on a higher level.

When a number of people work together in close harmony, it is understandable that they will be interested in one another's lives and will take advantage of opportunities to exchange information and confidences. A few moments can be allotted for this purpose before initiating the conference or while waiting for all members to arrive. Once the meeting has begun, however, participants will need to exercise discipline to keep their attention focused on the purpose for meeting. The leader can assist the group to hold to its mark by recognizing when diversion from the appointed task has occurred and bringing the discussion back into focus by using simple phrases such as "Can we return to . . . ," "You were saying that . . . ," or "Will you explore . . . a little further, please?"

Direction-giving conference

Direction-giving conferences are meetings called at the beginning of a work shift for the specific purpose of communicating job assignments, delineating areas of responsibility, and imparting information necessary for members to care for clients effectively.

PREDICTIVE PRINCIPLE: Obtaining the most recent data available prior to conference ensures the leader that imparted information is pertinent, inclusive, and accurate.

In settings where there is round-the-clock coverage the nurse-leader will receive a progress report from the person previously responsible for the groups of clients either by word of mouth or via tape recorder while the off-going nurse is completing the assignment. Additional information will be needed before giving instructions to caregivers. Leaders or managers will want to check pertinent data, such as preoperative orders, arrangements for tests, and so on, and to visit each client *before* the time of the conference. This will give the leader opportunity to make a personal assessment of the client's status.

In active units frequent attempts will be made to interrupt the time the managing nurse has reserved for personal visits to patients. Most interruptions can be handled by delegating tasks to others. Intercommunication systems prove invaluable to the leader making rounds, allowing the nurse to keep in touch with staff and yet proceed with the intended purpose of allowing client participation in the development of care plans and providing for client-nurse dialogue. Informal meetings will be conducted by primary care nurses, but the need for careful preparation is not lessened. In many instances the client and family will engage in preplanning activities by reading, experimenting with procedure, and investigating resources.

PREDICTIVE PRINCIPLE: Information that is paced, systematic, and inclusive allows participants time to assimilate the content and provides them with information necessary to function.

The success or failure of imparting pertinent information to an individual or a group depends on sufficient information and method of presentation. The leader must be sensitive to what information is needed and at what pace the members (clients or caregivers) are able to receive it. In a direction-giving conference, for example, members should not be avalanched with irrelevant information. They want to hear what will be most useful in the immediate situation.

Much of the information determining routine and time of performance is a part of core information. Routine care, time for meals, procedure for obtaining or imparting information, and the like are best omitted unless there is need for review. New members will require instruction in addition to routine information, but all members should not be subjected to the instructional part of the newcomer's orientation period.

Routine information that must be transmitted about patients, such as diet, activity, tests, and treatments, can be transcribed on caregivers' worksheets by the unit clerk prior to the work period. In group conferences use of serial order on individual worksheets allows the members to know the routine, thus enabling them to increase speed and effectiveness in writing the things they have just heard.

There is a direct relationship between the amount of information required and task difficulty. The amount of detail necessary in the "how" part of an order depends on how complicated the task is and how experienced the employee is in doing the job. For instance, there is no need to discuss nursing procedures familiar to the listener. But when the situation calls for new knowledge or skills or deeper understanding, the leader must allow time for a clear, understandable explanation.

In giving an order a leader may neglect to explain the reason for the directive. An explanation makes it possible for the worker to use sound judgment if there is a problem, and it often helps to eliminate misunderstanding. If, for example, the leader directs an aide to "ambulate Mrs. Sheppard for five minutes every hour," the aide may become so engrossed in the fulfillment of a heavy assignment that judgments must be made about priority and the aide may decide to omit Mrs. Sheppard's ambulation. A simple statement at the time of the directive will ensure proper consideration when priorities are established. For example, the leader could explain: "Mrs. Sheppard had a vein ligation of both legs yesterday. It is very important that she walk for five minutes every hour to avoid the formation of blood clots in her legs. If one were to form and become dislodged it could travel through the bloodstream directly to her lungs and cause her death."

Modern communication technology permits nurses to exchange information necessary to implement care plans in ways that provide for individual timing. Reports, directions, and communications about goal progress may be communicated via tape cassette. The oncoming staff may listen to short reports while off-going caregivers continue to work with patients. Any clarification may be done by individuals at their own convenience.

Client-centered conferences

Client-centered conferences are meetings in which problem-oriented care is discussed and evaluated. Client-centered conferences are designed to help overcome the decentralization of care. The focus of attention is usually on the analysis of one client or family situation for whom the nurse or group is caring. Client-centered conferences provide a means whereby all participants will benefit from the experiences of a few. Where possible, the client and other significant people are included in the sessions and the client is the focal point of discussion. The process is a dynamic, interactive, problem-oriented, sequenced approach (assessment, problem identification, formulating plans for nursing action, providing for evaluation and implementation).*

In utilizing the nursing process the leader opens the way for consideration of the needs of the whole patient—physiologic, psychologic, spiritual, social, and cultural—to acquire a rationale for nursing action and to devise ways to improve nursing care. The leader has an opportunity to guide members in recognizing individual patient or family needs and in formulating nursing principles that result in nursing prescriptions for action.

Separate meetings about clients or families, which are not in conjunction with another type of conference, allow time for discussion free from interruption. Participants will be more successful in keeping their commitment to purposes if meetings are planned at a time when the major share of the work load has been accomplished and if conferences are well spaced. Frequency of client-centered conferences depends on the situation. Intensive care units, for example, may not meet more than once a week, whereas an area with a slower pace might have the opportunity to meet more frequently. Thirty-minute to one-hour periods are usually sufficient for the average conference. Problem solving requires at least that much time, and little can be accomplished if the group must work under pressure.

*Bower, F.L.: The process of planning nursing care: a model for practice, ed. 2, St. Louis, 1977, The C.V. Mosby Co.

Use of principles of teaching, learning, and leadership will help the group to become increasingly more skilled in recognizing and solving specific problems as well as making appropriate generalizations in nursing care in similar, although different, nursing situations.

PREDICTIVE PRINCIPLE: Interaction of conference members on an equal basis encourages active participation and leads to usable solutions to the problem.

Conference participants have diverse cultural, educational, and experiential backgrounds. Acceptance of the philosophy that the group together has more knowledge about a subject than does any single member can serve to improve the productivity of the group.

In nursing care conference situations the members make decisions by consensus or majority so that the commitment to such decisions is corporate and not vested in any one individual.

The leader must provide a nonthreatening environment for members to feel free to share what they have done with others, engage in identification of problems, and give and receive suggestions for further action. By imposing personal opinions on the group prematurely, the leader, in effect, negates the potential benefits that can be derived from the participation of all members.

In a nursing care conference situation the leader opens the discussion, then invites members to make contributions to the discussion freely. The leader's role is primarily one of facilitating the group work in constructing plans that will benefit a patient or family. Some conferences will require little active participation from the leader, and others will demand a larger contribution. Regardless of who offers content in the conference, each contribution should be given careful consideration. The client or family and other significant persons may be an integral part of the process.

PREDICTIVE PRINCIPLE: Identification of the nursing problem to be considered expedites the formulation of nursing intervention.

The initial steps in a nursing care conference are (1) to assess the group interest and need, (2) to identify and delineate the problem, (3) to assess the group's knowledge about the problem or prior experiences that relate to the problem, (4) to select and utilize the appropriate content, and (5) to determine ways to evaluate the results of implemented plans.

The following is a sample discussion of a nursing care incident about which a client-centered conference was conducted. It is not intended to be all inclusive but is used to illustrate how a nurse-leader can conscientiously apply principles of teaching and learning (see Chapter 4) to bring about the desired goal of improving patient care through the use of client-centered conferences. The participants in the sample conference are members of the nursing team in a newborn nursery setting. Participation is commensurate with each person's role and capability. General introductory activities and other material and comments not specifically illustrative have been deleted. What remains is the process and structure.

> **LVN:** I am caring for Baby Lee in 317A. He was born at 2 AM, was full term, and weighed 7 pounds. Everything was going along well until this morning when he began to breathe in a strange way. He became very restless, began to breathe with jerky respirations, and his ribs pulled in with every breath. Right after that he started to grunt, cough, and then turned blue. I was scared to death; I did what I could and called the team leader. The baby is breathing better now.
>
> **Leader:** What do you believe are the problems in this situation?
>
> **LVN:** Well, I'd surely like to know what went wrong with him and I'd like to know if I did the right thing.
>
> **Leader:** Anything else?
>
> **Aide:** What I want to know is what do we do if a baby goes bad like that when we are taking care of it!
>
> **All:** (Indications of consensus.)
>
> **Leader:** (To LVN) What have you decided is the problem for the group to consider now?
>
> **LVN:** I think all of us should know what to do in case that happens again.

At this point the group has moved through the preliminary assessment period. The teaching and learning principle that *the learner's prevalent life needs determine what he or she will learn* was implemented by the leader (see chapter 4). The group was taken through a process that identified their need and readiness to learn.

The leader then implemented the principles that *participation of the learner in setting learning goals increases the number of learning activities meaningful and useful to the learner,* and *realistic behavioral goal setting enables selection of appropriate and meaningful content.* This was illustrated by the participation of the aide and LVN in stating and delineating the problem and in the group consensus about the topic for the conference. The established goal is realistic and behavioral and indicates to the leader the body of knowledge necessary to meet the goal. The teaching and learning principles about anxiety and motivation are implemented in this situation because the respiratory distress of Baby Lee has created the anxiety that members may not be able to meet a similar emergency situation.

PREDICTIVE PRINCIPLE: Analyzing nursing care given in the light of established goals enables members to validate their behavior and to devise ways to improve nursing care.

A member confronted with a problem while administering nursing care will react in some way. For an individual to describe his or her behavior in the nursing situation but be unable to give reasons for the care given is evidence of a lack of understanding. Nursing care situations are ideal for assisting members to increase knowledge and understanding without jeopardizing their sense of personal worth.

There is no better way to implement the teaching and learning principle that *an obvious relationship between learning activities and stated goals increases the motivational value of the activity* than to discuss what was done by the person involved in the situation at the time of the incident.

In the case of Baby Lee the group was well aware of the overall goal areas for the care of all infants—observation, prevention, comfort, and nurturing. When the LVN observed signs and symptoms that deviated from normal, she acted in an attempt to restore the infant to the desired state of being. The immediate crisis for her was over, but unanswered questions remained, causing her to experience anxiety. Through verbal interaction the LVN shared with coworkers her behavior at the time of crisis.

> **Aide:** (To LVN) What did you do when Baby Lee started having trouble?
> **LVN:** First, I made sure there was nothing obstructing the air from getting into his lungs.
> **Aide:** How did you do that?
> **LVN:** I pressed my thumb down on his chin and opened his mouth to look for any signs of obstruction. He had quite a bit of mucus but nothing more. Then I turned him on his side with his head brought forward to relax his throat as much as possible to allow the mucus to run out. By this time the team leader answered my call.
> **Leader:** You did the right thing: An open airway is the first thing to look for.

The LVN's actions were a result of her previous knowledge and experience. She acted maturely, demonstrated an ability to function well under stress, and carried out nursing activities based on previously learned materials about the emergency care of the infant with respiratory distress. The leader's comment on appropriate action implemented the teaching and learning principle that *rewards consistent with the value system of the learner, such as recognition, praise, peer status, or valued gains are motivating and reinforcing influences and thus facilitate learning rate, amount of retention, and degree of behavior change.* The recognition and praise validated and reinforced the appropriate action of the LVN and served as a vehicle for the members to devise ways to meet similar nursing emergencies and thus improve nursing care.

Validation helped the LVN to feel successful about handling the crisis, increased her confidence, lowered her anxiety, and readied the group to acquire additional information and move into the next stage of the learning process.

The LVN has completed the account of her experience. The leader's role now is that of teacher, because the LVN is unable to render the nursing care required in this situation.

Leader: When I arrived, I percussed the baby's posterior chest (illustrates the procedure with hands) before I suctioned him to loosen the secretions. He had quite a lot of thick material in him. This procedure will have to be done every 20 minutes or so.

Aide: Can we do that procedure?

Leader: No, the LVN and I will. Your part is to note if he appears to be in trouble again with his breathing; then call us right away. He is now in an Isolette with oxygen and an IV.

LVN: Baby Lee is suspected of having hyaline membrane disease, which is a condition affecting the lungs. I know that it occurs mostly with premature babies. Baby Lee is full term. I would like to know more about the disease. Can we take it as our subject for the content conference?

Leader: All agreed? Fine. I will get some reading material together and make it available to you. Find out as much as you can before Thursday. In the meantime, I will tell you that Baby Lee's critical period is the next 48 hours. It is very important that he (1) be kept in the warmed Isolette with 40% oxygen, (2) be percussed and suctioned every 20 minutes, (3) have his umbilical catheter kept intact, (4) be watched carefully to see that his IV goes at 10 drops per minute, (5) have his respirations recorded and graphed every 15 minutes (more often if necessary), and (6) be observed for signs of change in color or severe distress.

The LVN and I will assume responsibility for the treatments. We want everyone to help us with observation. Each time you go by the Isolette, will you have a look at him with these things in mind? Should you have occasion to note these same symptoms that the LVN has described in an infant you are caring for, do just as she did. Make sure there is no obstruction, then turn the child on his side, bring his head forward, and call for help.

The leader has given new information and set limits describing the patient's immediate needs and who is responsible for meeting those needs. This implements the teaching and learning principle that *structure, limits, and feedback provide an environment that promotes security and trust.*

The LVN now takes the lead by giving information she has acquired about the baby but that is less important than the immediate problem of compromised respirations.

The group has requested an opportunity to learn more about hyaline membrane disease. The leader has applied the principle that *the more congruent and relevant that goals are to the life needs of the learner-client, the more likely the goals are to be achieved* and has been consistent in the philosophy of the value of learner participation in goal setting. The leader (1) made sure the group had enough information to function safely immediately, (2) set group expectations of nursing responsibilities for the next 48 hours to allay anxiety about the course of events before the more long-range goals could be met, and (3) established goals commensurate with group need for the next meeting.

Since the objective for the patient-centered conference was a behavioral goal, the evaluation of the conference is built into the objective itself. If group members demonstrate in their subsequent care of Baby Lee that they can function effectively within the limits and expectations discussed in the conference, learning will have occurred.

PREDICTIVE PRINCIPLE: Formation of written nursing orders or care plans from client-centered conferences provides a central, continuous source of information.

Nursing orders or care plans are written expressions of the nursing process. They are essential for consistent care. Where advisable, a copy of the care plans may be left with the client, since, ideally at least, the client participated in their development. Nursing care plans are best formulated from client-centered, problem-oriented conferences. Although conceivably the nurse could write a nursing care plan without consulting other persons, it is not recommended. Synthesis of ideas of several people ensures a more comprehensive and accurate care plan. Furthermore, the care plan is more apt to be followed by client and caregivers if they participate in its formation.

The client-centered conference concerning Baby Lee is used as an example of transposing verbal communication into written form where vital content becomes accessible to all personnel involved with his care. Only those headings that have bearing on the case will be explored.

PHYSICIAN'S ORDERS

Warmed Isolette with 40% oxygen
Percuss and suction every 20 minutes or as needed
Heparin-saline solution through umbilical catheter as needed
Sodium bicarbonate, 3.75 gm or 44.6 mEq in 50 ml IV, 10 gtts/minute
Bennett respirator
Record and graph respiratory rate every 15 minutes, every half hour or as needed

NURSE'S ORDERS
Protective measures

Maintain controlled temperature of Isolette
Keep open airway (observe for excessive mucus)
Maintain prescribed flow of IV fluid
Keep arterial catheter in place (may need to inject heparin quickly)
Carefully observe color and breathing
Keep on either side

Physical care

Position on either side with head in forward position
Percuss and suction as needed every 20 minutes or as needed
Observe closely for cyanosis (blueness), dyspnea (difficult breathing)

Family

Mother is highly anxious about child (is hospitalized postpartum in room 342)

Mother may sit by Isolette as desired (physician's permission granted)

Father anxious. Work phone, 282-5486; home, 369-1182. Answer his questions and offer detailed descriptions of baby's progress. Avoid "doing as well as can be expected."

Grandmother, Mrs. Baxter, keeping three small children in their home

It is quite likely that an infant in critical condition might require some religious ritual; in this event the notations would be made under the appropriate heading. Later, as the infant progressed, referrals might be made and other family needs, such as parental teaching, identified that would be worked out through the care plan.

Nursing orders, developed on a systematic basis, derived from careful analysis of patient needs, and structured in collaboration with all concerned individuals and groups, enable clients and agencies to make better use of nursing personnel. The economics involved in planning and implementing client care are just as important to the agency and client as is the planning of personnel time and duties. Every coordinator of nursing services expends a considerable amount of time planning time schedules for employees, patients, and families. The efficient use of the full abilities and potential of each employee with client and family will result in maximum services for monies paid.

Content conferences

Constant input of knowledge enables client and caregivers to perform the tasks expected of them more effectively. One way of ensuring participants the opportunity to increase their learning is to provide them with time to meet for the sole purpose of exploring content. Traditionally, content conferences have been reserved for the novice, based on the premise that novices need time set aside to concentrate on specific content. However, when an aide, LVN, or RN has completed the appropriate basic course, education has just begun. Planned classes or content conferences furnish a vital and necessary link in the continuing growth and education of nursing personnel.

The practice of nursing can be improved in an environment that encourages individuals and groups to investigate ways to prevent problems. The opportunity to improve care entices the member with an inquiring mind and a creative spirit to grow and to innovate better nursing practices. Nursing practiced in a setting where learning is treated as exciting as well as useful reaps the benefits of such an attitude through a continued upgrading of the quality of care given. Individuals who become interested in developing better nursing practices will not only improve in ability but also will, by example, generate interest in others to follow suit.

Content conferences, like client-centered sessions, are usually held about once a week for a period of thirty minutes to one hour at any convenient time. The scheduling and length of time varies. However, adherence to the scheduled time indicates the importance of and commitment to the need for the conference. When pressures in the work situation occur or some member is not as well prepared as he would like to be, it may seem expedient to drop the meeting from the schedule with the intent of meeting at a "better time." Almost without exception, the more convenient time never arrives. Members who form the habit of keeping their commitments are usually productive.

The goal of a content conference is derived from any aspect of nursing that meets the need of the membership. The field is open to a broad range of subject matter. Medical concerns such as symptoms, pathology, laboratory results, clinical course of a disease, diagnostic tests, and pharmacologic data interest nursing personnel and influence nursing activities and judgments. Nursing content such as client care or comfort problems, client teaching needs, new technologic advancements, and preventive care are areas constantly in need of attention. Because of time allotment, all areas cannot be covered; if attempted, the conference would result in a general coverage of a number of problems with no appreciable gain in theoretical and practical understanding of what nursing involves. To ensure a successful content conference the subject matter must be (1) needed by the membership, (2) something that can be considered in the allotted time, and (3) adequately prepared prior to the meeting.

Leadership varies with each conference. As in the client-centered conference, the initiator of the subject matter usually takes the lead. The amount of guidance and assistance needed to prepare for the conference will depend on the individual's capabilities. Often the leader will suggest sharing the responsibility for presentation of content. All group members are expected to contribute to the discussion. Content conferences need not restrict contributions to the members of the group involved; participation from any person—coordinator of nursing services, physician, social worker, or therapist, the client or family—may be included when feasible and appropriate.

PREDICTIVE PRINCIPLE: Member participation in problem-solving processes during content conference results in more meaningful learning.

Participants come to content conferences having acquired a body of information beforehand. They are ready to fit their knowledge and understanding together to form predictive principles that can be used to prescribe nursing actions.

The need to learn more about hyaline membrane disease, expressed by the membership in the client-centered conference on Baby Lee, will be used as an example of the theory-building process in a content conference. The following is a model of a problem-solving process in a content conference:

LVN: (After giving a recall of background data about Baby Lee.) The definition of hyaline membrane disease is "a syndrome of neonatal distress, characterized by a hyaline-like material within the alveoli and bronchioles." This disease is very much like emphysema, in which bronchi in the lungs end in thin-walled air spaces (illustrates with chalk drawing).

The LVN has begun the conference by referring to content familiar to the group. Her next step is to introduce new information and then to make it meaningful by relating the facts to the more familiar condition (emphysema). Visual media assist the learning process. The LVN has applied the principle that *increasing the difficulty of learning material in small increments promotes learning success.*

Aide: Did you find out why the baby has this disease? I read that babies with hyaline membrane disease are usually premature, and Baby Lee is not.

LVN: Yes, I did. The specific cause of the disease is unknown, but it does occur frequently in two conditions. One is with premature babies, as we know, and the other occurs in babies born of mothers who have untreated diabetes mellitus.

Student: What about the mother? Has she been tested?

Leader: The doctor is working with her. She has had a glucose tolerance test, which was positive. Mrs. Lee was shocked, to say the least, but is now learning all she can about the problem.

Members in this conference are concerning themselves with a real situation, which is never simple. Extraneous factors will enter in and must be considered if they are pertinent to the subject. These activities actualize the principle that *learning episodes that contain input, operations, and feedback increase retention and utility of learning.*

LVN: Baby Lee's problems center around respirations. I have, with the help of the team leader, placed facts on the blackboard that will help us to see why Baby Lee is having problems. Will you help in deciding what they are? Anything you can add will be welcome.

Student: His carbon dioxide and oxygen combining powers indicate that acidosis is developing.

Aide: What does that mean?

Student: Interference with gas exchange in the lungs causes carbon dioxide retention.

The conference continues in an atmosphere of freedom, allowing facts and concepts to be exchanged and clarification of the learning structure to occur. The problem-solving process continues until the group has formulated principles pertinent to the situation and has developed nursing prescriptions supported by theory. The following is a sample of some of the formalizations as a result of group process.

Predictive principles	*Nursing prescription*
1. Poor heat regulation center prompts use of external control of temperature.	1. Warm Isolette.
2. Loosening tenacious pulmonary secretions facilitates breathing.	2. Percuss before suctioning to loosen pulmonary secretions.
3. Blood gas measurements indicate changing physiologic state.	3. Keep open arterial catheter (heparin-saline solution can be used).
4. Sodium bicarbonate IV combats acidosis.	4. Monitor closely.
5. In respiratory acidosis the use of positive pressure respirator promotes the blowing off of excessive CO_2.	5. Record and graph respiratory rate every half hour or as needed.

Nursing care conferences

PREDICTIVE PRINCIPLE: Conferences held between nurse and client as well as with significant others contribute to reciprocal development of care plans and lead to optimal health service for the client and satisfaction for the nurse.

Assessment and maintenance provide the causal elements for primary care conferences. Client-centered conferences are an effective means to bring together persons who can contribute to and profit from analysis of the care plan. Conferences are usually initiated by the nurse but may originate from any one of the involved persons. The time, place, and length of the meeting depend on several circumstances—needs, urgency, and availability of resources, materials, and personnel. The purpose is to plan together problem-oriented client care. The nursing conference is equally applicable to singular needs and problems of the client as it is to complex situations requiring multiple consideration. The conference may be concerned with an initial assessment process or with an ongoing appraisal of a health situation. Members discuss the health of the client to arrive at a decision of what must be done to help resolve the problem and to delegate responsibility for the maintenance of health, evaluation and management of symptoms, and appropriate referrals.

To function logically and responsibly in an assessment conference, the nurse must have knowledge and requisite skills in prescribing, providing care, and making referrals as appropriate.

The nurse-practitioner has direct access to clients and a one-to-one relationship with the client. Either the nurse or the client can initiate contact. Nursing responsibility includes history and physical examination, patient screening and referrals to appropriate physicians or other health workers, and nursing diagnosis and prescription, including counseling, care, and rehabilitation.

As health care is increasingly valued in our society, nurses are expected to take more responsibility for the delivery of health care, for coordinating preventive services, for initiating or participating in diagnostic screening, and for referring patients who require differential medical diagnoses and therapies.

A report submitted to the Secretary of Health, Education, and Welfare reviewing extended roles for nurses concluded that skills for the nurse-practitioner involve (1) eliciting and recording a health history; (2) making physical and psychosocial assessment, recognizing the range of "normal" and the manifestations of common abnormalities; (3) assessing the environment (family relationships and home, school, and work environments); (4) interpreting selected laboratory findings; (5) making diagnoses and choosing, initiating, and modifying selected therapies; (6) assessing community resources and needs for health care; (7) providing emergency treatment as appropriate, as in cardiac arrest, shock, or hemorrhage; and (8) providing appropriate information to the client and family about a diagnosis or plan of therapy.*

Primary care nursing, a concept different from the preceding, involves one nurse's being responsible for the total nursing management of a client or small group of clients. Nursing diagnosis and care plans based on a total and continuing assessment process are the vehicles for continuity and comprehensiveness. Primary care views the client as the center of action and focuses on him as a person, with the nurse having an increased opportunity for individual care.

In primary care nurses assume considerably greater responsibility for delivery of health care services. Primary care nursing establishes a one-to-one nurse-client relationship that can be experienced in any setting—home, community, or highly complex care context. The nurse assumes the role of client advocate. Primary care nursing is a self-maintaining care system, open to the environment, with adaptive mechanisms for the single purpose of providing quality services. In this system, direct conferences are held between nurse and client and any other member of significance to the client and care.

In present practice, utilization of the primary nurse varies extensively. Community health nurses have always functioned with relative independence, though with physician collaboration in assessing problems of individuals and families, treating minor illnesses, referring patients for differential medical diagnosis, arranging for referrals to social service agencies and organizations, giving advice and counsel to promote health and prevent illness, supervising health regimens of normal pregnant women and of children, and working with health-related community action programs.

Team nursing is one of the more common nursing care delivery systems and involves a group of people sharing responsibility for a number of clients. The team conference is the heart of this system. Nursing assessments, diagnosis, and care prescriptions are formulated by the group or team leader and furnish the guidelines for continuity and comprehensive practice. The team member assigned to a given client for a specified period of time is responsible for carrying out the plan and conferring with team members to revise the design.

PREDICTIVE PRINCIPLE: Periodic care review conferences with colleagues provide a mechanism for the nurse to validate care plans and maintain quality control.

---

*Nurs. Outlook **1:**50-51, 1972.

Each nurse, regardless of the system of nursing care delivery, is accountable for overall decisions about how the client is to receive attention. The nurse is a decision maker in control of the quality of nursing care administered to clients. Additionally, primary nurses are responsible in the caregiver's absence. With the burgeoning knowledge in nursing, medicine, and related fields, it is necessary to share the knowledge and skills of a number of health experts, each of whom is prepared in a particular area. Together these individuals attempt adequately to meet the comprehensive needs of the client.

Review conferences between the nurse and such colleagues as other caregivers, physician, nurse-specialist, and supervisory nurse provide an excellent avenue for collegial validation and advisement, with an informal network of peer control and dialogue. During the conference, each nurse presents the information on which the health plan is based and discusses the reasons for nursing prescriptions. Review conferences serve to increase the competency of the nurse, strengthen peer relationships, and maintain quality control necessary for the delivery of this health care system.

Nursing care conferences contribute to a sense of satisfaction in participants. Relationships necessary for a professional level of responsibility and for the comprehensive care of the patient are developed. The dual concept of individual responsibility for the delivery of nursing services and care, with each nurse functioning at her own level of performance and each client participating in the implementation of the care plan to the extent of his motivation and level of competence, makes the practice of nursing challenging and exciting.

Utilization of the problem-solving process has taken a form that allows the learners to compile their facts and concepts into a meaningful pattern that is logical and sensible. Definite guidelines for evaluation of behaviors have been established.

Reporting conferences

There is widespread agreement among nursing personnel as to the importance of keeping the leader informed about ongoing activities. No leader can operate efficiently without sufficient knowledge about member activities. One of the most logical sources of information is the reporting conference, where events of the workday are shared by all those engaged in the administration of care. Members bring to the conference the worksheets on which they have recorded the day's events. Verbally they share pertinent information with the group. The coordinator of nursing services attends these sessions; even though informed of major events throughout the shift, the coordinator usually has little opportunity to learn the many details discussed in the reporting conferences.

Reporting conferences have four major goals: (1) to report relevant information accurately and objectively, (2) to give reactions to situations when pertinent, (3) to evaluate the care in the light of objectives, and (4) to update the nursing care plans to ensure continuity of care for the client and family.

Listening is the primary task of the nurse-leader in reporting sessions. The leader must be a critical listener and be able to make judgments about the material being presented. The tools used to aid in this task are the leader's worksheet; a record of the physician's orders; awareness of each client's reactions and nursing prescriptions; and knowledge, understanding, and intuition. As with the instructional conference, members are encouraged to listen and record appropriate data about all patients or families for whom they are responsible.

The leader will utilize the information received in the reporting conference in finalizing action for the day, in recording data on clients' records, in giving the change-of-shift report to the oncoming staff, and in making plans for the next day.

Many predictive principles that have been proposed for all conferences have direct application to report giving. Prior preparation by all members, attention to behavioral messages, and paced and systematic presentation are of equal importance in the summarizing period.

PREDICTIVE PRINCIPLE: Directions given to conferees before report reveal expectations the leader has for the members.

Because situations vary in nursing, it is difficult to establish a set of criteria for reporting information. In primary care, for example, expectations for client and nurse will be mutually agreed on, with guidance from the leader. In acute situations the member must report many details, whereas in health care centers where the occupants' stay is long term or in the home, much routine information can be omitted. It is the leader's task to inform the members of the amount and kind of information desired. For example, a leader might begin by saying, "When I call on you, will you tell us please how the client ate, degree of ambulation, how he tolerated treatments, and anything you believe to be important for us to know?"

This procedure sounds simple, but complications may occur. The average staff member usually gives routine information but may not be clear on what additional data to report. In many cases the worker's past nursing experience and educational background limit the extent of the report. Just prior to the conference, for example, an aide may have noted casually one of the assigned clients looked pale while walking in the hall. The worker may not consider this to be significant enough to report. The next day, when the client is discovered slumped on the floor, the observation becomes significant to the aide and is reported.

There will be occasions when incidents that have proved troublesome to the member will be deleted from the report. The worker may not want to risk criticism, especially if the incident or problem may be perceived as a result of a mistake or poor judgment.

If something has been omitted from a report, the ultimate accountability lies with the leader. The leader's task is to prepare the members for their roles and to maintain an atmosphere in which free exchange of information can occur. Preoccupation with fixing blame consumes time and energy better spent on solving the problems.

Continuing training, practice, and review, as necessary, will help nurses and clients mature in ability to select appropriate information and to report clearly and accurately.

Reports lend themselves to the use of tape recorders. Clarification and elucidation can be made after listening to the tape and before the reporting nurse departs.

General problems conference

One of the more difficult roles for nurse-leaders in conference sessions is to cope with feelings, both their own and those expressed by members. Control of one's feelings is held in personal, social, and cultural esteem by North American society. The individual is expected to maintain "proper" control of feelings and also to act in a way that enables others to maintain theirs. Participants usually strive to convey precisely the feeling they believe others expect of them at a given time and place. Preoccupation with this can result in letting feelings go unresolved.

Any work assignment has problems and emergencies. The way problems are handled determines the amount and kind of feelings that will be built up in an individual. Many days are filled with one situation after another that builds up tension in the person until he "travels on his nerves."

Members in conference sessions do not always operate as a "happy family." Because of individual interests, clashes occur between the client, the health giving membership, and the management. The nurse is not expected to be a psychiatrist, but only to develop the ability to sense feelings and to understand and apply principles of effective interpersonal relationships when they are needed.

PREDICTIVE PRINCIPLE: Sharing of feelings through conferences unifies and integrates the membership and allows work to progress.

In work groups members sometimes have little in common except that they are drawn together by joint enterprise. The task of becoming spontaneously involved in conference activity when it is a job expectation places the individual in a delicate position. Expressions of feelings will be easier for some than for others.

Problems conferences are directly related to the administration of patient care. They should be scheduled often enough to keep the members in tune with one another. Interpersonal maintenance for goal accomplishment is a legitimate enterprise. A meeting should be called by the leader or any member anytime problems arise that hinder the communication process and therefore reduce work efficiency and effectiveness.

Reasons for tense situations may range from prejudice of one member against another to lack of consideration for the total membership by one individual. For example, problems may be created when a member announces openly that he plans to use all his accrued sick time because he is "never sick." His frequent absences without notice cause gaps in patient care and overloads for the remaining members, and hostility and anger result.

An alternative action for these situations is open expressions of feelings about the behavior and its consequences in a feelings conference. In this way, feelings are expressed openly and handled. Until these feelings are relieved, there will be barriers to communication. Positive relationships need recognition and reinforcement on a continual basis. It becomes easy to slip into the habit of dealing with crisis situations and to fail to acknowledge those behaviors that keep nursing practice on an even keel.

Expression of feelings becomes easier in the sharing process when one knows what the other is doing and feeling. The "feeling of knowing" is an emotional by-product of communication and makes the difference between the person who feels secure and the one who is anxious.

Development of a climate conducive to fostering collaborative interdependent and independent activity requires time, involvement, and concerted effort by each member. The operation of effective nursing process depends on the maintenance of open, trusting relationships among the participants. If problems are acknowledged and faced frankly, the chances for a remedy are far greater than if ignored and allowed to fester.

PREDICTIVE PRINCIPLE: Understanding and managing group behavior require ability to predict the processes through which feelings and meanings are transmitted among group members.

Investigators of small-group process have found group members address more communication to individuals whose opinions are extreme than to the more conforming members. For instance, an individual group member might believe that caregivers have an obligation to urge hospital management to serve patients their meals on request. If the majority opinion differs greatly from that of the dissenter, the group will exert pressure on the member in an effort to get him to change his opinion. Evidence shows that communication of feelings back to the instigator will reduce the intensity of feelings.

These findings make it possible for the members to pick up cues in behavior when they occur and to recognize the process as it unfolds. Another illustration will prove helpful. Probably the most common feeling expressed in conferences is that of pressure. Nurses seem to be particularly susceptible to pressure because the tasks are numerous, varied, and very often complex. The leader is frequently confronted with a member who is frustrated and angry and who vents feelings in negative terms. "I have to be everywhere at once and everything to everybody!" "There are not enough hours in the day; I have to do everything around here." "I'm still not caught up; I don't have time to sit in here and talk!" These feelings can be decreased if activities are put on a priority basis and the group shares the responsibility for the necessary ongoing work. Clear identification of anger and attempts to resolve the causes openly can effectively reduce member hostility and give the leader the opportunity to explore feelings with the individual concerned. If the discussion reveals duplication of effort, lack of organization, or, in fact, too large an assignment, adjustments can be made in the structure or perhaps even in the system of care. Failure to change the feelings may result in their intensification and transmission to other members.

The real significance of the "contagion" theory of feelings is that members recognize the impact they have on one another. Feelings of acceptance, caring, trust, and security will be transmitted when they exist, just as feelings of rejection, anger, hate, or hostility will be communicated despite attempts to hide them from the group. It is important to establish the rule among conferees that when feelings are interfering with the work of the group, they must be dealt with.

PREDICTIVE PRINCIPLE: Involvement in group process results in specific gains or losses for the individual member.

Rewards may take the form of such intangibles as prestige, recognition, or affection. The conditions or rules that govern the awarding of the payoff will have important motivational consequences for the members and for the functioning of the group as a whole.

Each person wants to feel that his individual contribution to cooperative endeavor is significant and identifiable. Group work, however, can subjugate some members to others unnecessarily unless steps are taken to offset this possibility.

In group process, "role blurring" is encouraged, in which emphasis is placed on outcomes of the group rather than on the status of the individual. The leader works with health care personnel to provide opportunity for each individual to expand his physical and mental energies to the fullest potential. In the process, personal achievements are recognized and the worth of the person is reinforced, but individual recognition does not take priority over group accomplishment.

If position or salary increments depend on such individual performances as the number of beds made or procedures accomplished, group effort is apt to diminish. If, on the other hand, a group is operating under a policy whereby each person's benefits depend directly on the group's performance, the members will want to engage in whatever behaviors they believe will contribute to this end (working hard, helping others, and making suggestions about ways to improve the group's efficiency).

In industry, a reward system of this kind operates most frequently in plant operations where salable items are the end result of effort and dividends include monetary gain. In nursing, patients are the end product; when they have benefited from the coordinated efforts of a group, tangible reward to all members, beyond established policy, are not forthcoming. The caregiver's motivation, then, centers around achievement of satisfaction in a job well done, acknowledgment by management, and patients' appreciation.

Involvement in group activity does not negate the autonomy and individual accountability reflected in the role of the primary care nurse. This nurse has the freedom to move in and out of groups as necessary to the needs of the client and the dynamics of the nursing care plan.

Application of predictive principles in communications

Mrs. Turner, an RN, recently joined a nursing group in the rehabilitative unit. Her former experience included ten years working with paraplegic patients in another part of the country. She is convinced that her knowledge and experience far surpass those of any other members. The RN completes her assignments by herself, communicating as little as possible with the members, who have countered with expressions of hostility.

Problem	Predictive principles	Prescriptions
Noncommunicative member	In retrospect: Preassessment of individual and group knowledge, skills, and expectations establishes baseline data for measuring progress or change.	
	Perceiving negative feedback enables group members to become aware of others' responses and to modify behavior accordingly.	Leader will have conference with RN; state observed behavior and problems that have arisen because of aloofness from others. Assist RN to recognize the influence one member's action has on the entire group and the responsibility of the group to discuss the problem.
	Understanding and managing group behavior require ability to predict the processes through which feelings and meanings are transmitted among group members.	
	The interdependent collaborating group facilitates accomplishment of its goals.	
	Circumstance and member capability determine the type of directions to be communicated.	Arrange meeting with all members; conduct so meeting will be a discussion of cause for behavior; encourage open communication (not a punitive session).
	Interaction of conference members on an equal basis encourages active participation and leads to usable solutions to the problem.	
	Integrative positive reinforcement increases individual identification with group goals and the participation level of the individual.	Make positive plans with member for reinforcing positive behavior.

BIBLIOGRAPHY
Books

Amidon, E.J., and Hough, J.B., editors: Interaction analysis: theory, research and application, Reading, Mass., 1967, Addison-Wesley Publishing Co., Inc.

Arndt, C., and Huckabay, L.M.D.: Nursing administration: theory for practice with a systems approach, ed. 2, St. Louis, 1980, The C.V. Mosby Co.

Bell, G.D.: Organizations and human behavior, Englewood Cliffs, N.J., 1967, Prentice-Hall, Inc.

Berne, E.: The structure and dynamics of organizations and groups, New York, 1966, Grove Press, Inc.

Bloom, B.S., et al.: Handbook on formative and summative evaluation of student learning, New York, 1971, McGraw-Hill Book Co.

Bower, F.L.: The process of planning nursing care: nursing practice models, ed. 3, St. Louis, 1977, The C.V. Mosby Co.

Carkhuff, R.R., and Berenson, B.G.: Beyond counseling and therapy, New York, 1967, Holt, Rinehart & Winston, Inc.

Cartwright, D., and Zander, A., editors: Group dynamics—research and theory, ed. 3, New York, 1968, Harper & Row, Publishers.

Combs, A., et al.: Helping relationships: basic concepts for the helping professions, Boston, 1972, Allyn & Bacon, Inc.

Coomb, A.W., et al.: Florida studies in the helping professions, University of Florida Social Science Monograph No. 37, 1969.

Fast, J.: Body language, New York, 1970, J.B. Lippincott Co.

Gagne, R.W.: The condition of learning, New York, 1965, Holt, Rinehart & Winston, Inc.

Glasser, W.: Schools without failure, New York, 1969, Harper & Row, Publishers.

Goffman, E.: Interaction ritual: essays on face-to-face behavior, New York, 1967, Anchor Press.

Gulley, H., and Leaters, D.: Communication and group process, ed. 3, New York, 1977, Holt, Rinehart & Winston, Inc.

Harris, T.A.: I'm OK—you're OK, New York, 1973, Harper & Row, Publishers.

Hodjetts, R.M.: Management: theory, process and practice, Philadelphia, 1975, W.B. Saunders Co.

Johnson, D.W., and Johnson, F.P.: Join in together: group theory and group skills, Englewood Cliffs, N.J., 1975, Prentice-Hall, Inc.

Krathwohl, D.R., et al.: Taxonomy of educational objectives: the classification of educational goals. Handbook II. Affective domain, New York, 1964, David McKay Co., Inc.

Litterer, J.A.: Organizations: systems, control and adaptation, ed. 3, New York, 1980, John Wiley & Sons, Inc., vol. 2.

Little, D., and Carnevali, D.: Nursing care planning, ed. 2, 1976, Philadelphia, J.B. Lippincott Co.

Luft, J.: Group processes, an introduction to group dynamics, ed. 2, Palo Alto, Calif., 1976, National Press Books.

Mager, R.F.: Preparing instructional objectives, Palo Alto, Calif., 1962, Fearon Publishers.

Marram, G.D.: The group approach in nursing practice, ed. 2, St. Louis, 1978, The C.V. Mosby Co.

McLemore, M., and Bevis, E.O.: Planned change. In Marriner, A., editor: Current perspectives in nursing management, St. Louis, 1979, The C.V. Mosby Co.

Ruesch, J.: The observer and the observed: human communication theory. In Grinker, R.R., editor: Toward a unified theory of human behavior, New York, 1956, Basic Books, Inc., Publishers.

Ruesch, J.: General theory of communication. In Arieti, S., editor: American handbook of psychiatry, New York, 1961, W.W. Norton & Co., Inc.

Ruesch, J., and Bateson, G.: Communication: the social matrix of psychiatry, New York, 1968, W.W. Norton & Co., Inc.

Steiner, C.: Scripts people live, New York, 1974, Grove Press, Inc.

Periodicals

Chopra, A.: Motivation in task oriented groups, J. Nurs. Admin., pp. 55-60, Jan.-Feb. 1973.

Cohen, M., and Ross, M.: Team building: a strategy for unit cohesiveness, J. Nurs. Admin. **12**(1): 29-34, 1982.

Chiavetta, L.: Group communication: when I speak no one listens, Nurs. Mgmt. **13**(5):36-41, 1982.

Dickoff, P., and Wiedenbach, J.: Theory in practice discipline, Part I, Practice oriented theory, Nurs. Res. **17**(5):415-435, 1968.

Duldt, B.: Helping nurses to cope with the anger-dismay syndrome, Nurs. Outlook **30**(3):168-174, 1982.

Gallagher, J.J., and Aschner, M.J.: A preliminary report on an analysis of classroom interaction, Merrill Palmer Quart. Behav. & Develop. **9**:3, 1963.

Gibb, J.: Defensive communication, J. Nurs. Admin. **12**(4):14-17, 1982.

Jehring, J.J.: Motivational problems in the modern hospital, J. Nurs. Admin., pp. 35-47, Nov.-Dec. 1972.

Lewis, G.K.: Communication, a factor in meeting

emotional crisis, Nurs. Outlook **13**:36-39, 1965.

Little, D., and Carnevali, D.: The nursing care planning system, Nurs. Outlook **19**:164-167, 1971.

Palmer, M.E.: Patient care conference: an opportunity for meeting staff needs, J. Nurs. Admin., pp. 47-53, March-April 1973.

Smullegon, M.: Teaching therapy groups, J. Nurs. Ed. **21**(1):23-31, Jan. 1982.

Stevens, L.F.: Nurse-patient discussion groups, Am. J. Nurs. **63**(12):67-69, 1963.

Teaching patients and use of the self in clinical practice, Nurs. Clin. North Am. **6**:4, Dec. 1971.

Vaill, P.B.: Management language and management action, Calif. Management Rev., pp. 51-58, Oct. 1967.

Veninga, R.: Communications: a patient's eye view, Am. J. Nurs. **73**(2):320-322, 1973.

Zander, A., et al.: Unity of group, identification with group and self-esteem of members, J. Pers. **28**:463-465, 1960.

chapter six

Predictive principles for delegation of assignments and authority

Scope and limitations of roles

Effective performance of assigned tasks depends on sufficient influence, power, and authority.

The nurse's belief that ultimate accountability lies with her determines the scope and limitations she sets for her leadership.

Decentralization of power allows for a greater amount of delegation.

Understanding the categories and roles of nursing personnel enables the delegator to select the type and number of personnel appropriate for the job.

Job descriptions, policies, and procedures

Written descriptions of policies, procedures, and guidelines by which an employee may handle situations promote ease of operation for the caregiver and control of the authority delegated by the nurse.

Staff member participation in the formulation of policies, job descriptions, and procedures increases use of policies and improves job satisfaction.

The philosophy and policies of a health agency determine the pattern of nursing care delivery system to be provided.

Guidelines such as established channels, methods, and provision for communication within an agency enable the nurse to delegate tasks and authority appropriately.

Responsibilities of direction giving

The number of workers and span of control depends upon consideration of factors that most affect the work group.

Formulation of objectives for care that are realistic for the health agency, clients, and nursing personnel assures successful goal accomplishment.

Utilization of nursing care plans provides the mechanism for making nurse assignments according to clients needs and the order of priorities.

A systematic planning process enables effective delegation for work implementation.

Assignment of client care and support services to increasing personnel depends upon the pattern or system of nursing care in force.

Consideration of safety factors and instructions regarding emergency situations prepare nursing staff to employ preventive measures and to cope with emergency situations.

The delegator's availability to staff members results in assistance, teaching, counsel, and evaluation where necessary.

Centralized control of incidental task requests prevents maldistribution of work loads.

A balance between variety and continuity of assignment increases motivation and productivity.

Consideration for each caregiver's preferences and areas of expertise influences morale.

Centralization of information storage and retrieval systems allows for efficient assessment, delegation, and implementation of tasks.

Clear and concise directions enhance task delegation.

Measuring results

Frequent evaluation of performance using criteria influences the quality of care and the level of actual performance of care activities.

Scope and limitation of roles

Delegation is the organizational process by which (1) a manager assigns specific duties to a worker and provides the worker with a grant of authority commensurate with the duties to be performed, and (2) the worker assumes responsibility for satisfactorily performing the duties and is held accountable for results (Fig. 6-1). Like most definitions this is an oversimplification. For example, it seems to imply that only authority is necessary for satisfactory performance of the assigned duties. But delegation is a highly complex and dynamic process involving a number of interacting variables. The amount of authority needed depends upon such factors as leadership style, attitudes of workers, the extent to which managers perceive themselves to have authority, and the extent to which managers possess the authority that comes from expertise and personality characteristics. (See Chapters 2 and 9.)

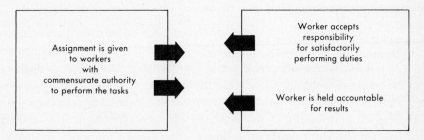

Fig. 6-1. The process of delegation.

Delegation is one of the most important functions of a nurse. The major responsibility of a nurse-delegator is to see that care is provided to a client or group of clients or to serve with other significant caregivers in the roles of validator, catalyst, decision maker, and controller of nursing care quality. The ability to perform these roles assumes that caregivers collaborate and accept appropriate shares of responsibility. Inherent in the philosophy of delegating authority is a commitment to the proposition that nursing caregivers be entrusted with some degree of responsibility for the tasks under their jurisdiction and that they have authority to act, thus making them accountable for their nursing actions (see Fig. 6-1). This assumes that the nurse-manager has the knowledge and skills commensurate with the responsibility of organizing and directing activities and making nursing care decisions that affect others. If the trial-and-error method in delegating work activities is employed, chaos, increase in costs, and worker dissatisfaction results. If, on the other hand, the nurse uses a conscious analysis of the delegation process to get members of the nursing team to perform, results will be more positive: organizational, group, and individual goals will be achieved more smoothly, work production and quality can be increased, cost effectiveness will occur, and workers will be more satisfied.

Delegation and responsibility. Delegation occurs any time a worker performs a task for which that person's manager is ultimately responsible. It occurs, for instance, every time a nurse administers a treatment or gives instruction to a client. The extent to which a nurse or an assistant is permitted to determine how the tasks will be performed varies, depending on the task and the preparation and abilities of the one assigned to perform the tasks. It is crucial to note that *responsibility can never be delegated.* Managers remain accountable to higher levels of management for all the tasks they delegate to others. The manager whose workers fail to produce or who make mistakes frequently cannot be absolved of responsibility by blaming the workers. One is always accountable to one's immediate supervisor.

PREDICTIVE PRINCIPLE: Effective performance of assigned tasks depends on sufficient influence, power, and authority.

PREDICTIVE PRINCIPLE: The nurse's belief that ultimate accountability lies with her determines the scope and limitations she sets for her leadership.

Influence is defined as a change in behavior or attitude resulting directly or indirectly from the actions or examples of another person or group. For instance, a hard-working team leader might, by setting an example, influence the other members of the team to increase their productivity. Or a head nurse might use influence to improve morale by recognizing individual accomplishments. The influence here would not necessarily change a behavior; it would simply bring about a change in work attitude.

Power is defined as the ability to exert influence. To have power is to be able to bring about a change in the behavior or attitudes of others. In the example above it is likely that the hard-working person would have more power to influence the work group if he or she were popular rather than disliked. The most powerful managers in an organization are invariably those who can most influence their associates. Power can be dominant and controlling and result in submission and acquiescence, but power can also be inspiring and benevolent. As discussed in Chapter 2, there are five categories of power: (1) legitimate, (2) reward, (3) coercive, (4) expert, and (5) referent. All of these types of power are acceptable and available to the nurse who delegates authority.

Authority is the right of an individual to use power. A manager employed by an institution is given formal authority to act contingent upon that person's position, for example, a director of nurses, a supervisor, or a staff nurse. Clues about the person's formal authority may be obtained from the job descriptions, observation of the behavior of previous occupants of the position, assessment of persons in comparable positions, statements made by one's supervisor, and scope and nature of management responsibilities. While workers in highly structured organizations have some freedoms, they are bound to obey the direction of their managers or face the consequences. Managers acquire power in different ways and in different degrees. Their success as delegators depends upon the recognition and value which those led give to the manager.

Earlier chapters have considered organization as a system, referring to the overall structure in a hospital or health facility in which all personnel relate to each other through specific channels. This chapter presents the organizational process of delegation at the lower or decentralized level, with the nurse working as a manager of a small group, coordinating personnel, equipment, and supplies in a designated environment for direction of some specific purpose or work.

PREDICTIVE PRINCIPLE: Decentralization of power allows for a greater amount of delegation.

The delegation of authority by individual managers is closely related to an organization's decentralization of authority. Delegation is the process of assigning authority from one level of management down to the next. The concepts of centralization and decentralization refer to the extent to which authority has been retained at the top of the organization (centralization) or has been passed down to the lower levels (decentralization). The greater the delegation of authority throughout the organization, the more decentralized the organization. For example, to the extent that lower level managers (head nurses, team leaders, primary caregivers) have freedom in carrying out their functions without first checking with middle level (coordinators or supervisors) or top level managers (director of nursing services), the organization is decentralized. Hospitals, for the most part, remain bureaucratic and centralized; however, there is a move toward

decentralization of nursing services within the formal structure. Top administrators are realizing the advantages of decentralization:

1. Top managers are unburdened.
2. Decision making is improved because decisions are made closer to
   the scene of action.
3. Better training occurs with a more personalized approach.
4. Morale is increased because of personal involvement.
5. Greater initiative is taken by nurses at the first or lower levels.
6. More flexibility and faster decision making are possible as environments change.

Total decentralization, however, with no coordination and leadership
from the top would be undesirable. Without some central authority and power,
the various parts of the organization would disintegrate into isolated subunits.
The very purpose of organization (efficient integration of various subunits for the
good of the whole) would be defeated without some centralized control. For this
reason the question for managers is not *if* an organization should be decentralized but *to what extent* it should be decentralized.

The extent to which delegation of authority is centralized is likely to be
influenced by the abilities of lower level managers, as perceived by top level
managers. This dimension is in part circular, as illustrated in Fig. 6-2. If authority
is not delegated because of lack of faith in the lower level managers, these people
will not have much opportunity to develop. In addition, the lack of internal training will make it more difficult to find and retain competent or ambitious people.
This, in turn, will make it more difficult to decentralize. One obvious solution is

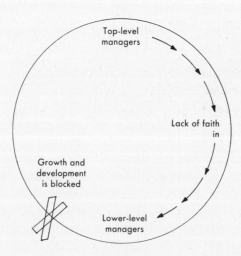

Fig. 6-2. Influence of top level managers upon lower level managers.

to avoid giving authority to nurses before they are ready to assume the role and to make provision for each individual's training, when the decision is made who is to be the leader. If training sponsored by the agency is not possible, then arrangements can be made for preparation elsewhere, such as in a nearby college or university, through workshops and seminars, or through individualized courses of instruction.

PREDICTIVE PRINCIPLE: Understanding the categories and roles of nursing personnel enables the delegator to select the type and number of personnel appropriate for the job.

Categories of nursing personnel are many and vary with each employing agency. It is impossible to delineate clearly among services rendered by each group because of differences in standards and requirements on the national, state, and local levels and the number of overlapping roles and functions. In general, nursing personnel comprise those who have had both formal and informal preparation. The three main categories of nursing personnel are (1) nurse's aide or assistant, (2) licensed practical (vocational) nurse, and (3) registered nurse.

Nurse's aides or assistants perform services directed at the safety, comfort, personal hygiene, and protection of patients and may be utilized as needed to assist with simple nursing functions as long as they do not presume to practice as licensed nurses. They are usually trained on the job, with a few weeks of instruction divided between the classroom, learning laboratory, and supervised experience. The extent of the training period depends on the philosophy of the educational program of the agency.

The scope of practice of *licensed practical nurses* (LPN) or *licensed vocational nurses* (LVN) is generally defined as the performance of services requiring the skills acquired at an accredited practical or vocational nursing school, under the direction of a registered nurse or physician. Licensed practical nurses are prepared to function as responsible members of the health care team concerned with therapeutic, rehabilitative, and preventive care for people of all ages in various stages of dependency. Graduates of practical/vocational nursing educational programs have completed courses offered through an adult education board, in a hospital, or under the auspices of a junior or community college. The LPN or LVN program varies in length from nine to eighteen months. Because of a shortage of RNs or as a cost control measure, LPN/LVNs are sometimes given assignments for which they are not prepared. This practice can jeopardize both the nurse and the patient.

Registered nurses (RN) are those who are licensed by their state to practice nursing skills in hospitals, military services, offices, clinics, private practice, homes, and the community. Minimal requirements for the RN are that preparation be in a school with an associate of arts or baccalaureate degree program in nursing accredited by the state. According to the National League for Nursing,* competencies expected of the *associate of arts degree graduates* on entry into practice include the role of provider of care through the application of the nursing process and management of nursing care for a group of clients with common, well-defined health problems in structured settings. In some places, collaboration with or supervision of an experienced professional nurse is required.

The beginning practitioner (1) carries out nursing functions directly related to patient care, including participation in implementing the physician's therapeutic plan (for example, by administering medications and treatments); (2) renders direct patient care in nursing situations requiring nursing judgment and recognizes those situations that require a higher degree of nursing expertise; (3) gives patient care that demonstrates knowledge of the nursing principles taught in all courses in the associate degree nursing program; (4) functions as a member of the nursing care team and as such may direct and guide other team members who have less education and experience; and (5) recognizes the client's need for instruction related to health and takes action to provide this instruction.

The graduate of *diploma programs* in nursing is eligible to seek licensure as a registered nurse and to function as a beginning practitioner in acute, intermediate, long-term, and ambulatory health care facilities. In order to fulfill such roles, graduates are expected to demonstrate competencies in assessment, planning, implementation, evaluation, and professionalism. Professionalism includes recognition of the legal limits of nursing practice, demonstrating ethical behavior in performance of nursing actions, not exercising discriminatory or judgmental behaviors, respecting the rights of others, accepting responsibility and accountability commensurate with the role, and demonstrating growth as a person.

Graduates of *baccalaureate programs* have completed study at a senior college or university where they were prepared as generalists to provide within the health care system a comprehensive service that assesses, promotes, and maintains the health of individuals and groups. These nurses are accountable for their own nursing practice and are qualified to provide nursing care through others, to serve in the advocacy role in relation to clients by acting in their behalf, and to apply interpersonal skills in working with other health professionals. Comprehensive care includes prevention, health promotion, and rehabilitation services, health counseling and education, and care in acute and long-term illness.

While findings indicate that registered nurses educated at all levels of nursing (diploma, associate, or baccalaureate) can and do perform the same ser-

---

*National League for Nursing: Competencies of the associate degree nurse on entry into practice, Nurs. Outlook **26**:346, June 1978. (Developed during workshops conducted in 1977 and 1978 by the Council of Associate Degree Programs.)

vices in a variety of health care settings, the interchange among nursing tasks and roles is not limited to the sphere of registered nurses. Other studies show that licensed practical nurses or licensed vocational nurses in hospital settings can and often do perform all the functions of registered nurses, and nurse's aides in many agencies often perform all the functions of licensed practical or vocational nurses, particularly on the night shift or at other times when registered nurses are in especially short supply.

One answer may be that the duties and responsibilities delegated to nurses in employment settings are frequently not related to their educational preparation. For example, registered nurses from two-, three-, four-, and five-year programs may all be employed as first level staff nurses functioning under the same entry level job descriptions, receiving the same orientation and initial salary, and being treated the same with regard to assignments and promotion. Nursing educators argue that overlap in function among registered nurse, licensed practical or vocational nurse, and nurse assistant is a result of hospital or agency exploitation, wherein the consumers of services suffer because the employer, in an effort to conserve funds, hires as few professional nurses as possible. Some employers counter that they cannot distinguish among graduates of the various nursing programs, as almost all are deficient in clinical skills and need intensive on-the-job training before they can meet agency expectations. There is great need for further clarification of categories of nurses and their use before the situation can be resolved.

Expanding roles for nurses. As far back as the early 1950s nurses were recognizing a need to accept greater responsibility for filling a serious gap in health care by helping to provide health care services to a greater number of persons at a reasonable cost. The explosion of medical knowledge had a profound effect upon medical procedures, patterns and organization of patient care, and increased effectiveness for the client. Similarly, the preparation and skills of registered nurses have expanded, allowing movement into primary health care roles with different and distinctive kinds of activities.

Primary health care by nurses takes many forms in and out of hospitals. Nurses have assumed increasing responsibility for direct observation of the client, recognizing illness and deciding what must be done to prevent illness and maintain health, control of nursing decisions, accountability for quality of nursing care, and development of a colleague or peer relationship with the physician.

Legal coverage for the expansion of nursing has required enactment of nursing legislation in many states. One survey* reveals that virtually all states have made some effort to accommodate the expanded role. The most significant action has been the revision or amendment of nurse practice acts. The usual

---

*Trandel-Korenchuk, D., and Trandel-Korenchuk, K.: How state laws recognize advanced nursing practice, Nurs. Outlook **26**(11):713-727, 1978.

approach is to expand the basic definition of professional nursing to include more autonomous functions, particularly in the areas of diagnosis and treatment. Another strategy is to change the nurse practice act to establish new nursing roles, using guidelines drawn up by nursing boards. A further step is enactment of legislation to create a separate category of nurses, such as nurse-midwife, nurse-anesthetist, or nurse-practitioner. Functions not covered by legal language are possible in many states through establishing standardized procedures and protocols jointly developed by nurses and physicians in the agency. California, Idaho, and Tennessee have adopted this approach.

There are two postgraduate designations for nurses who practice— *nurse-practitioner* and *clinical nurse-specialist*. In general, the nurse-practitioner has completed a generic nursing program, is licensed to practice nursing, and has completed either a degree or a nondegree-oriented course structured to provide skills and expanded roles. On the other hand, the clinical nurse-specialist is a registered nurse from a generic program who has completed a special program of study leading to a masters degree with an area of concentration designated "clinical nurse-specialist." Both of these programs of study prepare the nurse to assume versatile roles with clients with specific nursing and medical problems. These include the following:

1. Obtaining a nursing history
2. Assessing health-illness status
3. Making nursing diagnoses and writing nursing care prescriptions
4. Entering clients into the health care system
5. Providing sustenance, support, counseling, and therapy for clients who are impaired, infirm, or ill and who may be under treatment by others
6. Managing a medical care regime for acutely and chronically ill patients within the protocols of care provided by a licensed physician
7. Preventing illness and teaching how to maintain wellness
8. Teaching and counseling others about health and prevention of illness
9. Supervising and managing care regimens of normal pregnant women
10. Helping clients in the guidance of children with a view to their optimal physical and emotional development
11. Educating, counseling, and supporting people with regard to the aging process
12. Providing aid and support to clients and their families during the dying process
13. Supervising and teaching other professional people in areas unfamiliar to them

The difference in the practice of the nurse-practitioner and that of the clinical nurse-specialist is directly related to complexity, scope, and depth. The clinical nurse-specialist and the nurse-practitioner who has the benefit of the wider scope of education can be characterized as follows:

1. Can handle problems of greater complexity and containing more variables
2. Are able to provide more extensive services to families, groups, and communities
3. Practice with greater emphasis on the domain that is nursing rather than medicine
4. Tend to be more holistic in approach
5. Are better prepared to handle the unexpected and to work in unstructured settings

Naturally, individuals differ regardless of their academic preparations. But a broader and more diversified education usually produces a better qualified person able to meet the myriad demands of modern practice. In 1978 the U.S. Department of Health, Education and Welfare considered the impact of role expansion upon hospitals and community settings in the future. It was concluded that there will be nearly universal acceptance of all role changes discussed in this section. The optimal or "high" estimate is that about 80% of all in patient units will employ the primary nursing concept by 1985. In addition, all requirements for practitioner personnel in physician offices will be filled by nurse-practitioner personnel.*

Job descriptions, policies, and procedures

Clearly defining the exact nature and the limits of authority for each member in an agency not only provides structure for modes of operation but also promotes role identification by workers, sets boundaries, and avoids the possibility of task duplication.

PREDICTIVE PRINCIPLE: Written descriptions of policies, procedures, and guidelines by which an employee may handle situations promote ease of operation for the caregiver and control of the authority delegated by the nurse.

PREDICTIVE PRINCIPLE: Staff member participation in the formulation of policies, job descriptions, and procedures increases use of policies and improves job satisfaction.

A sense of personal involvement is created when individuals are given responsibility for participating in the formulation of policies that concern them. Personal involvement results in a feeling of belonging and a sense of power. Participation in the establishment of policies helps group members feel that their

---

*U.S. Department of Health, Education, and Welfare: The impact of health system changes on the nation's requirements for registered nurses in 1985, DHEW, publ. no. 78-9, Washington, D.C., Jan. 1978, Health Resources Administration.

contributions are of value and thus increases commitment. It is not feasible for a health agency to invite each employee to assist with the formulation of all issues, but through the various mechanisms, personnel representing all levels can have a part in most decisions. Each department within an agency can send members to policy and procedure meetings to represent the thinking of the group. Members who have had a part in determining both the qualifications required for a job and the procedure for implementing that job are better able to use their capabilities productively and with assurance.

The task of delegating responsibility is lightened when those affected have had a part in investing the leader with the right to guide them in the performance of their work. Job descriptions, policies, and procedures become dynamic for working groups when the content is reviewed on a regular basis and changes are made in accordance with increased knowledge and understanding. Investigating current practices and research in comparable settings and studying policies and procedures recommended by licensing associations for professional groups enable the establishment of guidelines to be an ongoing process, that is, one in which guidelines are constantly being revised to reflect current nursing care needs.

PREDICTIVE PRINCIPLE: The philosophy and policies of a health agency determine the pattern of nursing care delivery system to be provided.

PREDICTIVE PRINCIPLE: Guidelines such as established channels, methods, and provision for communication within an agency enable the nurse to delegate tasks and authority appropriately.

There are many ways to deliver nursing care. The effectiveness of the delivery system depends on such variables as setting, climate, abilities of the nurse, desires and needs of the client, and philosophy and conceptual framework of the agency.

Basically there are four systems for the delivery of nursing care: (1) functional, (2) team, (3) case, and (4) primary care. Combinations of these methods with new modes for provision of service are continually evolving.

Functional nursing is a system of care borrowed from industry that concentrates on duties or activities. In this pattern of care an assembly-line approach is utilized, with major tasks delegated by the charge nurse to individual members of the work group (Fig. 6-3). One member may be assigned to desk work, another to pass medications, another to administer all treatments and monitor IVs, another to give hygienic care, and so on. Each member of the working group is highly dependent upon the others for completion of the group's total assignments. Established protocol and procedural manuals are followed closely. Nursing care plans provide an important link between the workers and quality of care given, since there is limited opportunity for members of the nursing group to meet for coordination of efforts.

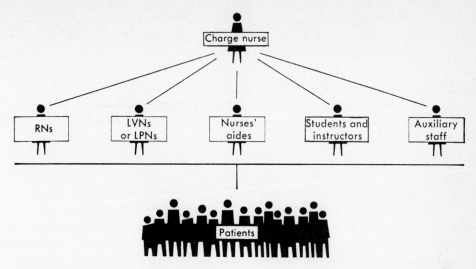

Fig. 6-3. Channels of communication in case and functional plans of nursing care.

Advantages and disadvantages of the functional system are controversial among nurses and hospital administrators. Many hospital administrators consider the functional system as the most economical way to deliver nursing services. This may be true if the goal is to meet minimal health care standards with as few nursing personnel as possible. Another factor is that greater control of work activities is maintained by the manager, commonly called the head nurse. In this autocratic system the manager bears responsibility for all activities of those persons assigned to provide care, as well as for the quality of care given. As chief of all activities the charge nurse is barraged with input from all sides: physicians, nursing staff, students, clients, visitors, and the public. In addition, the nurse-manager must complete administrative functions as well. This dichotomy of roles often becomes overwhelming, causing the nurse to be inadequate in the fulfillment of job expectations.

Some workers feel more secure in the dependent role necessary to functional care. The manager is adept at assigning activities, and workers are comfortable in following orders and in performing repetitive tasks. The more significant issue is that of client care. The functional design is aimed at work production with conservation of workers and cost. Psychological and sociological needs are often overlooked, thus defeating the very purpose of the care system.

Team nursing is a system of care in which a professional nurse leads a group of health care personnel in providing for the health needs of individuals or groups through collaborative and cooperative effort. Team nursing evolved in response to social and technological changes. World War II had drawn many nurses away from hospitals, leaving unfilled gaps. Services, procedures, and equipment had become more extensive and complicated, requiring specialization at every turn. Team nursing developed in the 1950s as an attempt to meet increased demands for nursing services, better utilization of the knowledge and skills of professional nurses, and increased satisfaction to both patient and workers.

Eleanor Lambertsen, with the aid of a Kellogg grant, studied the system of team nursing in a large hospital in New York City.* She concluded that team nursing, if properly utilized, could serve as one answer to the effective utilization of nursing personnel with diversified backgrounds and skills. Other authorities have contributed to the body of knowledge of team nursing. Team nursing has had wider application than any of the other methods described.

Team nursing is based on a philosophy of certain beliefs and values: (1) the worth of every individual, (2) the need for a qualified person to be overall coordinator and interpreter of plans for care, (3) emphasis on equal status with minimal hierarchical lines to separate the leader from followers, and (4) sensitivity and responsiveness to the need for adaptability and change.

Team nursing can be identified by specific characteristics. A nursing team (1) is always led by a nurse licensed to practice, (2) functions wherever there are health needs focusing on the client's total needs, (3) includes the client in the development and implementation of care plans whenever possible, (4) is changeable and adaptable, and (5) recognizes and appropriately utilizes each individual's talents, abilities, and interests to the fullest.

Team nursing is one form of decentralization. The intent is to bring decision making, authority, and accountability to an operational level. This is accomplished by reducing the degree of vertical control held at the top level and by developing increased horizontal communications at lower levels (Fig. 6-4). In this system the team leader can employ any or all patterns of nursing care according to the needs of the patients and the capabilities and desires of the caregivers.

The size of a nursing team depends upon the setting. Quantity and mix of staff needed to assure quality care to a group of clients is determined by the specific group and its nursing needs. In general units of most hospitals a nursing team cares for from ten to twenty clients, with three to five nursing staff members assigned to their care.

A nurse's task is more complex with team nursing than with the functional approach, as more managerial skills are required. The team leader is challenged to include all members of the team in the problem-solving approach according to their abilities. Inherent in the philosophy of team nursing is a belief that all members have the right to be entrusted with responsibility, to be given authority to act, and to be accountable for their actions. At the heart of team

---

*Lambertsen, E.: Nursing team—organizational and functional, New York, 1953, Columbia University Press.

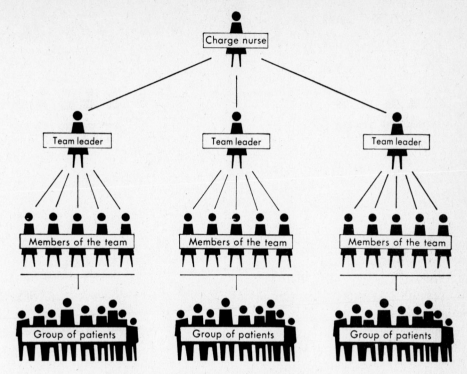

Fig. 6-4. Channels of communication in team nursing.

nursing is the communication system, which is important for providing direction, giving reports of assignments in progress and those completed, focusing on client care, acquiring information, and assessing team relationships. Team nursing has the advantage of involvement of all team members in planning, executing, and evaluating care. When the parts are working satisfactorily this involvement provides job enrichment and job expansion to all workers, especially at lower levels on the team.

Disadvantages of team nursing are viewed from different perspectives. Some believe this method of assignment to be more costly because the overall efficiency of the nursing unit is reduced by fragmented distribution of personnel. Others point to the increased time necessary for several team leaders to perform similar managerial tasks of assessing, delegating, and controlling work groups. The element of error is another factor to consider. There are risks with decentralization of authority, such as the confusion that may occur when several people are receiving orders (for example, from head nurse to team leader to nursing staff members). Also, some nurses may not wish the responsibility of leading a group, preferring a more independent or dependent system.

Primary nursing is decentralization of decision making at the bedside. It

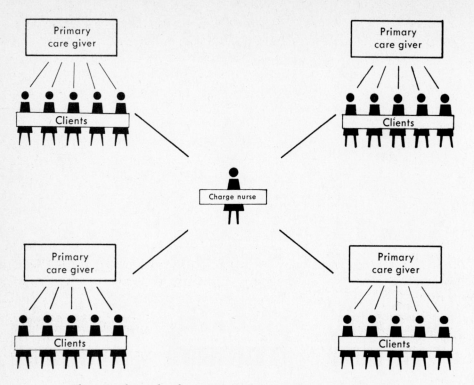

Fig. 6-5. Channels of communication in primary care nursing.

refers to the assessment and care of the individual upon entry to the health care
system. Primary nursing in hospitals is defined as a continuous and coordinated
nursing process in which a primary nurse provides the initial client care assessment and assumes accountability for planning comprehensive twenty-four hour
care for the client for as long as care is needed. The primary nurse has autonomy
and authority to function and is accountable for results. Primary nurses assess
and coordinate care provided by other members of the health care team, make
referrals for follow-up care, and consult with physicians and others to provide
individualized care.

     The primary nurse may provide nursing care services to the patient both
individually and through coordination of care with associates (Fig. 6-5). This is
accomplished through direct communication (on the job or by telephone), nursing care plans, notes, and other records. The primary nurse, physician, and head
nurse control the quality of care the client receives by maintaining an effective
communication system. This system is accomplished through regular meetings
to discuss and agree on the rationale for care, to plan comprehensive care, to
solve problems, and to evaluate and coordinate care. The quality of care depends
on the ongoing nursing care plans, clarity of directions, and the ability of the

primary care nurse. Selection of nurses qualified to function in the primary pattern of care is an important factor to successful achievement of purposes. For greatest results the primary nurse should be a registered professional nurse prepared for the role. Primary nurses are expected to be clinically competent to take nursing histories, to problem solve effectively, and to accept a new role of independence in contracting with clients for planning and providing their comprehensive care.

Primary nursing was begun in the early 1970s and is still in the beginning stage of development. About 10% of health facilities in the nation utilize primary care fully or in part as a system for delivery of nursing care. There are both strengths and limitations to consider. Primary nursing focuses on clients, in knowing their needs and providing increased care and effectiveness. This leads to greater satisfaction on the part of the clients, as they can identify with one nurse who they believe has a vested interest in their welfare. The communication system is improved between clients and nurse, and between nurse and physician or other health team members, since there are fewer channels to go through to get things done. Nurses have the opportunity to utilize their capacities and function as professionals, which may lead to greater satisfaction with hospital nursing and therefore result in less employee turnover. One primary nurse in an oncology unit was overheard to say, "I could never go back to any other system. I just love coming to work and seeing my patients. I know them and they know me. We work things out together—sort of like a family. I care about them and the feeling is mutual."

Disadvantages of primary nursing are related to cost, administrative efficiency, and personnel. Cost becomes an issue wherever primary care nursing is considered since primary nursing requires a major change in the organization of nursing care affecting related personnel and systems within the organization. Some top level administrators, physicians, and nurses feel that the changeover to primary nursing increases costs, while others counter that it can be accomplished without an increase in the budget. Overall administrative efficiency may be reduced with primary nursing, as each nurse's leadership is restricted to a small group of patients (usually three or four). There is also the factor of nurses' preparation for and interest in primary nursing. If inadequacies are present or motivation is lacking, the corresponding behaviors of the nurses may destroy the system.

• • •

All systems designed for the provision of nursing care have strengths and weaknesses that influence achievement of the goals of continuity and comprehensiveness of client care. Factors such as economics, communication, needs of clients, and needs of personnel are to be considered when a system for delivery of nursing care is selected.

Responsibilities of direction giving

There are certain managerial responsibilities common to community general hospitals: (1) *regulatory*, designed to preserve existing arrangements (by far the major type utilized), (2) *corrective*, intended to correct trouble or dysfunction in the system after it has occurred, (3) *preventive*, which anticipates problems and difficulties, and (4) *promotive*, designed to improve the system's ability to achieve. These four types of managerial responsibility are applied by nurses according to the individual situation.

Development of an assignment-making plan may be rational, deliberative, habitual, purposeful, random, or any combination of these, depending on the knowledge, experience, and skill of the delegator. The crux of the delegation process is the issuance of assignments, orders, and instructions that permit the worker to understand what is expected as well as the guidance and monitoring necessary to enable the worker to contribute efficiently and effectively to goal achievement. In the case method, assignments change from shift to shift and often from day to day or week to week and are delegated usually by territory. For example, the nurse is directed to take one patient in room 419 or to care for three patients in rooms 420 and 421. In the functional method, assignments are delegated by the tasks to be completed. For example, one is instructed to make beds and another to pass medications. In the team system, groups are divided by territory, and within that territory assignments are made according to difficulty of patient care and the preparation and the abilities of the nurse often in combination with territory. These assignments also tend to change at least weekly.

Primary nursing has no territory. In this system the caregiver either contracts for or is assigned by a nurse-leader to clients according to the client's needs and wishes and the nurse's abilities, special interests, and specific areas of expertise, as well as according to the individual case load. All care is planned on a twenty-four—hour basis. The nurse works with the client for the duration of his stay in the hospital and sometimes when he returns at some later date. In some agencies, care is continued into the home.

PREDICTIVE PRINCIPLE: The number of workers and span of control depends upon consideration of factors that most affect the work group.

Effective evaluation requires selection of an appropriate number of people for the nurse to lead as well as an appropriate span of management. In certain cases a wider or narrower span can make it more difficult for the nurse to integrate the activities of group members or to integrate their activities with those of other personnel. Following are factors that most affect the numbers of workers and choice of span.

Standards for care adopted by the health care agency. To assure provision of quality care to a specific group of patients, criteria for care are stated in standards and objectives by accrediting agencies. Whatever the circumstances, enough staff needs to be employed so that (1) the needs of the patients are met, (2) all time periods are covered adequately, (3) patient care does not suffer seriously if any member is absent, and (4) enough latitude is allowed for growth and development of the nursing staff.

Number and similarity of patients and functions supervised. The degree to which the care and support services for which the nurse is responsible are alike or different (for example, long-term care versus immediate postsurgical care) must be considered.

Number and mix of nursing personnel and the degree of supervision that group members require. Because of the number of variables associated with provision of care, there is no definitive statement of optimal nurse-client ratio. Delegators have a responsibility to determine the nurse-client ratio they believe necessary for the administration of safe, quality care and then to work for the maintenance of that essential ratio.

Complexity of functions supervised. A good reason for strategic delegation for nurses is that it enables them to prepare for and deal with the complex and rapidly changing environment of the organization. Delegators must make provision for such factors as a shift of clients (dismissals, admissions, transfers) and the complexity of the nursing problems and their resolution (monitors, special procedures, isolation precautions, and schedules such as dietary, operating room, physical therapist, and physicians).

Planning required. Consideration is given to the degree to which the manager must program and review the activities of the subunit involved, such as responsibility for daily, weekly, or monthly schedules, audits of care, evaluation of personnel, budget, and participation in committees.

Coordination. Coordination is the degree to which the nurse must try to integrate functions or tasks within the subunit or between the subunit and other parts of the organization. Examples are dietary, pharmacy, x-ray, recovery room, OT, and PT.

Organizational assistance. The amount of help received by the nurse in terms of assistants and other support personnel influences the delegation function greatly. For example, the nurse who can rely on the head nurse, unit manager, desk clerk, and auxiliary services for assistance can accept a greater span of control than can the nurse who is responsible for all functions affecting the assignment.

Physical support system. Work organization and direction giving are affected by the space, equipment, and physical environment available for support of nursing care. Some facilities are barely adequate, while others have every possible convenience and innovation. Resources range from cramped quarters with simple necessities such as beds, other furniture, linens, and wheelchairs to large, airy, and attractive surroundings filled with modern equipment and automated devices that lift, turn, breathe, move, and monitor almost every bodily function. Installation of computerized equipment influences the delegation process also.

Location and purpose of care provided. In many cases the location and purpose of care provides the answer to staffing size and span of control. A six-bed intensive care unit, a ten-bed recovery room, or a fifteen-bed pediatric area are cases in point. In some general care areas of a hospital, however, the span of management is usually less definitive. For example, a forty-five bed medical unit could have a number of possible spans of control. The unit could be treated as one large entity or could be divided into two, three, or more subunits. One of the care delivery systems or any combination of them could be applied—case, functional, team, or primary care. Smaller groupings have been found to bring the general results in terms of nursing care, with the directional process occurring as near the point of action as possible.

Regardless of the nature of the health care agency or nursing care setting, the intent is to work with prevailing circumstances while working toward adaptations or changes as desired.

PREDICTIVE PRINCIPLE: Formulation of objectives for care that are realistic for the health agency, clients, and nursing personnel assures successful goal accomplishment.

Previous discussions in this text have emphasized the importance of agency, subunits, and nursing personnel managing by objectives, based upon mutually acceptable standards. Guidelines for formulating objectives for care that may apply to a nursing group at the lower or first level include the following:

1. Provide a holistic approach to care that is comprehensive and continuous. The client is the central focus for assessing, planning, implementing, and evaluating care.
2. Initiate and keep current a written nursing care plan that includes physical, emotional, psychosocial, and religious needs and problems, assignment of priorities of care, and alternatives to meet needs for each client.
3. Assign staff to clients according to accepted criteria.
4. Ensure safety of clients.

PREDICTIVE PRINCIPLE: Utilization of nursing care plans provides the mechanism for making nurse assignments according to client needs and the order of priorities.

The nurse is responsible for the care of a number of clients and therefore needs to determine what should be done in order of importance. To achieve the primary goal of nursing the providers of nursing must come to terms with what constitutes quality of care. After nursing standards are accepted by the agency, each nursing department subunit determines how they will be implemented. Nursing care plans offer the best way for assurance of quality care. Assessing needs and problems, deciding how they can be met, controlling the process, and evaluating the results provide the mechanism for adherence to priority.

Through nursing care plans the manager benefits from input of all who have participated in the formation of the plans since the clients' admission: the recipient of care, medical and nursing staff, and supportive services. Having a means for centralizing information (the nursing care plan) offers a definite advantage to the nurse whose time for direction giving is often limited. Nursing care plans constitute the basis for work assignments. The nurse can check through the plans quickly for needs and priorities pertinent to direction giving. The delegator then ranks the needs in order of priority from life-threatening problems to ones of lesser importance and from long-term needs to short-term immediate needs. Through assessment of problems and formulating nursing care plans, priority setting helps the nurse to organize, delegate, direct, and evaluate care with a rational and realistic approach.

PREDICTIVE PRINCIPLE: A systematic planning process enables effective delegation for work implementation.

The nurse-delegator first must know the clients assigned for care and the workers available to provide that care, grasp the nursing situation as a whole, determine what needs to be done, and subdivide the whole into manageable parts. The leader assigns tasks in such a way that cooperation is reciprocal, high standards of performance and conduct are possible, and sound decisions are made.

Effective direction is best carried out by one person for one group. In situations where nursing service is given through a group of personnel with varied preparation and backgrounds, such as a nursing team, the leader is the centralizing force. This leader receives directions from the charge nurse as to the client load, staff appropriation, group responsibilities, and special assignments, and in turn routes these directions to the team or group members for implementation. It is important that the team leader maintain control of activities of the group assigned. Nurse-leaders are the closest professional link between the clients and the caregivers and should be able to determine the most ideal client-staff relationships.

Group members receive instructions from their leader and are accountable to that leader for their enactment. Care providers expect to be given the information needed regarding quantity, quality, and time limits of work. Group members expect the information to tell *what* is to be done, *who* is to do it, *when* and *where* the activity will take place, and when necessary, *how* and *why*. Assignments are expected to be within the workers' skills and abilities, and materials are to be provided necessary to complete the task.

PREDICTIVE PRINCIPLE: Assignment of client care and support services to nursing personnel depends upon the pattern or system of nursing care in force.

Assignment making considers two general categories: provision of client care and support services. Determination of who gives care to whom in nursing depends on the pattern or system of care in effect. The *one-to-one pattern of nursing care* (case or primary care) may be utilized effectively by either the head nurse assigning clients to nurses or by contractual agreement between the nurse and the client. One method for nurse-client assignment in primary nursing is to post new admissions on a blackboard in the nurses' charting room or other secluded area. Information is provided such as diagnosis, age, sex, and attending physician. Primary care nurses have opportunity to investigate the case (visit the client, review the records, collaborate with the physician) before accepting the client as their responsibility. A problem exists when there are no "takers" for a client. In this event it becomes the responsibility of the head nurse to make the assignment and the responsibility of the primary nurse assigned to accept the directive.

Because functional and team nursing are the most commonly used systems, the following discussion will focus primarily upon these; however, principles of effective assignment making and direction giving can be applied to all nursing care delivery situations.

In *functional nursing* the head nurse or charge nurse assigns the work for all nursing personnel in the department or subunit. Work organization and personnel assignment are simplified with a specialty or task-oriented approach. Personnel are programmed into fixed slots of role designation (for example, medication or treatment nurse) or assigned to blocks of rooms for production efficiency. The charge nurse first assigns the RNs or LPNs/LVNs to those tasks that require licensure for fulfillment, as with medications and some treatments. The RN or LPN/LVN may be assigned some desk work or major care to critical patients.

The next step is to assign hygienic care. The client load is divided among the number of remaining staff. For example, if there are forty-five clients in a nursing unit with seven nursing personnel to give hygienic care, three workers would be assigned six clients and three workers would be assigned seven. Usually the division of labor is not exact, necessitating a decision as to which worker should be assigned more and which less. The nursing staff is assigned to rooms primarily by territory; that is, each assignment covers as little space as possible to avoid expenditure of excessive energy and waste of time. Additional general areas of responsibility and times for coffee and lunch breaks are posted at the top of the assignment sheet, with specific room assignments given. Assignments should be posted in a place easily accessible to the staff. Fig. 6-6 provides an illustration of assignments made by a charge nurse for nursing staff appropriated to one department utilizing the functional system.

A fairly rigid plan for assignment making has been presented for study. Note that this task-centered plan considers coverage from the vantage of roles

Nurse	Assignment	Break		Lunch
RN X	Medication nurse	RN X	9:40-10	12-12:30
RN Y	Treatments and	RN Y	10-10:20	12:30-1
	rooms 1 and 3	LPN A	9:40-10	11:30-12
Nursing assistant 2	Treatment room	LPN B	10:10-10:30	12-12:30
Nursing assistant 3	Kitchen	NA 1	9:30-9:50	11:30-12
Nursing assistant 4	2 PM TPRs/BPs	NA 2	9:50-10:10	12-12:30
		NA 3	9:30-9:50	11:30-12
		NA 4	9:30-9:50	12-12:30
		NA 5	9:50-10:10	11:30-12

Nurse	Rm. no.	No. pts./rm.	Nurse	Rm. no.	No. pts./rm.
RN X	1	1	RN Y	2	1
LPN A	3	1	LPN B	4	1
LPN A	5	1	LPN B	6	1
LPN A	7	2	LPN B	8	2
NA 1	9	4	NA 5	10	4
LPN A	11	2	NA 5	12	4
NA 1	13	2	NA 4	14	2
NA 1	15	2	NA 4	16	2
NA 2	17	2	NA 4	18	2
NA 2	19	2	NA 3	20	2
NA 2	21	2	NA 3	22	2
NA 3	23	2			

Fig. 6-6. Sample assignment made by a charge nurse, utilizing the functional system for delivery of nursing care. (From Douglass, L.M.: The effective nurse: leader and manager, St. Louis, 1980, The C.V. Mosby Co.)

(RNs, LPNs, nursing assistants) and geographic location. It attempts to divide the categories of workers as equally as possible, with equal coverage during break times. Registered nurse activities are confined to administration of medications for forty-five patients. The charge nurse considered the RN's work load and assigned to her the administration of treatments and care of two patients, as administering treatment would not require the nurse's full attention. Dividing the number of clients remaining (forty-three) by the number of nursing personnel left to give hygienic care (seven), the nurse-client ratio is 1:6, with one nurse having seven clients. Because circumstances in health care delivery are not fixed, there will be some deviation from the formula, as with the sample provided below. The nurse-client ratio (divide number of clients by number of nursing staff) is as follows:

RN	None	NA 1	1:8
RN	1:2	NA 2	1:6
LPN A	1:6	NA 3	1:6
LPN B	1:4	NA 4	1:6
		NA 5	1:8

The charge nurse begins assignment making with the formula in mind. Then judgment enters in. The delegator rationalizes that clients in private rooms generally have critical needs or special problems that require special competencies or more time than normal. Conversely, when several clients share a room, the care provider is usually able to complete the assignment more quickly. Licensed practical nurse A and nurse assistant 1 have their assignments distributed over a wider territory than do other staff members. The charge nurse wanted the LPN to care for the more critical patients in rooms 3 and 5. If the assignment ended with room 7, the LPN would have had only four patients assigned; if room 9 were added, the load would have increased to eight. Not wishing to place two nurses in a four-bed unit and create unnecessary complications of vying for space and creating confusion as to who was assigned to whom, the choice was made to extend the parameter of the assignment for LPN A and nurse's aide 1. The staff members with lighter client loads are given the support assignments of keeping the kitchen and treatment room in order and taking afternoon vital sign readings.

Attention to individual needs of the clients and workers is possible but more difficult within the functional system than with utilization of a more personalized system. The charge nurse would have less opportunity and time to become aware of the many ramifications significant to a complex nursing situation.

In *team nursing*, rather than the charge nurse making assignments of patients to personnel, each team leader is given the responsibility for that team. Members receive directions from the team leader and are accountable to that leader for their implementation. The major responsibility of a team leader is to provide care to a group of clients, primarily through the work of others. This role of catalyst requires translating the needs of a nursing team into goals and objectives that are realistic, clearly defined, and reflect nursing and agency purposes.

When determining needs the nurse focuses on two major goals: (1) the provision of optimal nursing care for all clients through assessment, problem identification, formulation of plans for nursing action, implementation, and planning for evaluation of care; and (2) the provision of nursing care through an effective management process. Following are certain behavioral objectives the leader of a nursing team can follow to provide coordination and efficiency of service.

1. *Determine the number and characteristics of clients assigned to the nursing team.* This is accomplished by reviewing the orders and nursing care plans; consulting with individual clients, significant others, and physicians; reviewing records and listening to reports from nursing team members as they leave at the end of their shifts. At first this procedure may seem overwhelming to a novice leader, for the amount of data available can blur into meaningless content until the nurse learns to extract the information most relevant to the

Staff member to be assigned	Room no.	Name/physician	Age	Diagnosis	Diet	Activity	TPr Bp	I & O	IVs	Treatments and special meds	Needs and problems
	60	June Kingan / Dr. Jones	22	Tubal occlusion	Reg.	Amb.				Air studine 2 PM	Worried
	62	Laura Cobb / Dr. Fox	48	Sq. cell Ca of Rt. lung, Lt.-6	30° bed rest			I / O Foley		Personal care p.r.n., Irrig Foley 10	Force fl., No nicotine, Psych support
	64	Mrs. Heather / Dr. Fox	66	Cataract @ eye -6	Reg.	Bed rest				Eye shield (R) eye, 20% vision (R) eye	Skin fragile
	66	Roy Snell / Dr. Torre	41	Terminal Ca lung	As tol.	Bed rest, Rails, Lt. bd.		I / O		Maintain airway, Cough suction q.h., Turn q. 2 h.	No code, Fail, Encourage family
	68a	Mr. Fletcher / Dr. Able	71	Buerger's disease	Salt free 1000 cal.	Bed rest		I / O		Pedal pulse 10-2, Soak left... 10, Brian exercises 10-2	Toes necrosal, V for pain/med, Depressed, O'Bear, Needs help to turn
	68b	Jem Vargas / Dr. Kent	55	Aortic bypass graft -14	Lo fat	Bed rest		I / O	5% D.W. c̄ KCl 100 cc q h #3 Tube 300	Encour. fl., On Valium	
	70a	Elaine Motz / Dr. Barton	68	Ca colon	Lo fiber Kosher	Amb. Prep					Colostomy tomorrow, Pre-op teaching, Vrs refl.
	70b	Lela Smith / Dr. Salt	71	Gastric ulcer	Soft Force fl.	Amb.		I / O			Hard of hearing

Fig. 6-7. Sample of a partially completed worksheet used by a nurse leader to record pertinent information about patients on a nursing team in preparation for assignment making and for reference during guidance of team activities. (Adapted from Douglass, L.M.: The effective nurse: leader and manager, St. Louis, 1980, The C.V. Mosby Co.)

situation. An experienced nurse soon learns to accomplish this task quickly and well. A worksheet for this purpose is suggested in sorting information. Color coding priority activities helps the nurse to see them at a glance when making assignments. Fig. 6-7 offers a portion of one such worksheet that may be used by a team leader.

2. *Assess priority of care for all clients*, beginning with those who need the greatest amount of care to those who need the least. Establishing needs in order of priority serves as an indicator for action. Each need is considered as to its importance to the client and to the nursing work group using the criteria of (1) preservation of life, dignity, and integrity, (2) avoidance of destructive changes, and (3) continuance of normal growth and development.* The delegator can use distinguishing marks such as an X or * beside the client's name to indicate immediate or special attention. The team leader will scan a worksheet quickly and note the need for special tests and procedures and their specific times, such as reverse isolation or isolation technique, intravenous fluids, planning around routing of patients to other departments for special services, blood transfusions or lipids infusion, etc. The assigner will assess the number of total care clients, those who require intermediate help, and those who are fairly independent. Attention will be given to psychologic, sociologic, and spiritual needs that may be of highest priority with some clients.

3. *Review available staff and consider their roles, competencies, and preferences.* Delegation of roles and tasks is simplified if the nursing staff is comprised of all licensed personnel. However, many health agencies utilize the services of technical or semiskilled workers, such as nursing assistants. Ideally, team leaders participate in selection of all staff who serve on the nursing team, and, with time and attention, the team leader can become well acquainted with the nursing staff. Preparation and experience are weighed against the responsibilities of the assignment. Individual preferences are taken into account as much as possible. The team leader keeps in mind the matter of licensure requirements for activities such as administering medications, monitoring IVs, and certain treatments.

4. *Assign patients who require the most skilled attention to the most qualified staff members.* A major goal in assignment making is to divide the total load into a number of activities that can logically and comfortably be performed by one person. People cannot be assigned tasks for which they are not suited, nor should they carry too heavy or too light a work load. Too heavy a work load could mean the job would not be completed well or on time, while too light a work load could result in idle time and inefficiency. The philosophy of team nursing subscribes to "team" effort, of one helping the other to achieve

---

*Bower, F.: The process of planning nursing care, a model for practice, ed. 2, St. Louis, 1982, The C.V. Mosby Co.

common goals. While it is expected that underassigned personnel will help the overassigned members, problems are created that could be averted with careful preplanning.

The team leader may need to assume responsibility for administering medications and monitoring intravenous fluids. Assigning the leader to these activities provides additional opportunity for moving among the clients and nursing staff. Clients who need treatments that require licensed personnel may be assigned to a licensed member for care, or the team leader may assign the hygienic care to another person, if it is believed that the licensed member is needed more elsewhere. The leader attempts to match the greatest need with the team member most prepared to meet that need; then this same member is assigned to patients nearby in consideration of the geographic and physical setting. This system calls for some compromises in matching abilities of staff members to the needs of clients. If the criteria for assignment making were followed exactly, staff assignments might consist of one patient at the far end of a hall, two in the middle, and three on a side, with two or more staff members providing care in one room. Fragmented assignments are at odds with criteria for providing quality care and run the risk of client hostility because adequate attention is not given. In turn, the team member becomes overly tired because of confusion and unnecessary activity.

Some delegators advocate that the nurse leader administer care to the most acutely ill patient on the team, or that the leader care for the one who requires the most complex nursing care. Rationale for this suggestion is that the team leader is the most qualified for the task and the client will derive the greatest benefit from the leader's services. Also, the leader will be serving as a role model to the team members. When team functioning is viewed realistically, it becomes apparent that if the leader is assigned to an area that requires undivided attention, it then becomes impossible to fulfill other team commitments. A compromise in delegation of activities is suggested. The client with high priority needs is assigned to a qualified member of the team who has less skill than the team leader, and the team leader assists with the care at those times when special expertise is required. The nurse-leader is then available to the client needing special care as well as to all the others assigned to the team.

5. *Double-assign a client or groups of clients* if it is anticipated that assistance with care will be needed. Sometimes provision of care for a client requires help from more than one person (lifting, turning, treatments, and so on). If possible, the member who is working in an adjoining room or adjacent area is given the double assignment so that he or she is easily accessible and can provide the necessary help with minimal loss of time and energy.

6. *Note coverage for breaks from the work scene.* Times are coordinated for coffee breaks, meals, and conferences to ensure continued supervision and care

Date: _____
Charge nurse: _____

Team A

	AM break	Lunch	Conferences	Special assignment
RNT ldr: Marge Singer	9:45-10:05	12-12:30	7:30-7:50 2:00-2:30	
LPN: Ruth Telfer	9:30-9:50	11:30-12		
NA 1: Jean Rass	9:30-9:50	11:30-12		Kitchen NA 1
NA 2: Tam Spivey	9:50-10:10	12-12:30		Rx room

Meds _____ Rxs _____ Other _____

Assignment	Room no.	Patient	Diagnosis
	61		
	63		
	65		
	67		
	69a		
	69b		
	71a		
	71b		
	73a		
	73b		
	75a		
	75b		
	77a		
	77b		
	79a		
	79b		
	79c		
	79d		

Team B

	AM break	Lunch	Conferences	Special assignment
RNT ldr: Cleo Hastings	10:05-10:25	12:30-1:00	7:50-8:10 2:30-3:00	
LPN: Bea Kindall	9:30-9:50	12-12:30		
NA 1: Vici Wilson	9:50-10:10	11:30-12		Kitchen
NA 2: Linda Grace	10-10:20	12-12:30		Rx room NA 2

Meds _____ Rxs _____ Other _____

Assignment	Room no.	Patient	Diagnosis
RN	60	June Kerzan	Tube Occu.
LPN	62	Laura Cobb	Ca Cx
LPN	64	Mrs. Heather	Cat. (L)eye
LPN/NA 1	66	Roy Snell	Ca Lung
LPN/NA 1	68a	Mr. Fletcher	Buerger's
LPN	68b	Lem Vargas	Aortic ByPass Graft
NA 1	70a	Elaine Metz	Ca Colon
NA 1	70b	Lela Smith	Pneumonia
NA 1	72a	Reva Farrell	Mastectomy (R)
NA 1	72b	Barb Brink	Cholecystomy
NA 2	74a	Terry Erbb	Prostatectomy
NA 2	74b	John Baker	CHD
NA 2	76a	Angela Castro	Bunionectomy/Diabetes
NA 2	76b	Terry Meltzer	Hysterectomy
NA 2	78a	Bob Perry	Fx (L) Leg
NA 2	78b	Sam Frieson	x-rays BL Studies
NA 2	78c	David Cooper	Laminectomy
NA 2	78d	Larry Berg	Duodenal ulcer

Fig. 6-8. Sample assignment sheet for a nursing unit comprised of two nursing teams, indicating patient assignment for team B and cooperative assignments for breaks and other activities. (From Douglass, L.M.: The effective nurse: leader and manager, St. Louis, 1980, The C.V. Mosby Co.)

by qualified personnel. For example, there must be continuous coverage by a registered nurse, and each team should have equal staff coverage as much as possible. Planning with other team leaders and perhaps with the head nurse is necessary to see that adequate personnel are available to all teams continuously. Arrangements such as these take the leader's time, especially in a complex setting, but in the end staff time will be conserved, team functioning will be smoother, and patients will receive the necessary constant supervision.

In addition to patient care assignment, many health facilities expect nursing personnel to perform supportive services, such as keeping the unit in order, maintaining the kitchen and utility room, straightening linen closets, transporting patients, and prepared vacated rooms for new admissions. The requirements for this kind of ancillary service usually depend on the size of the hospital and the availability and distribution of personnel. It is certainly recommended that the nurses' time not be spent in these activities. Large hospitals and other health facilities usually maintain a separate staff for housekeeping duties and another for distributing supplies. Also, most hospitals have auxiliary groups who perform varied services such as caring for flowers, transporting patients, and running errands. Fig. 6-8 gives an example of an assignment of nursing personnel utilizing the team system to deliver nursing care to clients.

Fig. 6-8 demonstrates that major purposes of assignment making in team nursing have been carried out. At the top of the sheet is the name and role of each staff member, along with times for breaks. Continuous coverage for each team is provided, as well as assuring RN coverage for alternate teams for break, lunch, and conference times. Supportive services are assigned, with sharing of duties between teams. These responsibilities will be rotated between teams from week to week. The clients are not divided equally among the nursing staff, as consideration was given to established criteria. The RN will assume responsibility for medications and care of patient Kirzan in room 60. The patient is near the nurses' station, needs minimal nursing care, yet has need for teaching and emotional support. The LPN is assigned treatments and the care of the most critical patients, with assistance provided for care of patients Snell and Fletcher. Nursing assistant 2 has a greater number of patients, but the total work load is considered equitable. All workers are kept in as close proximity as possible. The team leader will be circulating during the shift to make observations and adjustments as necessary.

PREDICTIVE PRINCIPLE: Consideration of safety factors and instructions regarding emergency situations prepare nursing staff to employ preventive measures and to cope with emergency situations.

Each health care facility is required to meet minimal safety regulations established by law, as well as those adopted by the agency to meet its unique needs. The nurse learns of these regulations during job orientation, and assumes responsibility to assess at regular intervals each member's understanding of safety regulations should a fire, earthquake, tornado, or other disaster occur. Handling equipment, using proper procedures, and working with dangerous drugs require reinforcement, as unused knowledge and skills are quickly forgotten.

There are always some uncertainties in the nursing scene. This is particularly true in acute treatment areas, but no unit is exempt from crisis situations. Anything can happen such as an accident, hemorrhage, extreme reaction to a medication or treatment, or cardiac arrest. It is extremely important for the nursing staff members to know that *in times of emergency, autocratic rule prevails.* The nurse in charge (head nurse, team leader, or primary nurse) assumes command of the situation, directing activities until the crisis is past. If not available, the next best qualified person takes over. Other staff members are to remain in their assigned areas, ready to respond for service as needed. Excited personnel do little to alleviate already tense situations in patient care areas.

Members of the nursing staff need to know in advance what their responsibilities are in case of emergency. Specific instructions are given at regular intervals in conferences and in special sessions, such as fire and disaster drills. In times of emergency, the staff member present at the time of emergency calls for help by means of the intercommunication system. If there is no other way to get assistance, another person can be sent for aid, or the staff member can simply call out for help. In the meantime, that staff member will begin emergency measures as appropriate according to protocol and capability, especially where a life may be threatened for lack of action.

PREDICTIVE PRINCIPLE: The delegator's availability to staff members results in assistance, teaching, counsel, and evaluation where necessary.

The process of overseeing nursing activities requires the presence of the nurse in the area of action. For a leader, being available means being accessible and of some value to the situation. The leader is to be ready and willing to provide assistance whenever necessary, to delegate the needed help to another, to teach a procedure, to relay knowledge, to supervise a nursing function about which a member feels insecure, to offer advice with client or staff problems, and to evaluate the member's performance. It is for these reasons that the leader's personal assignment should be restricted to activities that will permit being in the mainstream of activity, such as administering medications or giving treatments.

PREDICTIVE PRINCIPLE: Centralized control of incidental task requests prevents maldistribution of work loads.

All tasks that require much time and have not already been delegated, such as incidental requests from physicians, special technicians, and other staff members, should be channeled through the charge nurse or team leader as appropriate for distribution. The practice of centralized control of these incidental requests by lower or first level managers (1) identifies a single channel for command to staff members, (2) keeps the nurse leader informed of all activities, (3) allows for allocation of tasks to the most capable or available person, and (4) protects the membership from excessive demands on their time and energy. A physician who asks a "favorite nurse" to assist with an extensive treatment for a client not assigned to that member provides an example of the disruption in completion of assignment that could occur if the nurse were to comply with the request without consulting with the charge nurse or team leader for response.

PREDICTIVE PRINCIPLE: A balance between variety and continuity of assignment increases motivation and productivity.

Ideally, a member should be given the same client assignment at least from one day off until the next. Studies show that assigning primary responsibility to a caregiver for the duration of the client's stay is more rewarding to the client and the nurse and ensures the client of better care, since there is more opportunity to know the person and to administer quality care on a continuous basis. The only times the client-nurse relationship should be broken are when the nurse and client have some basic inability to get along, when the caregiver cannot meet the client's needs, or when the nurse has time off. Consistency with assignment allows the worker time to become familiar with the clients and members of the nursing staff. It is well to rotate members from one geographic setting to another to ensure continued flexibility within the department. Occasionally, delegators receive requests from members to remain with the same group or in the same location for long periods of time with such statements as "I'm more comfortable on the east side," or "I work better with Miss Judd and Mrs. Sampson." Astute leaders will recognize participants' emotional needs but will work with the members to help them understand and accept the rationale of assignments.

Tasks assigned to members are best completed if they are palatable and stimulating. "The work isn't hard," one nurse's aide observed, "it's the never-ending monotony of the job." Routinization is often favored in an effort to facilitate getting the job done and to conserve expense. But too much sameness reduces the degree to which an individual can participate in the organizational affairs of the work and often prevents the worker from completing a task that is meaningful. A nurse assigned to giving preoperative medications day after day and week after week will lose the opportunity to experience the broader implications of nursing care.

If the delegator varies the member's assignments over a period of time to include the total spectrum of care, the members will grow and develop the ability to employ diverse physical, cognitive, and interpersonal skills. In addition, a limited assignment is not economically beneficial to an agency because the employee's training and potential are not being realized.

PREDICTIVE PRINCIPLE: Consideration for each caregiver's preferences and areas of expertise influences morale.

Giving thought to members' choices of one assignment over another fosters job satisfaction. Nothing makes a person feel as good about himself as being successful; one way to ensure success is to delegate assignments according to the caregiver's preferences and expertise, matching these with the needs of the client. Factors that have a bearing on the caregiver's preference of assignment include (1) physical characteristics of the job (such as the extent of walking, lifting, and standing) and the type of physical activity involved (such as hygienic care or working with specialized equipment), (2) the degree of independence permitted, (3) the fairness with which the member feels he or she is being treated, (4) whether the worker has had a part in policy and procedure making, (5) individual commitment to the decisions, and (6) the degree to which the assignment interests the worker.

Information concerning preferences should be acquired in a professional and systematic manner to ensure each member equal consideration. The leader can learn the desires of employees through observation, conferences, and evaluation. Knowledge of a worker's preference for a task does not imply that the member will be given priority. It may be that two or more members wish the same assignment, or an individual may express a desire to engage in work he or she is incapable of performing. Others may request assignments in which they excel, not wishing to extend their experience beyond what they know to be satisfying. The leader will consider the wishes of all members and make assignments in the best interests of client, staff, and agency.

PREDICTIVE PRINCIPLE: Centralization of information storage and retrieval systems allows for efficient assessment, delegation, and implementation of tasks.

The caregiver is in a key position to obtain and store information concerning the client. A variety of sources are tapped for information. Records, reports, orders, and messages—both written and verbal—provide input for processing information. People are not as efficient or as effective with storage and retrieval of information as are machines. For this reason, many nursing units are incorporating mechanical devices to facilitate the caregiving process. The cassette tape recorder is one medium widely used for transcribing messages and activities. Individual caregivers condense their reports to pertinent issues and record them as they have time. The nurse or group coming to the work scene listens to the tape while the worker or group going off completes the assignment. If there is need for clarification or additional information, reporting personnel are accessible for dialogue. New persons who need filling in on details seek out the caregiver after reading the client's record.

Computers are a major mode of storing information centrally. These are in operation in many health agencies and will become a common adjunct to most nursing arenas within the next few years. An individual can feed the client's data into the system and can receive whatever information concerning the client that is needed to facilitate the practice of nursing.

PREDICTIVE PRINCIPLE: Clear and concise directions enhance task delegation.

Assignments for caregivers should be both written and verbal. Definite plans should be devised to impart information. Staff members need to know such specifics as whom they will be caring for, where the patients are located, special tasks, coffee and lunch breaks, and any additional commitment. Assignments should be posted in an area easily accessible to staff members early enough to allow the personnel time to arrange individual schedules. Verbal directions can be given through prerecordings, on a one-to-one basis, or in a conference held early in the work period.

Members function better when they know the extent of their assignment. Managers who withhold part of the work assignment to spare the worker the pain of hearing a large assignment or who believe that delegating a task little by little is better than making one large assignment are operating on false assumptions. People who know what the work load for the day is tend to make the best use of their time.

Direction-giving conference

After the change of shift report has been heard and the worksheet prepared, the leader gathers those members who will be working together for a direction-giving conference. This is a time when the leader meets with the entire nursing group for fifteen or twenty minutes in a quiet, undisturbed environment to apprise the members more fully of their assignments for the day. These assignments have been posted as quickly as possible after coming on duty to allow staff members to begin the rudiments of their work while waiting for more specific instructions. Members of an alternate nursing team or group will cover for these members during their conference, as designated on the assignment sheet. The direction-giving conference is dominated primarily by the leader giving instructions to the group in preparation for the completion of individual and group assignments. Time is limited for this purpose; therefore the delegator must impart the necessary information to the members quickly and well so that understanding occurs concerning individual and group assignment. Following are guidelines the leader may follow to ensure a successful direction-giving conference:

1. Prepare thoroughly before meeting with the nursing personnel. Prepare a detailed worksheet that:
   a. contains all known pertinent information
   b. indicates areas of priority, special concerns, and need for additional information
   c. allows space for updating data as necessary (see Fig. 6-7)
2. Receive report from those workers who have had prior responsibility

for client services and update the worksheet (these reports may be incidental comments from nurses who are present and who are now assigned to a different team).

3. Check for pertinent data, such as tests, preoperative orders, and special treatments, or confer with head nurse or physician as needed; update worksheet.

4. Visit all clients briefly for individual assessment; make necessary notations on worksheet.

Conducting successful direction-giving conferences depends on accuracy, completeness of information, and conservation of time. The following guidelines work well for most direction-giving sessions:

1. *Keep to the same time schedule for at least a week at a time if possible.* Begin and end the meeting according to schedule. This plan provides for continuity of the work forces and gives all members opportunity to develop a routine.

2. *Select all members to provide for comfort and to encourage recording of information on individual worksheets.*

3. *Introduce self and group members to one another as needed.* Composition of nursing groups changes frequently in some settings, and giving names and role identification in a warm, friendly atmosphere promotes group morale and facilitates comprehension.

4. *Ask that each member record relevant information pertaining to all clients assigned to the nursing group*, not just that pertaining to individual assignments, to allow for informed coverage for one another. It is very helpful to have worksheets containing basic information (name, age, diagnosis, physician, diet, and activity) ready for nursing personnel when they report for duty. These sheets may be prepared by computer services or by clerical staff on the previous shift. Having basic information available reduces the amount of time spent in recording and enables the members to listen better and to clarify directions, thus reducing the high possibility of error when many people transcribe directions at one time.

5. *Use the procedure and pace that are right for the purpose and membership,* using direct, simple language. The more accurately words and phrases are tailored to the level of the receivers, the more effective the communication is likely to be. A certain amount of redundancy may be necessary in direction giving. If a message is very important or complicated, it is probably necessary to repeat it in a different way, possibly by adding the reason for the procedure. Unnecessary redundancy should be avoided because it will simply dull the receiver's attention. The direction giver should speak clearly, adjusting the pace to the receiver's preference and needs, allowing accurate recording of necessary information. Directions should proceed systematically. For example, it is most effective to offer information according to the format of the worksheet—name, age, physician, diagnosis, diet, activity, intake and output,

and so on—with instructions and explanations given after each item as needed. Irregularity in presentation increases the time spent in recording and also increases the probability of transcribing misinformation.

6. *Include all information necessary for individual and group members to hear.* The direction giver does not need to repeat all information already known or provided on the worksheet, as the time is better spent in reviewing items that require reinforcement or elaboration. Documented and well-written nursing care plans provide detailed information as to who, what, when, where, and how. However, enough information should be included to help the group understand what is needed in order to function together with purpose and harmony.

7. *Use feedback, looking for verbal and nonverbal cues from receivers.* The more complex the information, the more essential that receivers be encouraged to ask questions and indicate areas of confusion. For example, the direction-giving process breaks down when the delegator instructs, "Give Buerger's exercises to Mr. Fletcher for 15 minutes at 10 and 2," but the caregiver fails to follow through correctly for lack of understanding. Because of time limitations or lack of relevance to the total group, the leader may note the areas where clarification is needed and attend to these matters individually.

8. *Leave group members with the belief that the leader is available to them for assistance,* which allows the members to approach uncertainties about their assignments with assurance that support and help will be forthcoming if needed.

Informal direction giving by the delegator for clients assigned to the group is necessary from time to time. As the delivery of nursing care proceeds, matters arise that may not have been anticipated in time for the direction-giving conference, or they may simply have been overlooked. Nursing staff members should expect some interruptions in completion of assignments. The point to remember is, as far as possible, to give additional tasks to the staff member assigned to the area in which the action is to occur. For example, if a new treatment is ordered, the nurse assigned to care for the client will be asked to administer it, or if a client needs more assistance than one nurse can provide and there is no double coverage assigned to that client, the leader will ask the nurse nearest to that locale to provide assistance, keeping in mind other factors of assignment making, such as over- and underassignment.

Measuring results

Delegation enables one to assign roles, functions, duties, and authority to carry out those roles, functions, and duties. Responsibility can never be delegated; only roles, functions, duties, and authority can be delegated. Responsibility always remains with the delegator. This is why the art of delegation is so crucial to the art of management and leadership. It is in the quality of the decisions made around delegating work that one finds the seeds of success and failure of the enterprise. Evaluation, then, becomes a crucial element in the process of delegation. It is through evaluation that the manager determines whether or not the job was done according to specifications, carried out effectively, and implemented with the greatest possible comfort to the client. The manager attempts to evaluate both the process of doing the job and the product of the job itself. In other words, the evaluation process looks at both the process and the product in order to determine success or failure.

Process evaluation examines the plan itself and how that plan is carried out. Factors examined include the following:

1. Clarity of objectives, time limitations, and availability and use of the equipment
2. Organization of workers in performing jobs with efficiency and effectiveness
3. Degree of actualization of nursing care plans
4. Degree of inconvenience to clients or other workers
5. Compliance with safety rules and regulations
6. Use of skillful interpersonal communications
7. Performance of psychomotor skills

There are many other factors that could be considered in the process of delivering client care. These are but a few to provide the evaluator some indications about the process.

Product evaluation is looking at the consequences—the end product of the work. The evaluator goes into a unit, a home, or a nursing area and looks at the finished product. Is the client's bed made properly? Does the room look neat and clean? Is the client resting comfortably? Is the client safe? Is the environment arranged in the proper way? Is all the equipment restored to its proper place? Product evaluation looks only at the consequences, not at the process.

There are many sources of data for the evaluator. The evaluator may seek data as (1) from personal observations; (2) from clients' observations, feelings, and perceptions; and (3) from key others, for example, family, physicians, supervisors, and other health care providers. The more varied the sources of data for the evaluator, the more accurate the evaluation results are likely to be.

One cannot discuss assessment of goal achievement without speaking of mastery of the goal. In some instances, there is room for degree of accomplishment, as in the process of bed making, in learning an unsterile technique, or in various levels of communication. At other times no latitude can be allowed. Any break in sterile technique is untenable. Inappropriate counsel or action in crisis intervention may lead to disaster. The leader builds into the criteria all the contingencies necessary for desired practice and assesses outcomes accordingly. With a clear delineation in the nurse's role the leader can become the facilitator, validator, collaborator, resource person, and consultant. In this way the leader applies managerial skills largely to direct client care and is interested in that care and in the growing ability of people to provide such service rather than only using these skills to meet the logistical requirements of management. However, the leader retains the ability and authority to delegate those logistics to another person because logistics and direct client care are interwoven and influence each other.

Some leaders believe they must check personally on all details of an assignment if control of assignment is to be maintained. This autocratic manager feels confident only when he or she has witnessed the completion of all directions. Such restrictive measures usually result in (1) employee expectation of close supervision; (2) generation of subservient feelings; (3) exhibition of routine, compliant behavior patterns; and (4) lack of assumption of responsibility for the worker's own actions.

The effective leader will find it not only impossible but also undesirable to review all aspects of performance and consequently must select certain critical points that will provide an adequate indication of what is going on. In developing the checking process the leader must consider expenditure of time as well as employee reaction to the evaluative process.

In nursing operation the leader assumes responsibility for the overall functions but in the process of assignment making will delegate the duty of checking certain functions to caregivers capable of assuming the role. Responsibility for review of progress can be on an individual basis or may be extended to several members. For example, an experienced member may be given four patients to care for on a primary care basis. The member learns the major needs of the patients and is given freedom to devise the care plan and schedule for the day.

Another avenue of sharing responsibility for measurement of results is through group effort. The leader, for instance, may have been informed by group members of a belief that there is wasted effort in each worker's having to interrupt individual client assignment to run errands, such as transporting clients, calling for late trays, and locating special pieces of equipment. The delegator could request all caregivers to engage in a measuring procedure over a specific period of time to learn who was interrupted, for what purpose, and how frequently. The group could then study the results of the survey to develop a design for greater efficiency.

PREDICTIVE PRINCIPLE: Frequent evaluation of performance using criteria influences the quality of care and the level of actual performance of care activities.

Accurate identification and documentation of behaviors of caregivers is difficult. The problem of measurement of clinical competence is compounded because of (1) the variety of clinical problems encountered by the nurse, (2) the number of methods employed to deal with those problems, (3) the paucity of significant and useful research to validate the use of one methodology over another, (4) the difficulty of directly observing all activities, and (5) the tendency on the part of individuals to describe behavior through perceptions that vary greatly from individual to individual.

Evaluation that is left to be done until the end is always product evaluation and process evaluation by hearsay. Evaluation at the end does have value both for the manager and delegatee. However, its value is minimal when compared with frequent evaluations that take place during the process combined with evaluation at the end that views the end product. Frequent evaluation during actual performance of tasks enables the manager to provide supervision, teaching, and help to the worker so that corrections can be made during instead of after the activity. Evaluation after the activity can be costly in time, because a worker who is proceeding incorrectly can complete a whole series of tasks that must be redone.

Use of performance criteria enables a manager to determine with accuracy the level of skill being employed by a worker. Performance criteria can be highly specific or fairly general. In working with people who are lower level personnel, for example nurse's aides, orderlies, or other nonprofessional personnel, highly specific criteria are helpful both to the evaluator and to the person being evaluated. An example of this is the evaluation of an aide's ability to wrap an elastic bandage. A list of criteria for the safe wrapping of the bandage on a leg could provide points such as the following:

1. Tension is placed on the bandage
2. Bandage is wrinkle-free
3. Below-the-knee wrap terminates three fingers below the bend of the knee to prevent compression of the popliteal vein
4. Metal clips holding the end of the bandage are terminated on the shin or the outer lateral portion of the calf, not on the inner aspect or posterior section of the calf

A checklist of points such as these comprising highly specific criteria enables the manager to know how safe or unsafe a caregiver is. Other criteria, such as gathering all the equipment before a procedure, leaving the area neat and clean, providing comfort for the client during the procedure, and maintaining quality interpersonal relationships during the procedure, enable the manager to provide specific feedback to workers for both process and product.

Application of predictive principles in the delegation of assignments and authority

As the nurse-leader, you are responsible for planning and directing the work being done on the unit. You have made the work assignments for the day, and an LVN comes to you with the following statement: "I have had the same assignment for three weeks and I am tired of it. I would like to learn how to assist with the debridement of burns."

Problem	*Predictive principles*	*Prescription*
The LVN is dissatisfied with the work assignment and wishes to increase in knowledge and skills.	The delegator's availability to staff members results in assistance, teaching, counsel, and evaluations where necessary.	Encourage LVN to express feelings by listening and giving encouraging motions and words.
	Understanding the categories and roles of nursing personnel enables the delegator to select the type and number of personnel appropriate for the job.	Confirm with LVN that request is legitimate and that the assignment for the day will be unchanged but that plans will be made for change.
	A balance between variety and continuity of assignment increases motivation and productivity.	
	Written descriptions of policies, procedures, and guidelines by which an employee may handle situations promote ease of operation for the caregiver and control of the authority delegated by the nurse.	Help LVN locate material and resources that will prepare her for the learning episode, for example, procedure manual, books, other nurses.
	Consideration for each caregiver's preferences and areas of expertise influences morale.	Schedule LVN to assist in the care of a burn patient. Arrange for double coverage until LVN is competent.
	Clear and concise directions enhance task delegation.	Inform LVN when and with whom she will be working.
		Trust LVN to fulfill responsibilities.
	Frequent evaluation of performance using criteria influences the quality of care and the level of actual performance of care activities.	Observe procedure periodically and at strategic times. Obtain feedback from patient, nurse-teacher, physician, and LVN.
	Consideration for each caregiver's preferences and areas of expertise influences morale.	Be observant for other interests and expertise of LVN. Build into future assignments opportunities for variation.

BIBLIOGRAPHY
Books

Argyris, C.: Management and organizational development, New York, 1971, McGraw-Hill Book Co.

Berne, E.: Structure and dynamics of organizations and groups, Philadelphia, 1963, J.B. Lippincott Co.

Bower, F.: The process of planning nursing care, a model for practice, ed. 2, St. Louis, 1982, The C.V. Mosby Co.

Bullough, B., and Bullough, V.: Expanding horizons for nurses, New York, 1977, The Macmillan Publishing Co.

Douglass, L.: The effective nurse: leader and manager, St. Louis, 1980, The C.V. Mosby Co.

Ganong, J., and Ganong, W.: Nursing management: concepts, functions, techniques and skills, Germantown, Md., 1976, Aspen Systems Corp.

Glueck, W.: Management, Hinsdale, Ill., 1977, The Drysden Press.

Marram, G., Schlegel, M., and Bevis, E.: Primary nursing: a model for individualized care, St. Louis, 1974, The C.V. Mosby Co.

Stoner, A.: Management, Englewood Cliffs, N.J., 1978, Prentice-Hall, Inc.

Periodicals

Brown, J., and Kanter, R.: Empowerment—key to effectiveness, Hosp. Forum **25**(3):6-14, May-June 1982.

Bullough, B.: Nurse practice acts: how they affect your expanding role, Nursing '77 **7**(2):73-81, 1977.

Chinn, P. (editor): Accountability in practice, Adv. Nurs. Sci. **4**(2):1-94, Jan. 1982.

Chopra, A.: Motivation in task oriented groups, J. Nurs. Admin. **5**(2-3):55-60, 1973.

Ciske, K.: Accountability—the essence of primary nursing, Am. J. Nurs. **79**(5):891-894, 1979.

Department of Health, Education and Welfare, Secretary's Committee to Study Extended Roles for Nurses: Extending the scope of nursing practice, Nurs. Outlook **20**(1):46-52, 1972.

Fair, E.: Be sure they're listening, Superv. Nurse **11**(7):26-28, 1980.

Manthey, M.: A theoretical framework for primary nursing, J. Nurs. Admin. **10**(6):11-15, 1980.

Martin, R.: Identifying problems in the motivation, performance, and retention of nursing staff, publ. no. 52-1802, New York, 1979, The National League for Nursing.

McCarthy, M.: Managing your own time: the most important task, J. Nurs. Admin. **11**(11,12):61-65, 1981.

McConnell, E.: What kind of delegator are you? Nursing '78 **8**(10):105-111, 1978.

Millis, J.: Primary care: definition of, and access to, Nurs. Outlook **25**:443-444, 1977.

Monanco, R., and Smith, T.: How supervisors can put systems to work in day-to-day management, Hosp. Topics, Sept.-Oct. 1977, pp. 36-41.

National League for Nursing: Competencies of graduates of educational programs in practical nursing, publ. no. 38-1686, New York, 1977, The League.

National League for Nursing: Role and competencies of diploma programs in nursing, publ. no. 16-1735, 06-78-5M, New York, 1978, The League.

National League for Nursing, Council of Associate Degree Program, Task Force on Licensing: Task force report on licensing, New York, March 1976, The League.

National League for Nursing, Division of Associate Degree Programs: Competencies of the associate degree nurse on entry into practice, publ. no. 23-1731, 05-78-5M, New York, 1978, The League.

National League for Nursing, Council of Baccalaureate and Higher Degree Programs: Characteristics of baccalaureate education in nursing, New York, Nov. 1978, The League.

Scully, R.: Staff support groups: helping nurses to help themselves, J. Nurs. Admin. **11**(3):48-51, 1981.

Stevens, B.: Improving nurses' managerial skills, Nurs. Outlook **27**(12):774-777, 1979.

Swartz, E., and Mackenzie, R.: Time-management strategy for women, J. Nurs. Admin. **9**(3):22-26, 1979.

Trandel-Korenchuk, D., and Trandel-Korenchuk, K.: How state laws recognize advanced nursing practice, Nurs. Outlook **26**(11):713-727, 1978.

chapter seven

Predictive principles for evaluation of nursing personnel

Legal responsibilities

Conceptual framework for evaluation

Commitment of all concerned

> Involvement of personnel in all phases of the evaluative process increases belief in the fairness and accuracy of the evaluation, establishes a commitment to the evaluation, and increases motivation to utilize the results.

Standards of practice and criteria of evaluation

> Clear and concise role delineation and job descriptions enable employee, employer, and client to know the duties and responsibilities of the job.
>
> Clear standards and criteria for measuring performance increase the objectivity and validity of evaluation.
>
> Use of appropriate assessment tools and sufficient evaluative data gathered from varied situations increases the validity of the conclusions in the assessment of work performance.
>
> Use of the self-evaluation process promotes growth and development of the appraiser and contributes to better quality of care.
>
> A limited number of incidental observations jeopardizes the accuracy of evaluations.
>
> Informal and formal assessments that are noted and recorded systematically provide significant input to the evaluation process.
>
> Valid interpretation of data depends on fair evaluation of input.
>
> The evaluator who establishes mutual trust and confidence with the person evaluated and who is familiar with the criteria of evaluation increases the accuracy and usefulness of the evaluation.
>
> The degree to which the value systems of the evaluator and the person evaluated coincide influences their interpersonal relationships and directly affects the evaluation process.
>
> Use of evaluative information serves both incidental and formal purposes.

Performance review session

A well-planned performance review session increases the worker's effectiveness and promotes satisfaction.

Self-improvement strategies and coaching by management leads to improvement of worker competence.

Staff evaluation of nurse-managers reveals general areas of strengths and weaknesses in the leader as perceived by the evaluators and provides the nurse-manager with one means of validation for the effectiveness of the managerial practice.

An evaluation process that includes reciprocal participation both vertically and horizontally provides an avenue for high level morale and job satisfaction.

Evaluation is the means or method whereby one determines whether goals or desired outcomes have been achieved, and if not, how close to the mark one has come. In personal evaluation the single most important aspect is having a clear picture of the desired performance, either through written goals or established criteria. Chapter 2 deals with evaluation of quality control of organizational structure, agency policies and procedures, and record keeping. This chapter is devoted to the evaluation of personnel.

Traditionally in nursing, evaluation has been associated with unpleasant experiences during student days when the threat of failure was ever present. Negative judgments were all too often made with no help given to remedy the behaviors under criticism, leaving the recipient feeling nervous and confused.

Confusion of evaluation with establishing a grade and the negative experiences most nurses have had with activities called "evaluation" have given this experience a distasteful aura that is difficult to alter. Some agencies have modified the terminology used to remove negative connotations from the process. The evaluative procedure is sometimes referred to as "efficiency ratings," "performance assessment," and "appraisal." Whatever the term, all nurses evaluate, consciously or unconsciously, and the more leaders know about what personnel evaluation is and how to engage in the process, the more effective will be the use of this tool for improving patient care.

Quality control of nursing practice is highly significant, for an organization depends on its nursing personnel to provide the prescribed level of nursing care at reasonable cost and in a satisfactory environment. While performance appraisals are of importance to the employing agency, they have great significance to the personnel employed as well. From an organizational point of view, appraisals may be important for three reasons: (1) the maintenance of organizational control and direction, (2) the measurement of the efficiency with which human resources are utilized, and (3) the retrieval of meaningful information concerning development needs and improvement of human resources. From personnel's point of view the appraisal system may have significance in relation to: (1) determining whether the nurse should be left at the current level, transferred, promoted, demoted, or dismissed; (2) improvement of performance; (3) ascertaining potential and hidden or latent abilities; (4) identifying continuing education needs; (5) encouraging self-development; (6) providing a guide for salary advancement; and (7) testing the validity of the personnel selection process.

Traditionally the tendency has been to apply the evaluation procedure sporadically rather than continuously, as a result of pressure outside such as the Joint Commission on Accreditation of Hospitals rather than from within the system. Further, it is often done for expediency rather than as an expression of planning, and after the fact rather than as part of preplanned, cumulative, and integrated design. Furthermore, nurses tend to restrict their evaluative views to themselves and to the small functional areas in which nursing care is implemented.

The first recording of a performance appraisal system was made around 1800 by Owens of Scotland, who devised a plan using different-colored blocks to represent various levels of performance. Each day workers would find a colored block of wood at their place that best corresponded with Owen's assessment of their work performance for the previous day. Other studies continued until World War I (1914-1917) highlighted the need for a tool to identify and evaluate military leaders. However, it was not the military but business and industry which assumed the task of studying appraisal of managers. Many forms became available, still concentrating primarily on time and motion. During this period, rating scales were introduced. Individuals were graphed on a scale from "poor" or "unsatisfactory" to "good" or "excellent."

In the 1930s and the 1940s, appraisal forms concentrated on personality and behavioral characteristics in keeping with a surge of interest in human relations. By 1950, tools were available that included both work-related activities and human elements. During this decade management by objectives (MBO) was introduced. Emphasis was placed upon determination of objectives for both the total organization and individual managers and how to measure performance against these objectives.

Legal responsibilities

Performance appraisal has now become a legal matter. Court decisions finding physicians, nurses, or nursing services guilty of inadequate care, negligence, or even malpractice have reached an all time high. This underscores the need for protective measures for health professionals.

In earlier years a group called the Hospital Standardization Program attempted to evaluate institutions as to their quality of institutional care. The Joint

Commission on Accreditation of Hospitals (JCAH) became its successor, devoting its efforts to the visitation of hospitals to determine the degree of compliance with standards that were primarily oriented to the assessment of structure including facilities, equipment, and staff. The assessment of process, or the actual things done to and for the client, and the assessment of outcome, or the end results, were not included in their criteria. Compliance with these programs was voluntary.

The enactment of the Medicare Act in 1965 became the major force for compliance with standards for quality assurance. The Act contained certain conditions for hospitals to meet if they wished to receive federal benefits. As a result, the Joint Commission completely rewrote the language of its standards but still on the model of input and to a much lesser degree on the quality of care.

Law in relation to performance appraisal of nurses was further clarified by *Griggs vs Duke Power Company* in 1970. The United States Supreme Court decision mandated that any type of testing procedure for a particular job must relate directly to the job duties to be performed. Soon after this ultimatum the Equal Employment Opportunity Commission (EEOC) developed guidelines that reinforced the Supreme Court decision, stating "when used as tools for selection, promotion or transfer, performance appraisals are considered tests and the Supreme Court decision applies."*

In 1972 an amendment to the Social Security Act was mandated in Public Law 92-603, which caused the creation of quality assurance programs in health care. The act further provided that Professional Standards Review Organizations (PSROs) be established by July 1, 1978. The program was organized at the national level and is administered and controlled by local physicians and osteopaths on a state and local basis. While nurses were not successful in becoming a part of the planning organization, they serve on committees developing standards and criteria for assessment of implementation within health agencies on state and local levels. The American Nurses' Association fully supports the need to monitor quality care. This organization published standards for nursing practice in the major clinical areas in 1975; these can serve as guidelines for assessment of nursing practice in health agencies, as well as serving as a basis for decisions in courts of law.

In 1979 the JCAH issued a Program on Hospital Accreditation Standards, now published in the 1982 *Accreditation Manual for Hospitals.* This document contains criteria for evaluation of nursing services standards. Each criterion identifies the standards to which it relates. Following is an excerpt from the manual that relates to the requirement for evaluation of nursing personnel:

---

*Equal Employment Opportunity Commission: Guidelines of employment and selection procedure, Federal Register **35**(149):12333-12336, 1970.

In striving to assure optimal achievable quality nursing care and a safe patient environment, nursing personnel staffing and assignment shall be based at least on the following:
- a registered nurse plans, supervises, and evaluates the nursing care of each patient.
- to the extent possible, a registered nurse makes a patient assessment before delegating appropriate aspects of nursing care to nursing personnel.

Meeting these regulations requires a mechanism for validation of the services. In recognition of the need for continued improvement, plans are now underway for a major revision of the JCAH standards to include more specific criteria for evaluation; this is scheduled for publication in 1984.

Legal duty is another factor considered in resolution of nursing issues that reach litigation. Health agencies depend upon standards and procedures and criteria for meeting them to assess degree of performance of duty in their agencies. Courts of law rely upon these standards in addition to legal duty or the "reasonable person" standard. (That standard is the duty to conduct oneself with the same degree of care that a reasonably prudent person would exercise in a comparable situation.) It is not possible for an agency to have guidelines written for every action, therefore before a decision is reached, formal standards and criteria are reviewed and authorities in the field under discussion are queried as to their opinion of the nurse's reasonableness of action—assessment, conclusions, and actions. It behooves nurses to be aware of standards and the criteria for meeting them that exist in the agency in which they are employed. Further the nurse needs to know to what extent support is given for nurses making independent judgment in situations where written guidelines or other resource persons are unavailable.

Conceptual framework for evaluation

Evaluation of client care and quality control programs is a process and as such requires adoption of a conceptual framework in which to operate. The conceptual bases of all review activities for client care and quality control programs are structure, process, and outcomes of care (Fig. 7-1). Evaluation of the *structure* framework involves the study of the agency, concentrating on its mission, organizational characteristics, financial base, management practices, physical facilities and equipment, and status with regard to accreditation, certification, or approval by voluntary or government bodies. Assessment of structure assumes there is a positive relationship between good structural attributes and good care.

Examination of the *process* framework of care inspects and judges what is actually done by the provider of care on behalf of a client. The decision-making process is studied along with therapeutic interventions employed. Major and

STUDY OF STRUCTURE (agency)	STUDY OF PROCESS	STUDY OF OUTCOME
Mission Organizational characteristics Financial base Management practices Physical facilities Formal status	What is actually done by the provider on behalf of the client	Results or product of care

Fig. 7-1. Conceptual framework for evaluation.

minor steps taken in the care of a client are reviewed with attention to the rationale for the sequence of the steps taken as well as the degree to which these measures help the client reach specified goals.

The process of care is evaluated according to general or specific outcomes of care for the clients. Examples of process criteria would be as follows:

1. To examine a client's record using an instrument that contains specific questions to answer: Are any changes in skin tone noted? Are respiratory rate and quality recorded? Does the record indicate the type and quantity of food eaten?
2. To interview the nurse: Do staff check with one another to ensure that clients are ambulated on schedule? Are precautions taken to protect a client who is in reverse isolation from undue exposure to infection?
3. To observe the care provided: Are clients consulted regarding their care? Are meals served hot and is necessary assistance provided? Are prescribed nursing interventions implemented?

A study of *outcome* refers to the results or product of care or the client's response in terms of changes that can be noted with reference to client-oriented objectives. Variables often tested are disease status, presence or absence of symptoms, physiologic measurements, and ability to engage in activities of daily living. Factors much less often tested are psychologic or emotional responses, knowledge of health status, and compliance with proposed treatment. Examples of outcome criteria for a client postoperatively that are based on client-oriented objectives might be as follows: ambulates without assistance after third postoperative day; surgical wound evidences opening and drainage; is able to void without distress after twenty-four hours; evacuates soft, brown stool between forty-two and seventy-two hours after surgery; verbalizes name of surgery; knows about medications he is taking, including side effects; describes restrictions when he returns to work; and expresses emotional and psychologic feelings.

It is very difficult to identify outcome criteria that can be solely attributed to nursing care because the client receives care from other providers, such as physicians and a variety of therapists. Serious work has been in progress among nurses to develop nursing care outcome criteria for the past fifteen years. There are fine reviews in the literature, but the work has just begun. Individual nurses need to apply the process of evaluation that has been developed in their own work settings, make adaptations as necessary, and report their findings so that results can be shared and progress accelerated.

Dr. D. Bloch,* Chief of the Research Grants Section of the Nursing Research Branch, Division of Nursing of the Department of Health, Education, and Welfare, has a vital interest in evaluation of nursing care in terms of process and outcome. She has developed a model of the factors that bear on client care evaluation.

Four types of problems are proposed: (1) cognitive, such as an obese patient who does not understand the principles of nutrition; (2) psychosocial, such as problems of motivation, attitude, or poverty; (3) behavior, such as excessive drinking or smoking; and (4) health state, such as ulcerative colitis. In this model, these four categories of client problems make up the basis for evaluation of outcome.

Care providers constitute the structural framework or the system within which all care is provided. Housed between care providers (structure) and care recipient (outcome) is the care given by providers (process). In giving care the problem-solving process is employed, data are collected, the problem is defined, intervention is planned and implemented, and evaluation of the intervention takes place. Bloch believes that process should be related to outcome in every type of health care evaluation because it provides for review of how providers' actions relate to changes in the recipient of care.

In order for process-outcome evaluation to occur in nursing, certain tasks must be achieved: (1) measurable outcome criteria specific to nursing care provided must be developed (outcomes); (2) reliable and valid methods for measurement of outcomes must be developed (outcomes); (3) measurable process criteria must be known (process); (4) reliable and valid methods for measuring the process of nursing care in all forms, including physical, psychosocial, and cognitive aspects, must be formulated (process); and (5) testing of the various aspects of nursing practice in relation to patient outcomes by applying process as well as outcome measurement must occur (process-outcome).

Bloch states that the first four steps can be differentiated between process and outcome, but that all five tasks refer to the more inclusive and comprehensive process-outcome type of evaluation. Extensive work with outcome evaluation has been carried out since 1975. Inzer and Aspernall, nurses at the Veterans Administration Hospital in Long Beach, California, have developed an innovative model for use in assessing patient outcome; however, there is much work yet to be done, and the goal should be to work toward achievement

---

*Bloch, D.: Evaluation of nursing care in terms of process and outcome: issues in research and quality assurance, Nurs. Res. **24**(4):257-258, 1975.

of these tasks through a sound conceptual framework so that the scientific foundation for nursing can be strengthened.

Commitment of all concerned

Commitment means the act of pledging or binding oneself to a certain course or action. Commitment first requires a conscious choice among alternatives, then a belief in the ideals that spawned that choice, and finally behaviors that actualize the choice. The strength or degree of the commitment of an individual depends on the amount of belief or faith he has in the choice he made to produce a result he values. *Choice* is one of the key activities of commitment. Agencies with policies on personnel evaluation that have been previously established either by the administration or by employees do not offer a choice between "to evaluate" or "not to evaluate." However, within every situation is some element of choice. The choices may be about how evaluations shall be done, who will participate, or the procedure to be used. Within the prescribed policy restrictions, choices made in full knowledge of limits of the choices and options available give the individual or group the beginnings of commitment. Commitment grows through seeing the choices implemented and feeling that the outcome of evaluation will be worthwhile.

PREDICTIVE PRINCIPLE: Involvement of personnel in all phases of the evaluative process increases belief in the fairness and accuracy of the evaluation, establishes a commitment to the evaluation, and increases motivation to utilize the results.

Within agency structure, each employee cannot be involved in every phase of the evaluation process, but can participate in the process by giving input and receiving feedback informally and formally. Informal appraisal is conducted on a day-to-day basis. The nurse-manager spontaneously mentions that a particular piece of work was performed well or poorly, or the staff member may ask the nurse-manager how well she is doing. Because of the close involvement between the ones who assess the behavior and the feedback about the behavior, informal appraisal quickly encourages desirable performance and discourages undesirable performance before it becomes ingrained. Formal appraisal is a systematic procedure in which employers usually classify personnel positions based on administrative organization and defined client and fiscal policies. Job descriptions are usually initially drafted by administrative personnel, but employees join professional performance committees to participate in writing or revising job descriptions, establishing standards of practice, and developing criteria to determine if those standards have been met. In their studies of performance appraisal process, Meyer and his colleagues* have found that formal

---

*Meyer, H., Meyer, E., and French, J.: Split roles in performance appraisal, Harvard Bus. Rev., pp. 123-129, Jan.-Feb., 1965.

appraisals by managers are often ineffective in improving the performance of employees when they are formally given criticism about their job performance once or twice a year. It was discovered that without any other involvement in the appraisal process than this, performance tended to decline. This problem can be corrected by involvement of personnel who are to be affected by the committee's endeavors at all levels of evaluation. This kind of involvement will give the committee a wider base of support and will enable the committee to receive the necessary feedback to make valid decisions.

Employees can be involved in the formalized process of evaluation through participation activities using prescribed agency tools.

Standards of practice and criteria for evaluation

As quality assurance efforts have progressed, many individuals and groups have become increasingly active in the area of establishing standards to upgrade the quality of care. The most obvious milestone in setting minimum standards of practice was the instigation of the licensure examination, a measure for allowing an individual to practice nursing in a given state. Currently, most agencies have committees composed of representatives of the working group that establishes standards of practice and exercises control over the quality of nursing care in an agency. Quality assurance, criteria, standards of practice and norms for all levels of nursing service personnel, and the methods necessary to measure behavior by those standards are the subject of this section.

Isobel Stewart in 1919 first developed guidelines by which a procedure could be effectively standardized. Since that time, these have been modified and adapted by nurses and hospital associations for use in evaluating procedures and personnel. Stewart's criteria are modified here and slightly expanded, but they remain basically as she developed them. These criteria may be applied to any nursing activity and can be useful as guides to develop standards of practice and methods of evaluation for the measurement of quality. *Stewart's criteria (modified)** are as follows:

1. Safe and comfortable for the patient, nurse, and others
2. Technologically and therapeutically as advanced care as modern technology and science permits
3. Efficient and economical in time, energy, and supplies (the degree and priority of economy of time, energy, and supplies are legislated by the demands of criteria 1 and 2)
4. Legally, ethically, and morally acceptable
5. Culturally and ethnically biased for the client

The four key words, "safe," "advanced," "efficient," and "acceptable,"

---

*Stewart, I.M.: Possibilities of standardization in nursing techniques, Mod. Hosp., June 1919.

must be defined meaningfully for practical everyday use in evaluation. Each evaluating group may wish to discuss and define these words to its own satisfaction. A brief definition for each is suggested here:

1. Safe—will not harm the client or nurse physically or emotionally; does not violate the client's physiologic, emotional, religious, or cultural integrity. Safety implies that the nurse will choose among available alternative actions. These actions will have the greatest potential for accomplishing the desired goal with the least risk of an undesirable consequence.

2. Advanced—uses updated skills and modern equipment and involves making decisions or exercising judgment based on the latest available knowledge in physical, biologic, behavioral, and social sciences.

3. Efficient—produces the greatest amount of results with the least waste. Efficient does not mean merely "fast." It means effective, productive, and adequately fulfilling a purpose with the best possible use of the energy, time, and materials available.

4. Acceptable—is legal and meets the "reasonable person standard" of legal duty and violates the ethics of neither the client nor the nurse.

PREDICTIVE PRINCIPLE: Clear and concise role delineation and job descriptions enable employee, employer, and client to know the duties and responsibilities of the job.

Role delineation and job descriptions are discussed in Chapter 6 and will not be repeated here.

Employees need copies of job descriptions available to them for all job classifications. Job descriptions help all employees know what every other employee was hired to do. It is equally important for a caregiver to know what the job *is not* as well as to know what it *is*. Nursing roles and job descriptions, clearly described in terms of relevance of each item to nursing practice, provide an objective way to ascertain if goals have been reached. If the job description is vague or if it ends with "and such other duties as may be required," the employee will not know what direction to take or what goals and objectives will be considered as most significant when outcomes are surveyed.

In addition to role delineation and job description, where management by objectives (MBO) is in effect, individuals will be appraised on the basis of individual objectives mutually set by the participant(s) and the immediate supervisor. Usually these objectives fall into the categories of routine duties, problem-solving goals, creative goals, and personal goals. They are always consistent with the larger goals of the agency.

Vagueness in setting up job descriptions leads to a guessing game. Participants need to know areas of overlapping responsibility and areas of differing responsibility. Clear job descriptions and objectives are the nucleus of all subsequent evaluative activities.

PREDICTIVE PRINCIPLE: Clear standards and criteria for measuring performance increase the objectivity and validity of evaluation.

A *standard* is a desired and achievable level of performance that can be compared with a criterion. Before a standard can be tested the method to be used must be identified and spelled out as to the precise means for measurement by experts. *Performance standards* are usually generally minimal standards established to govern the quality of nursing care. These standards definitively describe safety and expertise necessary for acceptable performance of the job. *Evaluation criteria* enable the evaluator (caregiver, client, nurse-leader, supervisor, or worker) to establish categories for review and to determine the *degree* and *extent* to which the person evaluated is performing in relationship to the established minimal standard.

Objectivity and validity in evaluation of performance are ideals that are never completely attained. *Objectivity* means unprejudiced, based on real evidence, and uninvolved with self or at least minimally influenced by subjective involvement. Objectivity, although not completely attainable, can be controlled to some extent through the use of criteria as guides for making judgments and by remaining sensitive to and aware of biases and feelings.

Validity is the degree and extent to which the evaluation tool measures what it was intended to measure. Validity has two basic elements: (1) *reliability*, the degree and extent that an evaluation measures something, and (2) *relevance*, the degree and extent that it actually does measure what it is intended to measure.

An example of reliability and relevance follows:

Reliability: Standard: The nurse has the ability to develop a written schedule to assure administration of medications to an assigned group of patients for the shift designated.

Relevance: The schedule indicates each patient's room number and the number of medications to be given for each patient within hourly time frames, as illustrated:

	Time									
Room no.	6a	7	8	9	10	11	12	1	2	3
1		X		XX				XX		
2			X				X			
3	X Pre-op									

A criterion (a standard, responsibility, or rule) can measure reliability without measuring relevance, and vice versa. However, a criterion must be both reliable and relevant for it to be valid.

Norm is defined as a level or range of performance regarded as typical or normal for any individual or situation. It refers to a conclusion reached as a result of empiric study of present conditions or circumstances.

The following are examples in which job classification, job description, standards of practice, and criteria for evaluation for a head nurse and a team leader are followed through for general areas of nursing responsibility.*

EXAMPLE 1:
Job classification: Head nurse
Job qualifications: R.N., bachelor's degree in nursing; management training
Job description: To fulfill the basic objectives of the Good Samaritan Hospital for a specific unit through effective management functions

Standards of practice	*Criteria for evaluation*
Major performances:	Performance satisfactory when:
Responsibilities to Supervisor:	
Reports to supervisor all pertinent information.	Supervisor is kept informed of pertinent information at appropriate times.
Seeks counsel as necessary.	
Responsibilities to nursing staff:	
Acts as resource person in problem solving.	Makes self available to staff.
Provides staff with tools to achieve the job for which she is responsible.	Evidence that problem-solving has occurred. Staff oriented and educated as to the use of policies, standards, procedures, forms, and equipment.
Communicates current information regarding patient care, policies, procedures, and goals.	Regular, scheduled staff meetings occur with written minutes. Communication book is kept current.
Provides ongoing and yearly communication, for those under direct supervision, regarding performance.	Ongoing evaluative communication occurs; yearly performance evaluation is written with criteria for growth defined.
Assists to develop autonomy and decision-making skills regarding patient care.	Staff takes responsibility for own decision making; seeks help when needed.
Initiates planning for training to correct skill deficiencies when necessary.	Notifies Nursing Education Department when training is needed. Takes initiative for personal growth on-the-job, and through outside sources.
Promotes mutually supportive behaviors among nursing staff and between nursing staff and associates.	Collaborative relationships exist among nursing staff and between nursing staff and associates.
Affirms jobs well done, individually and by public recognition.	Gives positive "strokes" to staff; sends memorandums to appropriate people for jobs well done.
Provides time schedules one month in advance; informs staff of procedure for making special requests regarding time.	Staff know what their work schedule is one month in advance, and understand the system for making special requests.

---

*Modified excerpts from the policy manual of The Good Samaritan Hospital of Santa Clara Valley, 1982, San Jose, California. Used by permission.

EXAMPLE 2:

Job classification: Team leader

Job qualifications: Current registration as issued by the California Board of Registered Nursing or Board of Licensed Vocational Nursing. Preferably a graduate of an accredited school of professional or vocational nursing

Job description: A team leader is a professional registered nurse or licensed vocational nurse who is responsible for assessing, planning, delegating, supervising, participating in, and evaluating patient care for a specific group of patients

Standards of practice	*Criteria for evaluation**
Major duties:	
Reports to head nurse all pertinent information and activities; seeks assistance when needed.	Head nurse is kept informed of pertinent matters at appropriate times (when problems are unresolved, emergency situations, or anticipated trouble).
Uses nursing process in the performance of duties.	Evidence that nursing process has been employed in all activities relating to nursing care.
Plans for nursing care through team conferences, nursing care plans, and individual contact.	Hold conference prior to care-giving and before shift change, using care plans as a guide.
Maintains an open, two-way communication system with team members.	Is available as a resource person to team members.
Directs, supervises, participates in care, teaches, and evaluates nursing care.	Team is functioning smoothly, and meets quality assurance standards for nursing care.
Develops autonomy and decision-making skills among team members regarding client care.	Team members show growth and development in initiative and problem solving.
Initiates planning for correction of skill deficiencies in self and in team members.	Contacts Nursing Education Department for help, and seeks to improve self on the job and through outside resources.
Participates in evaluation of team members with day-to-day observations and suggestions, and by participating in the preparation of performance appraisals.	Team members show growth and development as a result of team leader's assistance.
Promotes mutually supportive behaviors between self and team members, among nursing staff, and between nursing staff and associates.	There is harmony in the nursing team; clients give evidence of being satisfied with care provided.
Prepares clients physically and psychologically for treatments, surgical procedures, and diagnostic studies.	Clients give evidence of understanding what is happening to them and accept prescriptions.
Maintains accurate and complete records of nursing care and observation of the patient.	Nursing records reflect completeness.

The appraisal system for personnel should consider such criteria as job knowledge, ability to carry through on assignments, judgments, attitude, cooperation, dependability, production, and creation of a positive environment. Carefully thought-out criteria and standards for performance help the evaluator and

---

*Criteria for evaluation of the team leader is the work of the authors.

the person evaluated take all relevant factors into account when assessing performance, thus minimizing the effect of personal bias. Use of a model similar to these presented for all nursing activities provide participants with evaluative criteria. (Note that when the criteria for evaluation are spelled out in behavioral terms the assessment process is facilitated.)

The examples given for assessing performance of a head nurse and team leader define standards and general criteria for evaluation; however, more definitive criteria are necessary if the nurse-manager wishes to identify specific areas of practice for appraisal. The nursing process criteria provide an excellent model for this purpose. They can be developed on the basis of assessing, planning, implementing, and evaluating nursing care, with components of each part of the process delineated in detail. Data can be acquired from numerous sources and methods: (1) information from client records, (2) observation of the client, (3) interview with the client, (4) interview with the nursing personnel, (5) observation of the nursing personnel, (6) observation of the client's environment, (7) observation of unit management, and (8) observer inference.

To illustrate how the nurse-manager can translate the more general criteria for evaluation into more definitive language, one standard of practice is used:

Major duty	*Criteria for evaluation*
Delegates and coordinates the team member activities in the care they perform for assigned patients.	Assigns patients according to acuity and ability of staff to meet needs; is available to staff members for ongoing activities.

Both planning and implementing activities are included in this single standard. In nursing process, each component is considered separately. A sample is provided below of more specific criteria for the delegation of activities, a part of the planning process:

Standard of practice: Delegates team member activities for the performance of client care.

Criteria for evaluation: Performance is satisfactory when the team leader:

1. Makes tentative assignments based on numbers and kinds of clients, and numbers and kinds of personnel assigned to the team.
2. Considers all workers assigned to team in terms of nursing care plans and caregivers' preferences, knowledge, and ability.
3. Considers physical factors (extent of walking, lifting, standing, distance between rooms, use of special equipment, etc.).
4. Makes necessary adjustments in assignments after receiving change of shift report and conducting initial rounds and prior to direction-giving conference.
5. Indicates on the assignment sheet the date, shift, team member's name, team member's position, meal hours and coffee breaks, client's name and room number, time of team conferences.
6. Writes on the assignment sheet routine duties to be performed (TPRs, BPs, I&Os, water, meal cards, and treatments) by specific team members.

7. Writes legibly and completely.
8. Gives verbal direction clearly and succinctly; encourages feedback for clarification of direction.
9. Posts the assignment in time for team members to adequately prepare for their assignments.
10. Holds to the assignment as posted unless there is an imperative need for change.
11. Adjusts assignments to meet emergency situations.
12. Provides for a balance of variety and consistency in team members' assignments.
13. Provides opportunities for team members' growth and development through incidental and planned teaching.

Stated behaviorally, these criteria can be used by the evaluator and the team leader to validate the degree to which the standard is being carried out. A checklist with a rating scale can be devised for use by both persons.

This kind of structure provides a measure of safety for both the evaluator and the person evaluated by making objectivity more achievable. A leader can have positive or negative feelings about the nurse but if the procedure has been performed and the criteria met as written, personal feelings are less likely to influence evaluative judgment.

PREDICTIVE PRINCIPLE: Use of appropriate assessment tools and sufficient evaluative data gathered from varied situations increases the validity of the conclusions in the assessment of work performance.

The modern theory of performance appraisal is based on the following important concepts: (1) that the foundation of performance appraisal rests on the criteria and standards established for various health care positions, (2) that there is participation in the process by all concerned, (3) that there is emphasis on obtaining factual information about specific achievements as they relate to criteria and standards, and (4) that the appraisal process can facilitate change in individual behavior in order to achieve personal and organizational goals.

Nursing practice is validated through informal and formal means. No single style has been found to be consistently superior to another. Most individuals and health agencies utilize more than one technique, depending on (1) the purpose of the evaluation, (2) the availability of resources, and (3) the expertise and preference of those involved in the appraisal process.

Evaluation is both intuitive and subjective. The evaluation process takes the form of informal and formal evaluation. *Informal evaluation* may consist of (1) observation of an individual's work performance while engaged in nursing functions; (2) on the job, incidental face-to-face work or collaboration; (3) reflections offered during a meeting or conference; (4) reactions of an involved person, such as a client, family member, or staff person; or (5) notation of the effects of a worker's actions on clients, families, personnel, or environment. *Formal as-*

sessment includes many methods. Nurses most often utilize (1) anecdotal recordings, (2) critical incident technique, (3) checklists based on preestablished criteria, (4) dialogue based on one-to-one and group exchange, (5) rating scales, (6) cumulative records of activities engaged in for professional growth and advancement; and (7) self-evaluation using criteria. Nurses may avail themselves of other methods, such as written and computer tests and other technologic testing devices. Practitioners can test their evaluative skills individually and collectively by viewing a filmed or taped nursing action and then assessing the situation. Videotaping with instant replay is an appropriate device for the assessment of some nursing activities. Microtelevision or videotape can be used in actual or simulated settings. Evaluation of verbal and nonverbal interaction is particularly subject to this method.

All these avenues are most effective when there is commitment to the evaluation process by the evaluator, the person being evaluated, and the receiver of the information.

Anecdotal recording. The anecdotal note is a means for describing a nurse's experience with a person or group. It is useful for recording and evaluating client progress. Essentially, nurses' notes are one form of anecdotal record, since they outline serially factual information with definite reference to the client's progress. Other uses for this mode include validating technical skills, dialogue, and interpersonal relationships.

An example of an interpersonal anecdote follows:

Nurse L. was confronted in the hall of the pediatric unit at 10 A.M. on 11-9 by an angry parent who shouted, "My son is left to starve and it is your fault!" Nurse L. guided the mother into a secluded area and, with calm assurance, used the problem-solving process to determine the facts and to solve the problem. Nurse L. acted in a commendable manner. (Signature of observer.)

The anecdotal note has both advantages and disadvantages. The device is useful for frequent brief observations where variations in situations and personalities preclude advance determination of behavior. With this mechanism, it is possible to discover trends of conditions and behavior over a period of time. In many ways the anecdotal notes are superior to checklists or rating scales because observers are not forced into rigid structure in describing behavior.

In any of these areas the behavioral pattern may vary from person to person and situation to situation. Although the general conditions and behaviors can be prescribed beforehand, the specific activities will be determined by circumstances incident to the occasion.

For maximum clarity, an anecdotal notation should include (1) a description of the particular occasion; (2) a delineation of the behavior noted, indicating who, what, why, when, where, and how; and (3) the evaluator's opinion or estimate of the incident or behavior. Decisions concerning what to observe and record are made on the basis of previously determined criteria, formal and informal. For expediency the evaluator will develop a code or an abbreviated system for recording to facilitate speedy and accurate memorandums.

Perhaps the greatest difficulty in the use of anecdotal notes is the matter of developing some relationship among the various notations. Before it is possible to get impressions of the overall behavior in a given period of time, it is necessary to organize the descriptive notes. Often the notes bear little or no relationship to one another, and for this reason it is difficult to use them. The burden of organizing the notes falls on the observer or on the person who is attempting to interpret the meaning of the notes in relation to the behavior of the person evaluated.

Critical incident. The critical incident technique is a method for collecting purely factual information. A critical incident is any important observable bit of human behavior sufficiently complete in itself to permit inferences to be made about the person performing the act. It differs from the anecdotal recording in that no evaluative or judgmental statements are made. Psychologist John Flanagan first introduced use of critical incident during World War II while attempting to evaluate men in the armed forces. Flanagan has since worked with nurse-educators testing the use of critical incident technique to evaluate nursing performance of students.* He believes the critical incident method can be of great value in helping nurses achieve and maintain a high level of performance in all areas of practice. A collection of critical incidents is made on the basis of day-to-day observation of nurses in providing nursing care, as soon as possible after they occur. The following procedure may help in keeping records of critical incidents that are relevant and useful:

1. Determine whether the incident observed was critical.
2. Decide if the behavior was effective or ineffective.
3. Relate the behavior noted to a specific standard and objective for the performance of the activity surveyed. (For convenience, use a number or letter code.)
4. Record the incident on the back of the worksheet, a slip of paper, or on small cards, indicating date, time, and a brief description of the incident. Use as few words as possible.

Following are examples of critical incidents recorded by a nurse manager:

Positive behavior
5/6   2:20 P.M.
Robin telephoned pharmacy at 9 A.M. to assure preparation of previously ordered solution. She picked the solution up at 1 P.M., verified its contents with the doctor's order, and allowed the bottle to stand at room temperature to cool. She changed the tubing and hung the bottle, using proper procedure.

---

*Flanagan, J.: The critical incidence technique, Psychol. Bull. **51:**327-358, 1954.

Negative behavior

7/8   7 A.M.

Nancy reported to me as soon as I came on duty that at 6 A.M. she misread an order for heparin and gave 10,000 units instead of the prescribed 5,000. She immediately notified the physician in charge, who ordered laboratory studies.

Use of critical incidents has the advantage of focusing entirely on behaviors and can be used as one means of discussing performance with a worker during times of feedback. There is a problem of time involved in observing and recording a sufficient number of incidents and the greater difficulty of the appraiser observing a representative sample of the member's performance. Certainly critical incidents can be recorded whenever possible and used as a means of documentation of reports. If it is noted that positive or negative patterns are emerging, further observations and follow-up can occur.

Checklist. By definition a checklist is a grouping of items by which something may be confirmed or verified. The checklist could be called a behavioral inventory. The checking process implies that standards and criteria are available for gauging items. The inspection procedure requires scrutiny of behavior under investigation. Checklists are most useful for determining the status of tangible items, such as inventory and maintenance of equipment and supplies. They have the advantage that items to be observed can be determined in advance and will be the same criteria used in each situation. Checklists are of some use as yardsticks for appraisal of nursing skills and techniques. There is no guarantee, however, that the observed behavior is a persistent one and that the procedure will provide a representative picture of the individual being evaluated.

Checklists applied in nursing attempt to itemize behaviors that are considered important elements of a task. One approach is to list satisfactory behaviors in a column, then determine the worker's overall performance on the basis of the items. For example, in observing administration of medications, the evaluator looks to see if the person being evaluated:

1. Checks physician's orders against nursing medication cards
2. Prepares the medication accurately using prescribed procedure
3. Identifies the client and checks the medication card (or sheet) against the client's identification band
4. Administers the medication
5. Documents medication given accurately

It is recommended that only significant behaviors essential for a successful performance be included on the checklist. Only those behaviors that, if omitted or performed incorrectly, would make the difference between successful and unsuccessful performance should be included. The checklist does not lend itself well to evaluating client progress, dialogue, or interpersonal relationships.

Rating scale. The rating scale, quite similar to the checklist, is another type of evaluation tool used in describing observed skills and performance commonly used in nursing appraisals. The basis of the rating device consists of such items as descriptive paragraphs, sentences, or phrases to serve as guidelines for the evaluator. Unlike the checklist, the rating scale may involve judgments as to quantitative and qualitative abilities. Such rating scales at the lower end might range from "incapable of performing a given task" to "poor" or "unsatisfactory." The scale will at its higher limits use such descriptive terms as "excellent," "outstanding," or "exceptional."

Some scales for the rating of performance employ the numeric system, using 1 to indicate the lowest behavioral pattern and 10 or more to indicate the highest. The evaluator may fabricate a scale according to his own design and check behavioral patterns as occurring "consistently," "frequently," "sometimes," or "never." These numbers or words are ill defined, and only the evaluator may know what an individual's level of performance and achievement is. Rating scales indicating frequency evaluate quantity only and have little ability to assess quality.

Rating scales where the numbers represent qualitative descriptions are more effective. Following are samples of descriptions that clarify categories in terms of quality and quantity:

Category	Qualitative statement (description of behavior)	Quantity (degree of accomplishment)				
		Poor				Excellent
Manual dexterity	Manipulates catheter into opening without contamination.	1	2	3	4	5
Attendance	Reports to work as assigned on time.	1	2	3	4	5
	If going to be absent, notifies proper person in time for a replacement to be obtained.	1	2	3	4	5
Safe practitioner	If procedure unfamiliar, reviews procedure manual or other resource.	1	2	3	4	5
	Proceeds carefully with procedure according to hospital guidelines.	1	2	3	4	5

The rating scale is usually reserved for formal evaluation procedures, such as periodic assessment of an employee and is frequently associated with retention, promotion, and tenure. The device is comparative in nature. The rating is based on retrospective recordings and observations and is subject to human errors associated with recall and interpretation. This tool is most useful when each unit on the rating scale is identified and listed in terms of specific behaviors or circumstances.

A well-calibrated rating scale will (1) consider all major items included in the job description, (2) include such measures as safety, comfort, responsiveness to the client, knowledge and its application, use of nursing process, (3) test for qualities, not just quantity or frequency, and (4) have no more than five degrees of achievement on the scale.

Maximal utilization of the assessment tool depends on involved individuals having prior knowledge of, participation in, acceptance of, and commitment to the content and use of the rating scale.

PREDICTIVE PRINCIPLE: Use of the self-evaluation process promotes growth and development of the appraiser and contributes to better quality of care.

Self-evaluation is used by everyone from childhood to senescence. The ability to be critical in assessing one's own performance is a mark of maturity and an integral part of nursing practice. Self-evaluation is implicit and continuous in the nursing process at every level of care giving. Self-evaluation has many valuable effects. The one engaged in introspection seeks to (1) obtain estimates of his or her level of achievement; (2) acquire meaningful information to assist with improvement in nursing practice; (3) gain information for self-improvement, growth and development, and the achievement of personal goals in a socially acceptable manner; and (4) enhance and improve human relations.

Self-rating can be heavily influenced by the individual's tendencies to over- or underestimate his own capabilities or achievements. Much success of self-evaluation programs depends on the preliminary preparation of the participants to recognize their own strengths and weaknesses and to be as objective as possible in rating personal performance. One hospital in California utilizes a nursing skills inventory, which includes the orientees in the evaluation process by giving them responsibility for assessing their own skill levels, then having the skills validated by the preceptor or clinical nursing instructor. Following are introductory instructions given to all new RNs, LVNs, nursing assistants, and orderlies:

Nursing skills inventory*

This inventory is a compilation of skills considered fundamental to clinical nursing practice at Good Samaritan Hospital.

Nurses come to this hospital from a variety of educations and backgrounds. This tool assists you as a new employee or as a long-term employee in identifying those skills in which you are proficient and those skills in which you have limited or no experience, subsequently, appropriate learning experience can be planned.

The Nursing Skills Inventory provides a mechanism through which all nurses take an active part in self-evaluation and in planning for skill training experience.

The Skills Inventory is divided into a number of sections which include: Basic Nursing Skills, Clinical Nursing Skills, Nursing Process, Advanced Nursing Skills, ACU Nursing Skills, Maternal-Child Nursing Skills, and Operating Room—Recovery Room Nursing Skills.

You will be asked to complete those sections required for your job description,

---

*Developed by The Good Samaritan Hospital of Santa Clara Valley, San Jose, California, 1978, and revised 1980. Part of the materials was originally developed by El Camino Hospital in Palo Alto, California. Used by permission.

clinical area, and educational background. You are responsible for attaining and maintaining those skills covered in the sections assigned.

The following procedure is used in identifying skills level and planning for skill training experience.

1. Indicate with pencil check in one of the A, B, C, D sections of the "self-assessment" column to indicate your present skill level.

   A—Was never taught

   B—Was taught but have never done

   C—Have done but need review

   D—Feel competent to do

2. Plan with preceptor or other appropriate person (clinical instructor, head nurse, co-worker) for skill training experience for any skill checked.

3. A check in the "GSH policy & procedure" column means you have read the Procedure Manual and may or may not have had the opportunity to perform the skill.

4. "Validated by preceptor" means that you have had supervised experience on those skills checked in the A, B, or C column.

5. Review Skills Inventory with your clinical instructor and preceptor at the end of your two-week orientation and with your head nurse or her designee as a part of your annual performance evaluation.

6. Checking off equipment in Skills Inventory implies that you know purpose for use, maintenance, and trouble-shooting techniques.

An example of a part of the section on Nursing Process Skill self-evaluation process validated by the Preceptor is given below.

	Self-assessment				GSH policy	Validated	
Skill	*A*	*B*	*C*	*D*	*and procedure*	*by preceptor*	*Remarks*
Nursing process skills A. Nursing interview/ history							
B. Assessment skills							
1. Physical systems a. Cardiovascular							
b. Respiratory							
c. Neurological							
d. Gastrointestinal							
e. Renal							

Continued.

Skill	Self-assessment				GSH policy and procedure	Validated by preceptor	Remarks
	A	B	C	D			
C. Nursing care planning: 1. Identifies problem areas							
2. Identifies expected outcomes							
3. Identifies deadlines and check-points							
4. Identifies nursing orders							
5. Identifies and documents patient response to care given							
6. Utilizes standard care plans; modifies as necessary							
7. Maintains current care plans							
D. Patient teaching: 1. Identifies patient learning needs							
2. Identifies available in-house educational resources, and uses as appropriate to need							

Provided with adequate and procedural criteria for the assessment process and with various other appropriate tools, the individual can evaluate progress in relation to these activities, subject to reexamination and feedback.

Self-evaluation is connected with personal goals, self-perception, self-confidence, and feelings of competence or incompetence. Most people have a fairly accurate picture of themselves and their abilities, but communication of self-evaluation is overlaid with many factors. Some of these are (1) who is reading the evaluation, (2) how the evaluation will be used, (3) the social acceptability of the self-judgment, and (4) peer pressures. If the caregiver's self-appraisal threatens a job, promotion, salary increase, or prestige or peer regard, it is likely, even though unintended, that the assessment will be articulated and communicated with a slant toward the "halo" effect, which enhances the individual's strengths and minimizes or overlooks weaknesses.

If, as is often the case, social pressure decries extremely high self-appraisals and the individual values social appraisal, the caregiver's self-evaluation is not likely to reflect areas of high competence. If (1) the evaluation is geared to citing goals for self, degrees to which goals have been realized, and plans for goal attainment, (2) the self-evaluation is to be used as a record of and provision for growth and not as a means for punishment or reward, and (3) the self-evaluation report is confidential within preestablished limits and constraints, then self-evaluation is an accurate and useful tool and is likely to be effective when used in conjunction with other devices.

PREDICTIVE PRINCIPLE: A limited number of incidental observations jeopardizes the accuracy of evaluations.

PREDICTIVE PRINCIPLE: Informal and formal assessments that are noted and recorded systematically provide significant input to the evaluation process.

Each of the actions carried out in the nursing role needs to be evaluated for its success and effectiveness. Concentration on some activities (for example, medication or treatment errors) and omission of others (for example, exceptionally well organized in completing work assignment) presents a false picture of the individual under surveillance. Observations of completed tasks can give an unreliable picture of performance. For example, the nurse-leader walks into a client's room one hour after the change of the morning shift and finds the client clean and neatly groomed, the bed freshly made, and the unit straight and uncluttered. Without additional data the nurse-leader could conclude that the nurse assigned to this patient was efficient and thorough. More complete data might reveal (1) that this client was first on the list and therefore was cared for first regardless of the fact that another client wanted early care so that he would be ready for a long-awaited visit from a loved one; (2) that the client's receiving such efficient and thorough care was at the expense of breakfast, which became cold while waiting for the nurse to complete the care; (3) that the linen was piled on the floor while the bed was being changed; or (4) that the client was bathed in one small pan of water, which was not changed during the bath.

Value judgments made on one performance, the end product of a performance without reference to the process, or on many performances in the same situation can be erroneous because of lack of a variety of observations that would validate or refute previous judgments. For instance, a practitioner may use aseptic technique smoothly, correctly, and consistently when emptying catheter bags but may contaminate unknowingly when changing a sterile dressing. The criterion "practices sterile technique with a high degree of skill" may be true when the nurse is performing one task and not true when performing another.

Both informal and formal feedback or evaluation becomes significant if noted systematically and recorded as consistently as possible. The evaluation process is a means of determining the professional characteristics of an individual or a group. Similar behaviors as recorded in the evaluator's notes or tabulations indicate that a set of actions is predominately exhibited. Desirable behaviors that are rarely manifested are not given high priority when assessments are made; however, isolated achievements might become significant when motivation and potential are discussed.

Undesirable behaviors are important to consider. Again, isolated incidences are not used as conclusive data unless they become significant to the safety or welfare of the client. The right to be "human" or to improve includes provision for making some mistakes without penalty or guilt. The evaluator's primary responsibility is to observe and note those behaviors exhibited most frequently and to deal with them. The aggregate of these samples gives a more reliable basis for determining a trend of behavior.

PREDICTIVE PRINCIPLE: Valid interpretation depends on fair evaluation of input.

Factors used in performance evaluation programs vary widely from one appraisal plan to another. Additional information gleaned from evaluation procedures may be meaningful only if it is used constructively and interpreted correctly. Judgments about the assignment of relative weight or value of each factor under consideration often become the responsibility of the evaluator, who will follow prescribed guidelines: (1) client and nurse safety, (2) advanced knowledge and technology, (3) client comfort, (4) efficient use of time, (5) cost effectiveness, and (6) legal acceptability.

Some hints leading to a balanced evaluation of input for consideration are as follows:

1. Whatever the specific criteria used, they should relate to the job description and performance standards.
2. Objective assessments should receive greater weight than subjective judgments.
3. When one person is evaluated and more than one individual is involved, the evaluators' impressions of the incident are diluted because it is difficult to determine the extent of each member's participation and the qualitative assistance obtained from extraneous sources.
4. Time may be a factor in calibrating certain skills.
5. No single evaluation should constitute the basis for success or failure in evaluating any nursing effort.

PREDICTIVE PRINCIPLE: The evaluator who establishes mutual trust and confidence with the person evaluated and who is familiar with the criteria of evaluation increases the accuracy and usefulness of the evaluation.

When the evaluator and the person evaluated have a trusting relationship, anxiety about evaluation is somewhat reduced. The extent to which evaluation activities cause anxiety, however, is directly related to what the person being evaluated stands to gain or lose. Evaluation that is constant and ongoing and has as its objective the improvement of client care through the upgrading of performance becomes so much a part of routine and everyday nursing relationships that threat is reduced.

Reasons individuals may resist attempts to evaluate or control them are (1) danger of being removed from the job, suspended, relieved of responsibilities, or demoted; (2) disruption of self-image; (3) incongruence in individual and organizational objectives; (4) belief that the expected standard of performance is absent, too low, too high, or not important; (5) dislike of designated leader or manager; and (6) existence of an informal individual or group control that is more important to the person being evaluated.

Evaluations resulting from cooperative effort and accompanied by qualitative explanations that make sense to the learner cause behavioral changes. Job descriptions, standards of practice, and criteria of evaluations all contribute to the ability to participate in evaluations. Employees who know what constitutes a "good" or "bad" activity can recognize their own success or failure and take the initiative in corrective action. Consistently accurate self-evaluation is the ultimate achievement of evaluative activities, for it enables self-perpetuating growth.

The effect of evaluative comments on the behavior of the employee is related to the manner in which the message is given as well as the content of the message. Positive comments such as "You did a very good job on that" or "That was a fine bit of work you just did" serve to boost the morale of the worker and encourage continued high level performance. Negative remarks create varied feelings ranging from the desire to improve to deep hostility toward the evaluator without a change in behavior. If negative critique is offered in a discounting manner the result is likely to be anger. Negative comments are very likely to be accompanied by an explanation of the reason for the criticism. For example, "Don't do it that way; hold the bottle up high so the fluid will run in faster." Whereas positive comments are seldom accompanied by explanation. It is important for the person being evaluated to have information about *why* a behavior is "good" or "bad" so that the characteristics of the behavior can be either identified and repeated or changed.

Whether the evaluation is informal or formal, the evaluator bears in mind the need to preserve the integrity of the person or group being evaluated. Positive feedback, earned and given appropriately, contributes to the morale of each individual involved in the evaluation procedure.

Negative feedback is also essential for growth, as is positive feedback, and although it is often more difficult to give and to receive, it provides necessary data. Withholding all feedback, whether positive or negative, is unhelpful because it robs another person of the data needed to make intelligent choices and behavioral changes. In terms of personal acceptance of evaluation procedures, it is generally true that the more familiar a person is with the criteria used for evaluation, the more likely it is that he will accept and support those criteria and fair evaluations derived from them.

PREDICTIVE PRINCIPLE: The degree to which the value systems of the evaluator and the person evaluated coincide influences their interpersonal relationships and directly affects the evaluation process.

The dynamics of personal interaction and decisions are not wholly shaped by policies, job descriptions, and agreements. The conditions under which an individual operates and his perception of self and others are the result of his value system. Value systems affect attitudes, which permeate and influence all contacts and have a direct effect on the task of evaluation. The bulk of administrative science literature in recent years emphasizes interpersonal relationships and the manner in which informal relations affected by values enhance or subvert interaction and organizational structure.

Interpersonal relationships are broad in scope, complex in nature, and constantly shifting. An attitudinal survey is a helpful part of the evaluation procedure. A cluster of attitudes recorded over a period of time assists the nurse-leader in guiding members toward positive directional goals. When guidelines are vague, evaluators may rely on discriminatory behaviors and may tend to introduce ascriptive criteria such as race, religion, sex, age, social background, personal connections, and friendships.

A study by Quinn and colleagues[*] supports the need for a well-defined and clearly understood policy to avoid discriminatory reaction. They conclude that interpersonal pressures have their greatest impact on a manager's decisions when he or she is not fully aware of policy; also, personality and values have their greatest impact on decisions when the manager is not certain of procedural format. Assessments become ability oriented when objective criteria are considered, and knowledge, creativity, and job performance take precedence. Values are a part of each person and therefore influence evaluation. Clarity about one's own standards and those of the person evaluated help keep value systems in perspective.

---

[*]Quinn, R.P., Tabor, J.M., and Gordon, L.K.: The decision to discriminate: a study of executive selection, Ann Arbor, Mich., 1968, Institute for Social Research, The University of Michigan Press.

PREDICTIVE PRINCIPLE: Use of evaluative information serves both incidental and formal purposes.

Incidental and formal evaluations provide data that promotes employee growth. Most evaluative feedback is verbal or behavioral and occurs between the evaluator and the person evaluated. This type of evaluation is incidental and occurs frequently throughout the working day; it is seldom translated into a formal report. Examples are a frown from a co-worker when a requested urine sample is obtained late, a smile when the laboratory results are obtained on time, or receiving the "cold shoulder" from peers for being late repeatedly. These kinds of behaviors are evaluative in nature and act as reinforcers of desired behaviors or inhibitors of undesirable acts.

Evaluations that are more formal, but still not written or reported, take place in the form of conferences. Unwritten and informal evaluations not reported to others should be based on the same criteria used for written reports. The evaluator has some purpose for scheduling such conferences, which necessitates planning of procedures that will facilitate accomplishment of the goal. The form and timing of the formal evaluative information depends on how the evaluation is to be used.

Evaluative information may be dispensed to any person involved in primary care, in independent nursing practice, or in the organization who has official access to the information. Among these may be any one or all of the following:
1. Client
2. Individual employee
3. Person evaluated
4. Head nurse
5. Supervisor or coordinator
6. Nursing service personnel
7. Official committees of the agency
   a. retention committee
   b. professional standards committees
   c. personnel promotion committees
   d. research or data collection committees
8. Personnel office

The form the dispositional activity takes can be in any one or a combination of the following:
1. Verbal feedback
2. Behavioral feedback
3. Written memo
4. Formal evaluation using prescribed form
5. Signed official or personal letter

All evaluations, regardless of the form used, must be substantiated and qualified with first-hand evidence of the application of established criteria. No person, unless directly and officially associated with the employing organization, has legal access to an employer's records without the employee's consent. However, a summary of evaluation or the evaluation itself may be given out on the written request of the employee.

Performance review session

The final step in the formal appraisal process is the review session between the leader and the individual being appraised. The review session is a crucial aspect of evaluation and must be treated accordingly. Primary purposes of a performance review are to *increase the effectiveness of the nursing staff member in the health care setting and to promote worker satisfaction.* Secondary purposes may be to determine whether or not the employee should receive a promotion, merit raise, or be retained in the organization. The formal performance appraisal provides tangible evidence for the evaluator and staff member to see and discuss.

PREDICTIVE PRINCIPLE: A well-planned performance review session increases the workers effectiveness and promotes satisfaction.

During the interview the immediate supervisor and worker discuss the progress of the worker through (1) clarification of goals and objectives of the agency and area to which the worker is assigned, (2) identification of strengths and weaknesses (if critical to the job), (3) promotion of a feeling of satisfaction about the work and the individual's part in its accomplishment, and (4) establishment of new goals for the worker's growth and improvement.

A key element in the review session is maintenance of an open, two-way communication system where give-and-take can occur. The principles of effective communication apply to the review process, however, there is a uniqueness about the review process. Any time an individual's progress is being reviewed, there is a certain amount of nervousness and apprehension. This is particularly true if the individual feels that performance is questionable or inadequate and the job is in jeopardy. Guidelines are offered which can help to ease the situation:

1. *Provide a comfortable environment.* Make certain the meeting place is private, with the participants seated side-by-side so that they can review the written form together.
2. *Assure freedom from work assignment.* Arrange for coverage during the time of meeting; begin and end the session on time.
3. *Establish rapport.* Indicate to the staff member the appraiser's concern for sharing the leader's evaluation with the member. Acting as if

the task is something forced on the appraiser tells the worker that appraisal is not considered an important part of the management process, or may create fear about the appraisal. A few brief exchanges of informal conversation are advisable, but the appraiser should move right on to the business at hand.

4. *Indicate the appraisal is tentative, pending feedback from the individual.* Without a response from the worker, the appraiser does not know how that person is reacting to the information. The final product must be one that is acceptable to both parties.

5. *Begin the session on positive terms.* Establishing a positive relationship during a performance review requires a past history of primarily positive interactions with the individual. If negative interaction between the appraiser and the individual under consideration has occurred just prior to the meeting, then the appraiser must take a few moments to reestablish a harmonious relationship. The nurse can say for example, "Marie, I know we have had a disagreement, but that disagreement does not affect this review. I am glad you are a member of our staff." Of course, the appraiser must be sincere, for if the message is untrue, trust will be destroyed.

6. *Include all important issues.* The degree of attention that is given to individual items or issues during the appraisal session depends on the time factor and the significance of the matter to the job situation. Preplan the session to allow for appropriate emphasis. The appraiser makes certain the member being evaluated understands the rules of the conference, standards and criteria for the evaluation, and that feedback is encouraged. Broad categories can be covered with a single statement such as, "You function well in these areas," giving a few examples to confirm the assessment. Persons under appraisal need to know that their entire contribution to the work scene is considered and not just a few isolated incidents. Most people respond readily to positive feedback and thereby are motivated to improve their performance.

7. *Present criticism sparingly and carefully.* The purpose of criticism is to effect constructive behavioral change and not to reduce the individual to tears or to cause anger and hostility. Negative reactions cannot be avoided in criticizing work, but they can be made mild enough so that the worker will seriously consider the criticism rather than withdrawing or attacking the appraiser. Some more aggressive managers believe in "telling it like it is" and readily criticize in a direct and blunt manner. Often these same managers are reluctant to compliment the worker with the same emotional force. It is suggested that before recording and offering criticism during an appraisal conference, the ap-

praiser address the same kind of issues as for noting critical incidents; that is, ask the questions, is the manner critical and does the behavior affect job performance? Then if the behavior is deemed important enough to highlight in a review conference, the following guides for presenting criticism to the worker should be considered:

a. *Use a concerned tone of voice.* Appraisers who are nervous about offering criticism to a fellow team member may raise their voices or speak in rapid, curt tones. A harsh, authoritative quality of voice has a decidedly negative impact on the listener.

b. *Never combine positive with negative comments.* "John, you are very conscious of patient safety, but you are consistently late" illustrates such a combination. Pairing turns both comments into a negative appraisal. Positive comments are handled alone, as are negative stimuli. In this kind of situation, it is advisable for the appraiser not to give a criticism and then move right into an example. The usual outcome of this approach is for the worker to become immediately defensive and to offer reasons or excuses for the incident mentioned. The conference can quickly deteriorate into a blame session; "If you had not done so and so, I would not have acted in this way." The behavior the manager is trying to get the employee to change becomes lost while attempts are made to justify one incident. The best plan is to discuss incidents considered by the manager to be significant as near to the time of occurrence as possible; then reserve the formal appraisal time for cumulative or summative statements. Then if the worker says, "Can you give me an example?" the manager might counter with, "No, I'm not thinking of one incident in particular. We have discussed your performance from time to time in the work setting. My impression is that you are not as thorough as you need to be in recording client reactions to medication. What do you think?"

c. *Encourage feedback immediately after criticism.* The simplest way is to use a direct question: "How do you feel about that?" Then listen for the response! Most appraisers are uncomfortable with silence and tend to interrupt the silence with another remark. By waiting quietly, the appriaser lets the worker know the issue is important and time has been set aside for discussion. The thrust of the conference can be in two directions: agreement, with consideration of how to change the behavior, or disagreement. If disagreement occurs, some positive reinforcement can be used: "Kathy, are you saying that you are often late in arriving for work, but that you do a terrific job once you are here? I agree that you are a fine worker. Could we discuss your feelings about the effects of your being late on those who are waiting for you to relieve them?" The manager is reinforcing the person's worth as a team member, but the focus of the conversation is returned to the behavior that needs correcting.

d. *After necessary criticism has been reviewed, always reinforce the positive:* "Kathy, as I mentioned before, I believe you are a fine nurse and I am pleased that you are a part of our team. I am interested in your improvement." When the criticism is fair, most people will respond favorably. "I know I should be more prompt. I'm going to try harder." This attitude can lead to planning for behavior modification.

8. *Establish new goals for modifying or improving behavior.* If the appraiser accepts the concepts that (a) human resources are the greatest asset to goal accomplishment, (b) each individual is unique, and (c) each person has potential for improvement, then efforts will be made to understand and help individuals meet their needs. A leader can greatly affect the quality of performance of the worker by using the review session as a means for planning for change. Simply stating that new goals are needed does not make them materialize. But too much structure can lead to undesirable outcomes. The effective leader maintains a balance between too much and too little control. In detecting important deviations and in guiding behavior in the desired direction, some structure and limits are necessary. Too much control causes workers to feel overcontrolled, and the environmental climate becomes a stiflling, inhibiting, and unsatisfying place to work. With too little control the environment becomes chaotic, and people become disorganized and ineffective in achieving goals. The appraiser works toward maintaining a balance of control by allowing enough freedom to exercise individual judgment and initiative, and yet provides structure by having enough checkpoints to assure goal-oriented activity.

   Prior to the review session with the staff member, the nurse leader will have planned methods to assist the worker in professional growth and development. At the close of the conference the appraiser and the worker will agree on a plan that best suits the individual's needs and organizational interests.

PREDICTIVE PRINCIPLE: Improvement of worker competence leads to self-improvement strategies and coaching by management.

There are several approaches that can be used to improve competence. One is *self-development* in which each worker assumes responsibility for his or her own improvement. This plan is commonly followed in seeking knowledge and skill based on individual desire or in meeting continuing education requirements for relicensure. A wealth of resources are available to the nurse for self-improvement. Lectures, workshops, seminars, and courses are but a few. While self-development is admirable and to be encouraged, the nurse-leader cannot depend on the self-development approach entirely, as those who need improvement most may be least willing to seek help. Time and cost factors may also be deterrents to self-development.

A second approach to improving professional competence is through *planned, continual, on-the-job education and experience for all employees*. Employees are exposed to a certain amount of continual information from which they receive training in policies and practices of their employing agency. Also, new developments in theory and technology necessitate regular updates. These functions are thought of as an integral part of the staffing function. Larger health agencies operate in-service education programs, to meet the needs of all workers.

A third approach to modifying and improving professional competence is through an *individual, on-the-job coaching and counseling program*. The nurse-leader who is in closest association to the worker plays a major role in the coaching and counseling program through identifying the need for behavioral changes in skills, abilities, and attitudes that have not been managed through routine offerings, and for planning ways to coach and counsel the individual member while engaging in daily activities. Following are key concepts to remember in planning an individual coaching program with a worker:

1. There must be *a reciprocal relationship of trust and security between the leader and the worker.* The optimal environment for discussing and effecting changes is fostered by: (a) freedom to question and discuss issues without feeling foolish or stupid or being afraid of punishment or recrimination; (b) freedom to participate in establishing goals for improvement, and (c) the freedom of choice if there is a choice. If both participants in the review conference feel comfortable in the process, then development of the worker can advance.

2. The individual *must be motivated to fulfill a felt need.* Maslow's* hierarchy illustrates that opportunities must be safeguarded for the member to feel safe and secure, to belong, to have self-esteem, and to become fulfilled or actualized; therefore the desired goals of the leader for change in the worker must coincide with needs of the worker. The worker must come to the realization that meeting minimal standards of nursing care is necessary for continued employment and for approval of the appraiser. Self-esteem needs are involved, in that poor performance leads to feelings of self-depreciation. Other ramifications can be easily explored.

3. *The goals for modifying and improving behavior are realistic and specific to the problems.* When a problem is identified, Mager and Pipe† suggest a systematic

---

*Maslow, A.: Motivation and personality, ed. 2, New York, 1970, Harper & Row, Publishers.

†Mager, R., and Pipe, P.: Analyzing performance problems or "You really oughta wanna," Belmont, Calif., 1970, Fearon Publishers, Inc.

approach. The appraiser first decides if the problem really matters (Does the nurse smile enough? Is she obese? Is her hair too long? Are her shoes dirty?). If the problem does not interfere with work performance, then let it be. On the other hand, the problem may be a performance discrepancy or skill deficiency. If a performance discrepancy, Mager and Pipe propose the appraiser decide if the performance is punishing (for example, a staff nurse offers to take an extra load to fill in for an ill team member until her return; when the nurse resumes her duties, the charge nurse continues to assign the helping staff nurse as heavily as before). If nonperformance or failure to meet job requirements is the issue, then the appraiser determines if noncompliance is rewarding to the nurse. (For example, the nurse rarely seems to have time to prepare and hang all necessary IVs; she has learned that if she does not do all of them, another nurse will pick up this responsibility for her.)

The solution to the performance that is punishing is to remove the punishment (return the helpful staff nurse to a reasonable work load after return of her peer.) The answer to the problem of reward for nonperformance is to remove the help provided by a well-meaning associate. If there is a skill deficiency, the appraiser determines the reason for the lack: (1)Did the nurse use to do it? (2) Has she forgotten how? (3) Has she never done it? (4) Is she not able to master the skill? With data in hand, the nurse-manager can arrange for formal training, practice with feedback, or counsel the individual into another area of work.

Some qualities are more difficult to classify. These are generally interpersonal characteristics. For instance, a nurse may be very efficient, technically expert, and creative in her nursing care. She may also be cold, uncaring, and mechanical instead of humanistic. She may be difficult to work with, causing trouble among the workers and be a generally disruptive influence. These characteristics do influence client care because they directly affect clients and because they affect the work environment.

4. The plan devised for modification or change of behavior *utilizes principles of learning:* (1) acquiring *input,* which may be in the form of theory, instruction, or any other thinking or reasoning process (cognitive), (2) *action,* putting thoughts into observable behaviors, and (3) *feedback,* which provides information regarding any part of the learning process. The entire procedure may occur with such speed that clear delineation among the steps is not always possible. The very act of thinking may trigger doing, which in turn elicits a reaction that calls for more input or correction. The most useful element about familiarity with the three phases of the learning process is that the likelihood of the learner modifying or changing behavior is increased.

5. If possible, *no more than one or two problems are handled at a time.* When the manager attempts to modify or change a number of behaviors in an individual, successful achievement is jeopardized. It is easier to learn one thing at a time than to try to cope with a list of things. For example, if the leader

concludes the review conference with the worker with the statement, "The way I see it, you need to improve in organization, pick up speed in administering medications, visit each client at least every hour, and help team members more with their work," the worker may be overwhelmed and angry. A better plan is for the leader to pick the problem areas that are most critical and begin with these. For example, it can be mutually agreed upon that the nurse will use specific behavioral objectives to help with organizational skills. Given top priority, the remaining problems may not even have to be addressed, as there will be time for them.

6. *The results of the nurse's efforts are reviewed together with the coaching nurse.* A system of positive reinforcement is provided. The "law of effect" that states that behavior followed directly by a rewarding consequence tends to be repeated; behavior that leads to a negative or punishing consequence tends not be be repeated.

7. *Accountability for learning modified or new behaviors rests with the learner.* The nurse leader is involved in the improvement program to such an extent that the leader and the worker plan together what changes are needed and how they will occur. Together they establish alternate ways the nurse might go about learning or modifying behavior and checkpoints for measuring progress. But ultimately the decision to learn information, to acquire new skills, or to change other behaviors rests with the individual.

An excellent coaching program was developed by Place and Lederer of El Camino Hospital in San Mateo, California, for the new worker employed in a hospital. Using the nursing process, they programmed activities in terms of behavioral objectives for the department manager, preceptor, nurse-educator, and orientee as shown in Fig. 7-2.

Each of the approaches given for maintaining, modifying, or improving behavior can be integrated into a plan for development of the nursing staff individually and collectively if the leader knows the personnel, is aware of elements that influence performance, and is committed to the task.

PREDICTIVE PRINCIPLE: Staff evaluation of nurse-managers reveals general areas of strengths and weaknesses in the leader as perceived by the evaluators and provides the nurse-manager with one means of validation for the effectiveness of the managerial practice.

Although many nurses in leadership and management positions believe wholeheartedly in the process of evaluation for their staff, it becomes an uncomfortable matter when their own performance is under scrutiny. The usual procedure is for the immediate supervisor to evaluate the leader or manager, with only incidental input from the staff supervised.

Staff evaluation of the leader occurs on an informal basis through many ways. The manager assumes that staff assessment is high when there is coopera-

ORIENTATION RESPONSIBILITIES GUIDELINES

	HEAD NURSE	PRECEPTOR	NURSE EDUCATOR	NEW EMPLOYEE
ASSESSMENT	1. Interviews and hires new employee with input from AHN. 2. Administers Clinical Unit Skills Inventory 3. Pretests for theory and clinical abilities 4. Compares new employee to competencies in CORE curriculum	1. Reviews results of and explains use of: • Clinical Skills Inventory • CORE curriculum • Objectives • Other tests given to new employee 2. Direct observation of new employee clinical performance	1. Reviews results of: • Clinical Skills Inventory • CORE curriculum • Other tests given 2. Direct observation of new employee performance	1. Completes and updates Clinical Skills Inventory self-assessment of current performance level 2. Identifies own learning needs
PLANNING	1. Selects Preceptor for new employee 2. Informs Nursing Education, Preceptor & Unit Staff of new employee's hire date and learning needs 3. Assigns new employee to orient day shift and/or off shift	1. Has planning conference with new employee first clinical day 2. Writes mutually agreed upon goals and objectives to increase skill and performance level of new employee	1. Informs Preceptor & Unit of first clinical day 2. Assists Preceptor in writing goals & objectives	1. Writes mutually agreed upon goals and objectives with Preceptor
IMPLEMENTATION	1. Provides orientation and Preceptor time for new employee	1. Is not "in charge" while precepting 2. Provides Learning Center time for new employee 3. Provides learning activities for new employee 4. Acts as clinical resource for new employee 5. Weekly conferences to review progress on technical and process skills 6. Gives ongoing feedback regarding performance 7. Validates skills according to protocol	1. Provides new employee with general hospital orientation 2. Provide Preceptors with Preceptor Training Program 3. Assists Preceptor in locating appropriate learning activities	1. Reads Procedure & Policy manuals 2. Initiates own learning experiences 3. Follows learning activities outline in CORE curriculum and follows "Guidelines for Integrating Nursing Process into Practice"
EVALUATION	1. Evaluates orientee's progress by obvservation & feedback from orientee and Preceptor 2. Conducts 3-month evaluation conference with Preceptor and new employee 3. Determines if orientation needs to be extended 4. Assigns new employee to permanent status	1. Conferences with new employees about progress at end of orientation 2. Give feedback to HN regarding new employee performance 3. Provides written evaluation to new employee using: • Goals & objectives • Direct observation • Clinical Unit Skills Inventory • Process to Practice Tool	1. Assists Preceptor & new employee in evaluating new employee's progress 2. Consults on any proposed extension of probation or orientation 3. Evaluates orientation and updates learning programs as needed 4. Reviews orientation evaluations and gives feedback to Preceptors and Head Nurses	1. Conferences with Head Nurse and Preceptor at end of orientation 2. Evaluates Preceptor program and orientation 3. Writes self-evaluation of progress with use of Clinical Unit Skills Inventory & mutually set goals & objectives

Fig. 7-2. Orientation responsibilities guidelines. (From Plase, J., and Lederer, R.: Preceptors: A resource for new nurses, Superv. Nurse **12**(6):40, 1981.)

tion, willingness to receive and follow orders, freedom to ask questions, and the goals of the group are achieved at a desired level. Conversely, the manager senses evaluation of the role is unsatisfactory when there is quarreling, distrust, unwillingness to participate in planning and implementing care, and evidence that goals are not achieved.

Objective reactions to the leader's performance cannot be obtained from staff members unless the staff are given the opportunity to respond anonymously. It is suggested that each staff member receive an evaluation form on which to rank items that pertain to the manager role. The tool should reflect the standards of care and criteria developed for the agency and the specified work area. Examples that may be included are "Gives appropriate answers to my questions," "Provides help when needed," and "Listens to me when I discuss nursing care problems." A scale of numeric responses is used sometimes, with an explanation as to their meaning. In addition to responses to items, comments and suggestions should always be asked for. The evaluations should be given to a person outside the clinical area for tabulation and typing of comments.

The results may then be given to the leader being evaluated. It is proposed that the evaluation not be shared with anyone other than the leader. This provides the nurse-manager with the opportunity to (1) obtain an overall assessment of herself in terms of strengths and weaknesses, (2) validate personal assessment with that of those led, (3) identify and deal with staff problems that might not otherwise have been known, and (4) make changes or adaptations in behavior.

Future evaluations by the staff could be included in the formal evaluation process of the nurse-leader.

There are many benefits derived from positive and problem-oriented feedback. Open communication between leader and followers fosters trust and respect. When workers feel their work, attitudes, and comments are considered important by their leader, they are better able to value themselves as persons and as contributing members of the enterprise. When appreciation of the person evaluated is incorporated into the formal evaluation process, there is tangible evidence that this individual is worthy of recognition and reward.

With continuous feedback the evaluator avoids surprises. There is opportunity to check out with the worker areas where there may be misunderstanding. This averts the painful circumstance wherein a member receives a poor evaluation without opportunity to offer defense or to make changes in behavior.

PREDICTIVE PRINCIPLE: An evaluation process that includes reciprocal participation both vertically and horizontally provides an avenue for high level morale and job satisfaction.

Assumption of responsibility for one's actions and individual growth and development requires feedback data. There is no way to equate the democratic process with secrecy. Employees want to know how they stand in the eyes of the evaluator and management because status in the organization, raises, promotion, and seniority depend to an extent on assessment of individual performance. Counseling after performance appraisal that invites a reciprocal process is an indispensable step in the evaluation process. Not only are the individual's strengths recognized and areas that need improvement identified, but a feeling of self-worth and value is nurtured that serves to promote a high level of job satisfaction.

The individual or group in question not only should see the progress report but also should actually be involved in the assessment process. The evaluator can then validate actions as they occur and are later discussed and recorded. Unresolved differences of opinion in appraisal may remain even after attempts at clarification. In a fair manner and with the right to appeal in due process, opportunity should be provided for opposing views to be heard and recorded. The group or person being reviewed may request a third party report in defense of stated opinion. The evaluator may also wish to elicit assistance from outside sources, such as an immediate supervisor, nurse-leader, or allied health personnel, in gathering data and preparing the report.

All written evaluations should be read and signed by the person evaluated in the presence of the evaluators, and any rebuttal or confimation that the person evaluated wishes to enclose can then be attached and forwarded to the appropriate agency official or committee.

Application of predictive principles in evaluation of personnel

A staff nurse, assigned to an oncology unit in a voluntary hospital, is scheduled for her year-end performance appraisal review. The head nurse has arranged for coverage of the staff nurse's assignment during the time she is in session, has taken her into her office and shut the door, and has reached this point in the discussion.

Problem	Predictive principles	Prescription
The staff nurse is taking "shortcuts" in nursing procedures.	A well-planned performance review session increases the worker's effectiveness and promotes satisfaction.	Prior to conference, head nurse reviews evaluative data accumulated, determines patterns of behavior, and outlines a tentative plan for correction of the problem.
	Clear standards and criteria for measuring performance increase the objectivity and validity of evaluation.	Head nurse presents the problem to the staff nurse indicating the behavior persists even though conferences have been held on the subject previously.

Problem	Predictive principles	Prescription
	An evaluation process that includes reciprocal participation both vertically and horizontally provides an avenue for high level morale and job satisfaction.	Head nurse refers to procedure manual; asks staff nurse to indicate those procedures in which she takes "shortcuts"; head nurse validates, rejects, or adds items to the list.

Head nurse reaffirms the need to adhere to fixed policy. Develops a plan with the staff nurse's participation to achieve compliance.

Suggests that in the meantime, if the staff nurse wants to do procedures another way, she can join the hospital procedure committee and try to effect changes.

If staff nurse agrees to comply with hospital procedure, end the conference on a positive note of reinforcement for the performances that are well done.

If the staff nurse feels she cannot comply, then apprise her of the outcome of such an attitude.

BIBLIOGRAPHY

Books

Alexander, E.: Nursing administration in the hospital health care system, ed. 2, St. Louis, 1978, The C.V. Mosby Co.

Armstrong, R., and others: The development and evaluation of behavioral objectives, Worthington, Ohio, 1970, Charles A. Jones Publishing Co.

Biehler, R.: Psychology applied to teaching, Boston, 1971, Houghton Mifflin Co.

Cazalas, M.: Nursing and the law, ed. 3, Germantown, Md., 1978, Aspen Systems Corp.

Creighton, H.: Law every nurse should know, ed. 3, Philadelphia, 1975, W.B. Saunders Co.

Durbin, R.L., and Springall, W.H.: Organization and administration of health care: theory, practice, environment, ed. 2, St. Louis, 1974, The C.V. Mosby Co.

Flanders, N.A.: Analyzing teaching behavior, Reading, Mass., 1970, Addison-Wesley Publishing Co., Inc.

Gagné, R.M.: Perspectives of curriculum evaluation, Chicago, 1967, Rand McNally & Co.

Haussman, R., and Hegyvary, S.: Monitoring quality of nursing care. Part III. Professional review for nursing: an empirical investigation, Washington, D.C., 1977, DHEW Pub. No. HRA, U.S. Government Printing Office.

Havelock, R.G.: A guide to innovation in education, Ann Arbor, Mich., 1970, Center for Research on Utilization of Scientific Knowledge, Institute for Social Research, The University of Michigan Press.

Mager, R.F.: Giving care through others, Belmont, Calif., 1975, Fearon Publishers, Inc.

Mager, R.F.: Goal Analysis, Belmont, Calif., 1972, Fearon Publishers, Inc.

Mager, R.F., and Pipe, P.: Analyzing performance problems, Belmont, Calif., 1970, Fearon Publishers, Inc.

Maslow, A.: Motivation and personality, ed. 2, New York, 1970, Harper & Row, Publishers.

Reilly, D.: Behavioral objectives evaluation in nursing, New York, 1980, Appleton-Century-Crofts.

Stevens, B.: The nurse evaluator in education and service, New York, 1978, McGraw-Hill Book Co.

Periodicals

Bell, D.: Effective evaluations, Nurs. Educ. **4**(6):6-15, 1979.

Bloch, D.: Evaluation of nursing care in terms of process and outcome: issues in research and quality assurance, Nurs. Res. **24**(4):256-263, 1975.

Bloch, D.: Criteria, standards, norms—crucial

terms in quality assurance, J. Nurs. Admin., pp. 20-30, Sept. 1977.

Bloch, D.; Interrelated issues in evaluation and evaluation research: a researcher's perspective ... an evaluator's perspective, Nurs. Res. **29**(2):69-77, 1980.

Breedon, S.: Participative employee evaluation, J. Nurs. Admin. **8**(5):13-19, 1978.

Brief, A.: Developing a usable performance appraisal system, J. Nurs. Admin. **9**(11):7-10, 1979.

Council, J., and Plachy, R.: Performance appraisal is not enough, J. Nurs. Admin. **10**(10):20-27, 1980.

Crisham, P.: Measuring moral judgment in nursing dilemmas, Nurs. Res. **30**(2):104-110, 1981.

Del Bueno, D.: Implementing a performance evaluation system, Superv. Nurse **10**(2):51-52, 1979.

Eichhorn, E.: Managing maladaptive attitudes, Superv. Nurse **12**(2):25-31, 1981.

Eimers, R., Blomgren, G., and Gubman, E.: How awards and incentives can help speed learning, Training **16**(7):A3, 1979.

Flanagan, J.: The critical incidence technique, Psychol. Bull. **51**:327-358, 1954.

Goody-Koontz, L.: Performance evaluation of staff nurses, Superv. Nurse **12**(8):39-43, 1981.

Gray, M.: Rating departmental tasks: a tool for accountability, Hosp. Progr. **61**(4):74, 1980.

Haar, L., and Hicks, J.: Performance appraisal: derivation of effective assessment tools, J. Nurs. Admin. **6**(7):20-29, 1976.

Hamric, A., Gresham, L., and Eccard, M.: Staff evaluation of clinical leaders, J. Nurs. Admin., pp. 18-26, Jan. 1978.

Hatton, J.: Performance evaluation in relation to psychosocial needs, Superv. Nurse **8**(7):30-37, 1977.

Hochman, G.: Continuing education: how can you make the most of it? Nursing '78 **8**(12):81-89, 1978.

Kabot, L.: Objective evaluation for clinical performance, Superv. Nurse **8**(11):16-19, 1977.

Kaelin, M., and Bliss, J.: Evaluating newly employed nurses' skills, Nurs. Outlook **9**(5):334-337, 1979.

Kaye, L.: Work evaluations: are they effective? Nurs. Mgmt. **13**(4):44-51, 1982.

McClure, M.: The long road to accountability, Nurs. Outlook **26**(1):47-50, 1978.

McGregor, D., and Smith, M.: An uneasy look at performance appraisal, J. Nurs. Admin., pp. 27-31, Sept. 1975.

Plase, J., and Lederer, R.: A resource for new nurses, Superv. Nurse **12**(6):35, 1981.

Regan, W.: Head nurse responsibility: legal aspects, Regan Rep. Nurs. Law **16**(7):1, 1975.

Schwirian, P.: Evaluating the performance of nurses: a multidimensional approach, Nurs. Res. **27**(6):347-351, 1978.

Sherman, V.: Communicating expectations, Health Serv. Man. **12**(7):6-8, 1979.

Silver, D.: Counseling and peer review are key disciplinary procedures, Hospitals **52**(15):189-196, 1978.

South, J.: The performance profile: a technique for using appraisals effectively, J. Nurs. Admin. **8**(1):29, 1978.

Wooley, A.: The long and tortured history of clinical evaluation, Nurs. Outlook **25**(5):308-315, 1977.

Predictive principles for changing

The context of nursing and its influence on nursing change

The process of changing

Basic ground rules

Using clear communication and ground rules facilitates the interpersonal exchanges necessary for planned changes to occur.

Sharing ideas and opinions and using interpersonal communication predictive principles develop trust in the group process and facilitate effective problem solving.

Conditions necessary to changing

Failure of a nursing care delivery system to meet the needs of its practitioners, clients, or employers ensures changes in or the death of the system.

The breakdown of effectiveness of standard procedures and traditional organization patterns causes an increase in anxiety of the individual nursing caregiver.

Experiencing high anxiety levels provides a need for change or adaptation accompanied by an increase in individual and collective energy.

Need for change or adaptation stimulates personal fantasies of solutions or anticipation of achieving objectives.

Free exchange of ideas about goals and subgoals enables the establishment of specific and legitimate goals and collaboration for their achievement.

Explicit participation in and support of the administration for change ensures that the changing group has the power and authority to implement plans for change.

Creating environmental and operational conditions that nurture the change process supports the potential success of the change effort.

Group commitment to the change process itself instead of to specific changes enables continuing investigation, growth, and improvement.

Basic organizational patterns for changing

Use of an organizational pattern for changing that utilizes a framework for guiding the logistics of human resources in a task-oriented system promotes effective and efficient use of energy toward attaining the goal.

Basic planning strategies for changing

An explicit and definitive task analysis supports the ability of the client system to have an overall view of the subgoals and tasks to accomplish these goals.

Formation and assignment of task groups according to the task, time limitations, and capabilities of the change participants enable each member to contribute optimally.

Organization of change participants around components of task analysis decreases power and increases goal orientation of work groups.

Feedback from an alter group during the planning phase increases the probability that the group product will meet the staff needs, fulfill the task charge, and be useful to the target system.

Generating several solutions to a problem to achieve a goal enables the group to select an option most nearly in keeping with group needs.

Explicit rewards or recognition of individual or group achievement reinforces changing behaviors and promotes continuing efforts toward realization of goals.

Stability is a mirage for which one yearns and dreams. Individuals move through life seeking stability as knights sought the mythical Holy Grail. But life consists of balancing forces that tug and push in powerful energy fields. Nurses often feel caught in these forces, tossed and helpless in their grasp. The feeling of loss of control is frightening, and the energy drain in simply attempting to cope is tremendous. Energy exerted toward controlling self and others is often wasted because the forces of life's changes buffet people like a volleyball floating on a river. The resultant sense of powerlessness is a devastating feeling, and anger, aggression, frustration, and depression are high correlates of this powerlessness.

Control is the key. To affect, influence, and facilitate changes rather than be tossed hopelessly by them, one must focus the energy of control on the *forces causing change, not the people who are buffeted* or caught in the forces. This strange paradox can be likened again to the volleyball on the river. The force, speed, direction, and temperature of the water in the river directly influence the inflation pressure within the ball and the direction and rapidity with which it moves. If the change agent wishes to control the ball, the most reasonable approach is to control the flow of water in the river. Volleyballs do not lend themselves to having rudders, sails, or engines placed on them for control of movement; neither do people. Volleyballs can be tethered to a rope or string, but such control severely limits their movement and orients them in a single direction. Real, free-moving direction is exerted by controlling the forces that regulate the flow of water. This can be accomplished by removing or adding rocks and boulders, leveling the terrain, smoothing the river bed, rechanneling a curve, damming up tributaries and reducing the water volume, or even altering the water temperature by adding a power plant. Similarly, energy directed toward identifying and isolating the forces causing change, examining the consequences of controlling each of these forces, wisely selecting which consequence is desirable, and manipulating the force field is energy that has a payoff in a directly controlled and effective change program.

An example more vivid to nurses is found in the following story.

Margo is a small town that sat for many years off the beaten path in an agricultural section of upper New York State. Its small 160-bed Hill Burton hospital poked along in its sleepy way. The policy and procedure books were mostly window dressing for the Joint Commission, and nurses were shifted around pretty much as needed. Doctors worked on the "good old boy" system, keeping newcomers out and the physician "club" small. The emergency room was run almost entirely by nurses who bothered the doctors as little as possible.

In the space of three months two major freeways were completed that intersected at Margo, and a large chemical plant attracting 2500 employees was located there. Construction boomed bringing in additional workers, and three new physicians moved to town. It was a setup for chaos in the emergency room. The E.R., long used by the local doctors as a "Band-aid" facility to take care of patients they did not want to see or felt they did not need to see quickly, found themselves inundated with real emergencies. The accident rate climbed from the new interstate, new construction, and new influx of people to the town. The two emergency rooms stayed full, people sat untreated in the halls, waiting areas, and on ambulance stretchers. Doctors unused to being summoned to the emergency room were slow to respond. Nurses unused to the new kinds of conditions they were being asked to treat were hesitant to act without a physician or nurse-practitioner present. No routines were established, no precedents were available, no policies were in place, no twenty-four-hour physicians were hired, and no nurse-practitioner was employed. Coping patterns just were not available. The nurses complained, then began to quit. The hospital administration blamed nursing service, nursing service blamed the E.R. nurses, and the E.R. nurses blamed the doctors. A good hard look at the factors causing the breakdown was needed. The nurses and patients were like the volleyballs in the river. The additional client load and different types of conditions were like the force, speed, and direction of the water. Measures to investigate how the influx of clients could be controlled, staffing problems solved, and new procedures and policies instituted needed to be developed so that effective change could be initiated.

The context of nursing and its influence on nursing change

Nursing is a process or system and is subject to influences of other processes. Alterations in other processes or systems act as stimuli to nursing, and nursing responds to them either adaptively or maladaptively. The system that does not respond will not remain viable. The system that responds maladaptively may cease to be functional and thus become outmoded or unused. Nursing is an open system and is linked with other living processes. Nursing is influenced by and is responsive to stresses from such other operant systems as the political system, the social system, and the technologic system.

1. *The political system.* Funding patterns, such legislated matters as national health insurance, licensure and accreditation laws, nurse and other health worker practice acts, and educational legislation affecting nursing care delivery, client receipt, and nursing manpower production and distribution constitute the political system or arena. This arena is the basic battleground for nursing care quality control, education and development, and delivery system funding. Nursing leaders need to address themselves to the politics of health care and the subsequent cash flow patterns, which are derived from legislation on the community, state, and federal levels. Management of nursing care delivery will be influenced by political trends.

2. *The social system.* The characteristics of populations in social systems influence their change. For instance, the values in the United States have shifted from the melting pot dream of complete amalgamation of ethnic and racial population to pridefully organized groups, with emphasis on cultural, racial, and ethnic uniqueness. The need system shifted when the value system changed. Population characteristics are constantly changing, both nationally and in the specific environment of any nursing care group. The shift may be to concentrations of senior citizens in particular locations as retirement villages become more popular. There may be high density areas for specific ethnic groups or for great numbers of young people, as around colleges and universities. As mental hospitals emptied and halfway houses, board and care homes, and other such group-living situations became more prevalent and preferred, concentrations of the disabled or socially maladapted became more common. Other alterations are evidenced by changes in marriage patterns, the role of women, family dynamics, organizations and power groups, and trends in social values.

3. *The technologic system.* The technologic system affects nursing through various avenues. The equipment developed for health care makes nursing care pattern changes necessary. Changes in transportation patterns are causing health care delivery modes to adapt. Mobile clinics, increasingly efficient urban transportation, satellite health care centers, and other nonhospital-oriented care systems such as home health agencies are the direct result of increased technology. *Computer technology* perhaps offers the largest untapped potential for influencing modifications in nursing care. This potential is being widely implemented in some health care centers. The near future will see computer banks used for central recording and instant retrieval of client information for solving nursing problems beyond hospital walls. The client's chart will be a disc in a computer. Social Security numbers will be the magic keys to cumulative health records, which can be easily transferred with the client's permission from one health agency to another, enabling health care to become integrated. Nurses needing information ranging from preoperative procedures to the order and sequence of diagnostic tests may obtain this information with greatest efficiency by computerized data control. Although used currently in individual health agencies, the technology is not yet used on a nationwide telemetry network.

Because of these and other forces, changes in nursing are gathering speed and nurses are learning to respond and control some of the variables influencing change; thus they are affecting the direction, speed, and quality of innovations. The problem with modification is that change is not permanent; each ensuing experience brings another set of circumstances to be viewed, dealt with, and recycled into the change format.

Nurses usually cannot affect all the forces that make up the context of nursing and thereby influence nursing response to those forces. Nurses, however, can attain enough influence over the immediate variables affecting nursing care to govern the direction, rate, and expression of change in nursing. This chapter addresses itself to those areas over which nursing leaders can exercise influence and effect change.

The process of changing*

The process of changing is a process of leadership and accountability. It is a method of organizational structure and management; a means of adaptation and problem solving. In the process of changing, the interdependent and mutually inclusive nature of all processes meaningful to nursing is obvious. Planned change is change with a purpose, devised to solve problems of nursing care through the use of behavioral science technologies. Planned change is a type of human engineering in which theories of human behavior are applied so that intelligent choices and actions are made. *The process of changing deals with making alterations by choice and deliberation and is distinctly different from change by indoctrination, coercion, natural growth, and accident. In all facets of nursing, appropriate application of behavioral science techniques can produce changes that are the result of collective and collaborative choice, that is, participatory changing.*

For any nursing care system to change and grow, practitioners must respond through participation and collaboration to the vast number of variables in the health needs system with constructive deliberate changes in ways and means of coping with health problems. The use of theories of change with all recipients of nursing care—individual client, family group, and community—is necessary to the creative element of nursing processes.

One of the most difficult problems facing change agents is the lack of a conclusive theory on how to implement changes. Many studies have been done on the mechanics—the dynamics—of change. According to Bennis,† there is no theory of changing. However, there are some propositions about effecting social change that can be used as guides for change in nursing.

---

*The remainder of this chapter is adapted from Bevis, E.O.: Curriculum building in nursing: a process, ed. 2, St. Louis, 1978, The C.V. Mosby Co., chap. 5 and 8.
†Bennis, W.G.: Changing organizations, New York, 1966, McGraw-Hill Book Co.

Change theorists commonly refer to the components of the change process as follows:

Agent: facilitator, social scientist, nurse (trained in the science of change)

Rate: speed at which change takes place (evolutionary, slow, revolutionary, galloping)

Arena: organization, institution (the place in which the change occurs, the environment of change)

Person: target of change (client system; may be an individual or a group)

The bureaucratic way in which nursing care agencies are organized—the use of authoritative patterns of organization, the use of committee structure, and the use of parliamentary law for decision making—locks nursing care systems into stable and sometimes inflexible patterns of behavior unproductive for change. These practices mitigate against optimal participation, generation of the most workable alternatives, and maximal use of all participants' talents in planning for changes.

Nursing agencies, like most institutions, are organized around the military model of authoritarian structure. Employees fit into a line organization that stacks in groups or units toward people with more and more power and authority.

All authoritarian organizations use some modification of this military pattern. There are many variations of format, but basically each person is responsible, at least in name, for all that occurs beneath his or her level in the hierarchical setup. In this way, decisions are delayed while they are passed up the line for someone who has more authority to make decisions to act on. When groups organized in the traditional bureaucratic or hierarchical form deny that the authoritarian pattern exists, managers are placed in the position of having to maintain the responsibility because of institutional organization but with little or no authority because of the nursing group organization. Attempting to change the bureaucratic system can absorb energy that would be better used in making changes in nursing care and can effectively delay work to that end. Since the objective is usually nursing care improvement rather than institutional reorganization, a group can (for that objective) create a nursing organization that will facilitate work; for example, the staff can agree to try a different organizational mode for planning, creating, building, and testing change. Formal lines of operation can be maintained for other business and activities. The organizational problem is twofold: (1) how to get maximum participation by the total group involved with change and (2) how to make the changes flexible and responsive to society's or clients' needs. There are four categories of change factors that facilitate the two goals listed: (1) basic ground rules, (2) conditions necessary to changing, (3) basic organizational patterns for changing, and (4) basic planning strategies for changing. The term "basic" is used because the suggestions here are beginning ones; for each phase of change activities, the group may wish to modify, add to, delete, or suspend some of the organizational modes, ground rules, or planning strategies suggested, depending on their own immediate needs.

Basic ground rules

During change, people become somewhat frightened of the future because it is an unknown. Participants in change easily become suspicious that something is being put over on them. People often feel isolated and powerless. Their usual power bases are dissolved, familiar landmarks disappear, and fear of having no influence over the changes often underlies some of the resistive behavior seen in groups. There are ways a change agent can avoid some of the difficulties resulting from the nebulosity of change. Ground rules for the group interaction involved in planning for and implementing changes can, when used consistently, help to decrease communication problems.

PREDICTIVE PRINCIPLE: Using clear communication and ground rules facilitates the interpersonal exchanges necessary for planned changes to occur.

Group work toward changing is facilitated if there are some basic operational ground rules for the accomplishment of objectives. Nurses working together for change need to develop ground rules that facilitate change and promote healthy group relationships. It is possible to achieve both ends. Most often, nursing staff working relationships have established patterns of interaction—some patterns that facilitate and some that inhibit functional communications. On any nursing staff there are committees or groups that are powerful. Immediately on the opening of an issue, groups for and against draw their battle lines and win-lose conflicts are generated. With people who have worked together for long periods of time, the "red flags" or "buttons" that will elicit known predictable reactions are familiar and assessable. Button pushing and red flag waving can be a favorite pastime or a smooth way to sidetrack an issue. There are no easy answers to the problem of establishing communication patterns that are more supportive, productive, and useful for facilitating change. An outside communication facilitator is invaluable to any group that considers approaching change. Neutral, uninvolved facilitators can help group members look at transactions and interactions, analyze the communication factors, and establish more effective ways of communicating. The following list provides a sample of items that groups might like to consider for operational ground rules. Each group will evolve its own list and supplement it as it is used. Following are some prescriptive interpersonal ground rules for communications regarding change:

1. Try to have no surprises. Let everyone know in advance plans that are underway; previews, preliminary reports, and agreements to check out rumors will keep surprises to a minimum.

2. Provide as much informational input as possible. Part of the backbone of any planned change is the collection-of-data phase. Handouts, consultation with experts, training sessions, television, movies, and other audiovisual materials, circulation of helpful articles, and data discussion sessions prior to the time the information must be used help to provide the data base necessary to planned changes.

3. Make conflicts explicit and legitimate. Bring out hidden agenda items so that real issues can be handled. Legitimacy of conflict makes it possible to look for alternatives that meet every group's goals rather than locking into win-lose power struggles.

4. Identify high investment areas (areas of high feelings) and elicit the help of a neutral facilitator either from within the group or from a source unrelated to the problem or issue. This enables all factions to struggle or "fight fair," for a facilitator will ensure each participant's rights.

5. Make risks legitimate and failure salvageable and acceptable. Operating in small task areas allows greater risks to be taken because if one small part fails, the whole system of changes is not likely to fall apart. Back-up systems are other options for handling the problem if an original plan fails.

6. Make change in the middle of a trial run acceptable. Then if a plan being instituted is not working, alterations in the plan can be made without violating the group's preconceived notion that a trial run *must* be made all the way through.

7. Try to make it necessary to analyze failure or the reasons a part of a program is not working so that alterations and changes are not precipitous or without fair trial and so that the parts of a plan that may be causing the problems can be changed.

8. Agree to respond to each other's contributions to the group—comments, needs, and behaviors. Acknowledgement of entering into the group process reinforces and encourages continuing contributions and provides feedback. To be unacknowledged or consistently ignored leaves one having few behavioral cues, having a feeling of impotence and powerlessness, and feeling very alone in the group. Other participants are aware of nonresponsiveness and are reluctant to risk contributing and not being responded to. A simple agreement to respond or use some body language that is an obvious acknowledgment is necessary to a developing sense of being important to the group.

9. When complete win-lose deadlocks occur, agree to some form of action that will allow unlocking and saving of pride. Delay the issue or shuttle it to another time if necessary so that the group can be explicitly charged to look for options to meet criteria for a solution that pleases everyone. One way is to say "What do we want in the solution that will fulfill the needs of both groups?" Then brainstorm for criteria. Try never to make a voting decision while in win-lose situations.

10. Delay making final decisions. Make tentative decisions, take a consensus, decide on a trial basis, accept something as a provisional or working copy. Voting and recording in the minutes create a feeling of finality that makes it more difficult for members of the change group to accept alterations. Minutes become "laws," and members refer to them to win battles. If records are needed, call them "notes on the conference" or "record of discussion."

PREDICTIVE PRINCIPLE: Sharing ideas and opinions and using interpersonal communication predictive principles develop trust in the group process and facilitate effective problem solving.

Free exchange of ideas is not possible without an atmosphere of trust. Trust is basic to the mechanisms of planned change and is developed through consistently respecting the rights and limits of others and through meeting the needs of individuals and the group as a whole. Continuing communication requires a set of changing, evolving, colleague-oriented, equally participative ground rules. In autocratic systems, loyalty is given to the institution or group, the employer, the boss, or the supervising personnel. Peer group relations are marked by competition and a win-lose attitude in setting goals or generating solutions.

In a group in which the safeguards of ground rules have been established, in which each group member assumes the responsibilities for the group's work and is accountable for the quality of the group's communications, several things occur:

1. Individual faith in the ability of the group to produce successfully increases.
2. Individual respect for members' ability to participate increases.
3. Trust in the group process increases.
4. Group skill in problem solving increases.
5. Win-lose discussions decrease as the group becomes increasingly skillful at designing a multiplicity of options that are win-win.
6. Essential support for individuals becomes possible without sacrificing the goals of the group.
7. Loyalty to the profession of nursing and to colleagues begins to replace loyalty to agency or authority people.

Conditions necessary to changing

The rapid changes occurring in society cause change waves that affect all facets of life. Rigid structures, like seawalls, take the brunt of change waves and crack under the constant battering. Flexibility enables people and institutions to survive battering by altered needs that make change inevitable.

PREDICTIVE PRINCIPLE: Failure of a nursing care delivery system to meet the needs of its practitioners, clients, or employers ensures changes in or the death of the system.

Change occurs when needs arise that standard procedures and modes of behavior cannot meet. When new factors appear and many variables become part of a formally stable organization, new adaptive mechanisms are necessary to ensure continuity, quality, and efficiency of nursing care responses. Organizations, institutions, and individuals, having found a modus operandi that works for them, tend to solidify that operational system, because the very fact that it works is reinforcing. Thus when factors in the environment or some of the needs of consumers of the nursing care delivery system change, the system fails to respond by modifying its standard mode of operation, causing a decrease in efficiency, unmet needs, and unachieved purposes, as well as a decrease in quality care and a reduction in nurse and employer satisfaction.

For instance, when the quality expectations of clients change, the nursing care delivery system may or may not respond to that change. If the system does not alter with each new need or new variable, the problems begin to accrue and affect the relevancy of the whole care system. Eventually the variables accrue—for example, changes in the ethnic composition of the client group, shifting emphasis in the numbers of clients cared for at home rather than in the hospital, the number of clients seeking nursing care, changing laws affecting nursing education and service, and greater participation of clients in their own health care. The system of nursing must either respond to these changes or remain rigidly unresponsive and thereby become increasingly irrelevant. Subsequently, the majority of the nurse's time is spent in coping with a series of crises generated by poor adaptation.

Nursing historically has had very few variables; in the past many factors were stable and dependable, and standard procedures and stylized care systems were the ways used to cope with those conditions. Now health care as a national concern is a focus of the energy of consumers, legislators, and health professionals. The variables are so many and the stable factors so few that standard, previously learned modes of operation will no longer serve. The cues in the nursing world that were formerly considered stable points of reference no longer exist. Nursing will either decline as a discipline or devise more flexible and versatile programs of service and education.

PREDICTIVE PRINCIPLE: The breakdown of effectiveness of standard procedures and traditional organization patterns causes an increase in anxiety of the individual nursing caregiver.

Anxiety is the signal of readiness to change. Even though mild anxiety is the natural state of an organism, a rise in the normal level of anxiety makes for discomfort, and nurses often seek to return to a more comfortable state of being. If change procedures that will enable better coping with the new factors are not instituted, anxiety will continue to increase until total efficiency is affected. Some nursing groups do not institute plans for changing until there are a limited number of choices; change is then a matter of crisis. In this instance, change in long-term goals must be delayed while crisis intervention occurs, panic is controlled, or extreme anxiety states are lowered.

Crisis is a time when intense learning can occur and rapid changes can be made. A change agent must be available during crisis to participate with the nursing group in crisis intervention activities. Changes are easier when nurses preplan and work out changes in advance. But when a care delivery crisis occurs because of legislation, administrative edict, client demands, or changes in the nursing care group composition, crisis can become the useful vehicle for change.

PREDICTIVE PRINCIPLE: Experiencing high anxiety levels provides a need for change or adaptation, accompanied by an increase in individual and collective energy.

People in the anxiety/need-to-change sequence exhibit greater work output. However, if there is no articulation of goals, the work output takes on the form of busy work, of trying to make the obsolete system work successfully, of vicious circles, or of activities designed to control self and others. If the next phase of planned change is instituted, energy is available for work toward planning change. Nurses experiencing anxiety are open to alternatives and can learn new behaviors both for planning and for implementing changes. Change agents who can provide options, models, cues, and stimulants, and otherwise facilitate solution-directed activities during anxiety help the group use their energy in positive ways. This phase of anxiety, when the energy output level is increased, is the prime time for changing.

PREDICTIVE PRINCIPLE: Need for change or adaptation stimulates personal fantasies of solutions or anticipation of achieving objectives.

Everyone who is troubled dreams of a trouble-free world. Fantasies occur, such as "If only this and that were so, all would be right with heaven and earth" and "If we had this or that in our agency, everything would fall into place." Everyone anticipates the achievement of a personal vision of how things could be better. One of the difficulties is that visions of improvement, visions of how things could be improved, and visions of objectives are *private*. As private objectives, they have the connotation of illegitimacy, or being unacceptable. People fear offending power people, vested interest groups, and friends. If the goals are shared at all, they are shared with a few chosen associates. When nurses share ideas and goals, they often find others in the group have common dreams and goals. Aloneness is decreased, and objectives become legitimate.

PREDICTIVE PRINCIPLE: Free exchange of ideas about goals and subgoals enables the establishment of specific and legitimate goals and collaboration for their achievement.

Visions of the future can be translated into group objectives only if the group provides a time or mechanism for articulating ideas and fantasies about the future so that goals for work and criteria for changes can be established.

Change can be just a product of chance. Chance brings many alterations—some toward a desired end, some away from it. The ability to talk freely together as a group involved in changing promotes the realization of group goals through the mechanism of *making goals and means for reaching them legitimate, explicit topics for discussion.* Participation of those affected by change at every level—administration, head nurses, staff nurses, LVNs, aides, and students—generates a commitment to the change process itself and makes collaboration for specific tasks possible and desirable. One way to help staff members verbalize their ideas is to distribute a small questionnaire. The wording will vary according to the agency's specific needs; however, the principle remains the same. An example can be seen in Fig. 8-1. Using a form such as this can be the basis for participation in change. It makes problems, goals, and ideas explicit and reduces isolation. It legitimizes the expressed feelings of the workers.

PREDICTIVE PRINCIPLE: Explicit participation in and support of the administration for change ensures that the changing group has the power and authority to implement plans for change.

Every nursing organization has an administrator, a supervisor, a chief, a chairman, or a director. This person, in the eyes of the institution, is accountable to a superior for the activities of the staff, the delivery of care, and the success or

The thing I worry about most is _____

_____

The thing I dislike most is _____

_____

What I like most about my job is _____

_____

What I hope happens around here is _____

_____

Some ideas I have about how to get this accomplished is _____

_____

Fig. 8-1. Sample of a questionnaire to assess nurses' feelings regarding their jobs.

failure of the developing change enterprise. Thus no changes of major dimensions can occur without the consent and participation of the ranking persons. Because authority figures have and can exercise veto power or can influence administrators up the line to exercise veto power, the veto ability needs to be made explicit to the planning group. Inclusion of high level management people in work (task groups, heuristics, findings) decreases surprise, keeps them involved with the changes being planned, and reduces the chance that vetoes will occur.

PREDICTIVE PRINCIPLE: Creating environmental and operational conditions that nurture the change process supports the potential success of the change effort.

For change to occur, certain conditions must be provided. The change agent or manager seeks, in collaboration with others, to establish these conditions so that planned change can proceed. These conditions are as follows:

1. *Key organizational people must support and participate in the change.* In nursing care delivery system change, administrators, directors, committee chairmen, in-service education coordinators, physicians, and other key power people must support the idea of planned change as a total group effort. Since this means relinquishing some power to the group and exposing oneself in the group on a peer basis, it is at first a beginning acquiescence but one designed to become a growing commitment. Dignified retirements, transfers, and resignations are not necessary except in rare instances. Trust, collaboration, peer relationships, and free exchange of ideas are *learned* phenomena; with a skilled change agent, any group can learn these behaviors.

2. *The processes employed in change must be congruent with the philosophy, processes, and goals of change.* The ends do not justify the means, and the means employed for change must be of the same kind and caliber as the desired change. People learn as much from models as from any other learning mode, and the means for obtaining change furnish a behavior model for groups in the process of change. If an authority figure resists change, and if subterfuge, underground tactics, deviousness, and dishonesty are used to obviate the authority structure, the planned change will contain the same group tactics; thus the seeds of failure for the new attainments are sown.

3. *Participation in change is a voluntary commitment, as is opposition to change, and the battle must be freely and overtly fought.* The implications of this condition are that (1) the only pressures existing on individual participants are peer group pressures and (2) only in discussions where differences are aired openly without authority pressure for a particular, previously determined outcome can there be true resolution through the examination of available alternatives. In addition, mutual agreement must be reached within the change group and not imposed by an authority figure.

4. *All relevant or interdependent units are involved or oriented to the fact that the*

process of change is occurring in one of the groups so that change does not damage, shock, or interrupt other contingent units. For instance, if nurses wish to change the delivery pattern in a section of an agency to make their care of better quality, then nurses of other sections, physicians, other departments (x-ray, laboratory, and dietary), and all authority people involved should be notified so that shock, threat, and articulation problems are anticipated and minimized. Organizational patterns undergoing change in a nursing care situation need to be communicated to other departments interconnected with nursing so that others can aid the change instead of blocking it and so that the changes do not interrupt or decrease the effectiveness of others or of services to the client. The administration could question the feasibility or workability of the new plan or the plan could fail, not because the change is ineffective but because the necessary people were not consulted, alerted, oriented, or included in the planning phase.

PREDICTIVE PRINCIPLE: Group commitment to the change process itself instead of to specific changes enables continuing investigation, growth, and improvement.

Groups who organize for change and who proceed to plan and implement change can devise a desired change that gets frozen into decisions of total commitment. Commitment to the specific change, rather than to changing, is a trap. Using words like "provisional," "tentative," "trial," and "interim" communicates the concept of change as a process—continuing and progressing forever. Nurse commitment to flexibility, innovation, and creativity becomes real only with use. The process-of-change concept is actualized by building a framework for change that provides for and necessitates constant use of feedback for making continuous alterations to the whole nursing care system. For instance, no public health nurse would make a plan for a visit to be acted on regardless of the conditions encountered on the visit. The conditions encountered on arriving at the client's home would become rapidly gathered data that would probably be utilized quickly to alter the preconceived plan. The same habit of gathering and utilizing data and feedback and altering plans becomes a habit, whether one is dealing with nursing care delivery system, individual patient care, or organizational structure.

Basic organizational patterns for changing

Most health care agencies are organized for stability. Standing committees, steering committees, executive committees, and ad hoc committees are the avenues through which the work of the agency is accomplished. Normal bureaucratic agencies are structured to change slowly. They do change, but their response to the forces causing change is slowed by the very mechanisms that provide them with stability and permanency. To speed change and make agen-

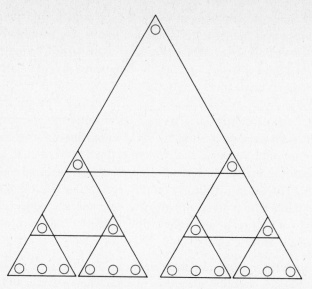

Fig. 8-2. Traditional pyramid type committee structure of bureaucracies.

cies more responsive to social forces, new, usually temporary but sometimes permanent, alterations must be made in the organizational structure.

PREDICTIVE PRINCIPLE: Use of an organizational pattern for changing that utilizes a framework for guiding the logistics of human resources in a task-oriented system promotes effective and efficient use of energy toward attaining the goal.

Organizations can take a variety of organizational patterns or structures. The types described here will be traditional (bureaucratic) nursing agency organization, modified traditional or "linking pin," collegia, and functional team.

Traditional or *bureaucratic* systems are typical of nursing service organizations. Hospitals, colleges, most businesses, and governmental agencies in the United States function under a hierarchical structure. Committee structure pyramids toward the top chairmanships, which are awarded by rank and tenure. A committee superstructure of chairmen meets and plans the work other committees are to do. Fig. 8-2 illustrates this organizational format. Changes are slow and difficult to make when using this organizational pattern. Response time is delayed while decisions are filtered through a maze of official channels.

Nursing organizations usually have six characteristics listed by Bennis* as typical of authoritarian organizations:

1. They have a division of work based on functional specialization (often medical model clinical specialization).
2. They have clear-cut channels of communication and hierarchy of authority and responsibility.

---

*Bennis, W.G.: Changing organizations, New York, 1966, McGraw-Hill Book Co.

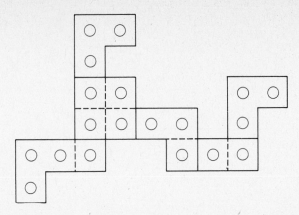

Fig. 8-3. Linking pin organizational structure. One person on a given task group serves on another task group working on a related task, thus furnishing a communication link and enabling the tasks to complement each other.

3. They are characterized by rules and bylaws and job descriptions that cover the rights, duties, responsibilities, and relationships of members.
4. They have specific and predetermined procedural specifications and directions for handling work situations.
5. There is a certain amount of impersonality in the relationships between levels of the hierarchy.
6. Tenure and promotion are based on job or technical competence.

The *modified traditional* or *"linking pin"* organizational system has many of the characteristics of the preceding list. It varies somewhat in that the groups within the organization have some autonomy; leaders may be appointed or elected and are not necessarily chosen because they are ranking members of the hierarchy; leadership can rotate periodically; and one or more members of each group belong either to another group or to a central executive or advisory board or group, thus linking each group and providing continuity, liaison, and communication. Procedure manuals, job descriptions, and other marks of bureaucratic organization are still in evidence. However, in linking pin organizational structure, committees are small, task oriented, and organized so that one member of a task committee serves on a related committee and is the communication pathway that enables work to be complementary and supportive toward goal attainment. Authority people may or may not be the link (Fig. 8-3).

On the opposite side of the continuum is a very loosely knit organizational pattern called a "collegium." Individual accountability is an earmark of a collegial organization; roles are almost completely blurred and can shift and change with the task to be accomplished (Fig. 8-4). Small groups assemble and shift in membership based on the needs of the group to accomplish an objective.

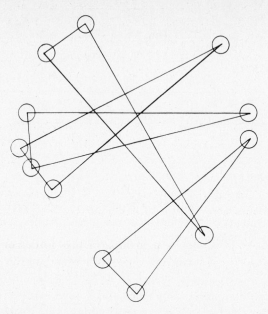

Fig. 8-4. Collegia. Objectives are clear cut. Participants collaborate with whom they need to at the time to achieve the goal. Lines are temporal. Membership in group is by ability. (From Bevis, E.O.: Curriculum building in nursing: a process, ed. 2, St. Louis, 1978, The C.V. Mosby Co.)

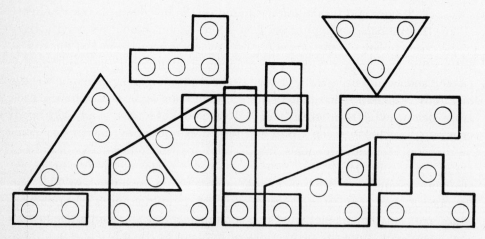

Fig. 8-5. Functional team. Groups are established and dissolved around tasks that need doing. Membership is by ability to contribute to the task. Role blurring occurs. Rank, position, and tenure are unimportant. All participate equally. (From Bevis, E.O.: Curriculum building in nursing: a process, ed. 2, St. Louis, 1978, The C.V. Mosby Co.)

Group membership is temporal, as is group leadership. Leadership is almost always by ability to facilitate the task, knowledge of the part of the task being worked on, or sudden inspiration or insights. Investment of energy is toward the task, and no energy is committed to stabilizing the group. The job or task to be accomplished can be envisioned as being like a basketball passed back and forth among the players according to their place on the court, the pattern of play, or their particular talents. The group moves the ball down the court, throwing it from one person or small group to another until at last someone puts it in the basket and the job is finished. If the ball hits the backboard and bounces back into play (feedback), reworking occurs until the ball is finally put through the basket and the goal is attained.

The type of organization that offers the most for change in nursing is a modification and synthesis of the collegium and linking pin approaches—the functional team or task group organization.

In *functional teams* (Fig. 8-5), groups or task forces of from two to five participants are organized around specific tasks. Membership on the task force

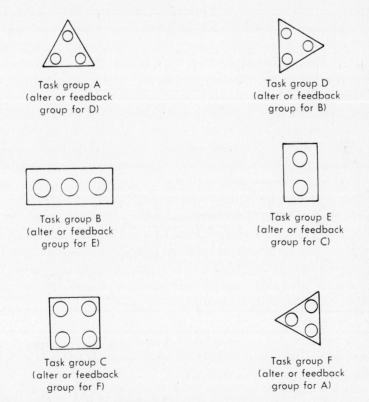

Task group A
(alter or feedback
group for D)

Task group D
(alter or feedback
group for B)

Task group B
(alter or feedback
group for E)

Task group E
(alter or feedback
group for C)

Task group C
(alter or feedback
group for F)

Task group F
(alter or feedback
group for A)

Fig. 8-6. Typical task group organization pattern with feedback or alter group assignments. (From Bevis, E.O.: Curriculum building in nursing: a process, ed. 2, St. Louis, 1978, The C.V. Mosby Co.)

lasts for the duration of the job. Once the job is accomplished, the task force dissolves. Role blurring occurs, and task force members contribute on equal footing according to their ability. Leadership in the group evolves from group needs and is not imposed on the group from without. Ground rules may change from task to task or from day to day within the same task force, for they, too, are generated in response to the needs of the task and not on a permanent basis. Completed work can either be sent to another task group for a critique—called an alter group or a feedback group (Fig. 8-6)—or submitted to the whole group. Reworking, revising, or altering based on the feedback may be done by the same task force or may be altered by the critiquing group, depending on the agreement between the groups. The difference between a collegium and a functional team is the degree of structure. Functional teams are highly structured, that is, they are given clear directions, time limits, checks and balances, a quality control or feedback mechanism, and a person or group with whom to communicate. Collegia work extemporaneously.

Basic planning strategies for changing

An altered organizational pattern for change preserves an altered way of looking at the task of changing. Often nursing care groups do not know what they wish to change to; they just know what they wish to change from. The goals and the content of changing can be separated from the process of changing. The change process can follow any number of patterns. The most effective patterns use a task analysis framework. Task analysis is a methodology that arose from systems analysis. Systems analysis was used during World War II to ensure the delivery of weapons to the fighting forces by specific times. Systems analysis has been most commonly associated with the space program and has been highly successful in enabling many companies manufacturing a small component of a space system to complete their work and deliver their component at the time specified with confidence that the component would work effectively when interlinked with the other components being produced. These same methods are now component tasks. These tasks are then assigned to small groups. The completed product is used as a basis for the next stage of work, forming a systemic linkage of work designed to achieve goals.

PREDICTIVE PRINCIPLE: An explicit and definitive task analysis supports the ability of the client system to have an overall view of the subgoals and tasks to accomplish these goals.

PREDICTIVE PRINCIPLE: Formation and assignment of task groups according to the task, time limitations, and capabilities of the change participants enable each member to contribute optimally.

PREDICTIVE PRINCIPLE: Organization of change participants around components of task analysis decreases power plays and increases goal orientation of work groups.

The traditional way of organizing for change involves the establishment of committees. Committees, subcommittees, and ad hoc committees are the modes used in most bureaucratic organizations that rely on parliamentary law, parliamentary procedures, and parliamentary organizational forms. Committees have several characteristics that make them poor means for achieving change:

1. Committees tend to be power bases for individuals and factions in an organization. Much effort then goes into maintaining the power group, obtaining more power, and exercising power.
2. Power struggles tend to develop over issues, and individuals lock into a win-lose situation. The parliamentary procedures then tend to inhibit the search for alternatives that are win-win. The very act of voting locks people into win-lose modes.
3. Once power struggles arise in a committee and power lines are drawn, each new issue perpetuates the power struggle. This causes compromises to be made in ways that may pull the teeth from changes. This is done over the issue of power and influence and not often over the issues inherent in change.
4. Committee membership becomes a prestige item, and changes that threaten the prestige, power, or existence of membership are resisted. Thus the committee tends to structure in order to perpetuate its own existence. Energy that could go into accomplishing goals is funneled off into committee maintenance.

The first major planning strategy for change is to opt for a structure that enables nurses and interested others to form small, loosely knit task groups. These groups are formed of individuals who have an interest in or expertise for a specific task to achieve a specific goal. A task group organizational pattern assumes a task analysis format. Task analysis, as mentioned earlier, is a method of taking a large goal and breaking it down into the steps, subgoals, or tasks that will ensure the reaching of the overall objective. Often the sheer size and magnitude of a change is frightening. Task analysis is reassuring in that groups can see the probability of succeeding in a small given task, whereas the overall job may seem overwhelming. Small tasks or jobs are easier to achieve, and success is fairly quick, clear, and definitive. Success then breeds successes, and the reinforcement of completing one small bit of the total job motivates and energizes the nursing group to go on to the next task group and the next task. New people, new working relationships, and a new task dissipate the potential for developing power plays that siphon energy from the job to be done.

Every change goal can be reached by the simple expedient measure of analyzing the steps necessary to reach the goal. In each of the steps or sequence components there is a group of tasks for that component that must occur before that phase of development can be successfully organized and accomplished. Each group will need to analyze the tasks that are necessary to the change patterns of each individual nursing group. The following is an example of a task analysis.

Example of a task analysis

Goal: To create a better nursing care record or charting form and system.

Task analysis:
1. Devise criteria for a desirable charting form.
2. Mentally create components of a format that would meet those criteria.
3. Generate two or three alternative plans for using the components.
4. Choose a plan or synthesize from the ones presented.
5. Measure synthesized plan against established criteria.
6. Plan and select ways and means for testing a sample run of the new charting forms.
7. Institute the test run.
8. Get feedback from testers and share with all work groups.
9. Alter plan, using feedback.
10. Retest.
11. Confirm and implement or revise and retest the plan until perfected.
12. Establish regular evaluation and review so change is ongoing.

Example of task analysis for task 1: Devise criteria for a desirable charting form.
1. List the purposes of the nursing care record.
2. List the content necessary to accomplish the purposes.
3. Survey target group: What do participants like about present forms? What is disliked about them? What would the members prefer in a form? Do the present forms accomplish the purposes as listed? Categorize and sort findings and provide summary.
4. Survey similar agencies over the country for sample forms and analyze for strengths and limitations. Categorize and sort findings; provide a summary.
5. Survey the literature on nursing record formats. Distribute useful articles or annotated notes or summaries to target group.
6. Obtain summaries and findings from all task groups. Ask three different task groups working independently to present the criteria by which they would evaluate a charting form and system.
7. Each of the three groups presents its criteria to three different alter groups for critique and feedback.
8. Select and use the feedback felt appropriate to improve criteria.
9. Present criteria of all three task groups to the target population. Obtain feedback and suggestions.
10. Assign one task group to use feedback to make one criteria list for a desirable charting form and system.

The task force organizational pattern allows implementation of a format for change that facilitates optimal participation by all people involved in change. A task analysis framework for organizing nursing care systems change enables tasks small enough to be handled in a short time span to be assigned to a specific group for a specific purpose. The tasks listed can be divided among small task forces and the work accomplished efficiently.

By using the task group format, power struggles have little time to develop and compromise is often delayed until adequate numbers of choices have been generated. Groups are small enough so that each member can generate possibilities and choices and bring them to the group for a critique. The group can then put together the desired product from individual contributions.

Task groups are transitory, membership expectations are for a temporary existence, work is task oriented with no energy given to maintaining the group, and dissolution is natural when the task is completed.

Working in task groups using a task analysis as a basis for organizing for change accomplishes some of the following:

1. Explicit and definitive task analysis provides client systems with an overall view of goals and steps that must be taken to reach the goals.
2. Established target dates enable change participants to pace their work realistically.
3. Temporary organization keeps participants job or task oriented and decreases focus on power.
4. Participating in task groups outside the area of immediate skill widens the horizon of individual members' views of nursing, decreases tunnel vision, provides scope, and brings fresh ideas from people not necessarily locked into a single system or way of accomplishing a goal or viewing a concept.
5. Working with people outside the usual committee structure broadens the base of working relationships and decreases fantasies about what colleagues are like; it establishes new communication habits and patterns.

PREDICTIVE PRINCIPLE: Feedback from an alter group during the planning phase increases the probability that the group product will meet the staff needs, fulfill the task charge, and be useful to the target system.

The second planning strategy that is most useful is to provide for feedback prior to total staff and management consideration. Feedback is provided by task groups called alter groups (Fig. 8-6). These critique groups provide checks and balances so that the creators of an idea, or task, can have the benefit of objective feedback, for example, a disinterested perspective for examining the work, asking questions, suggesting clarification of specific parts, looking at congruencies among parts, suggesting revision, addition, or deletion in the work, and any other functions of feedback. The use of an alter group not only improves the product of the task group and helps to prepare it for total group discussion, but also widens the base of support through investment. When the second group becomes involved, it has already participated in accomplishing the task and therefore is prepared to speak to it and to support, at least in some measure, the group originally assigned to that task. The more people who participate in the creation of an idea or completion of a task, the more balanced the discussion of that suggested alternative is likely to be.

PREDICTIVE PRINCIPLE: Generating several solutions to a problem to achieve a goal enables the group to select an option most nearly in keeping with group needs.

The third basic planning strategy suggested here is the generation of more than one choice for every phase of, or task in, change building (see example task analysis, p. 332). Choice is perhaps the most important aspect of facilitating change. One of the reasons preplanned change can be so effective is that groups need not be faced with having to accept an option solely because it is the only one available. Group planning for change includes, at every phase, the assigning of more than one task group to a task, with directions to work independently of each other, and the offering of more than one alternative plan to the total group. The consequences of having a choice are that (1) groups tend to be more stimulated as they look at options and discuss the potentialities and liabilities of each plan; (2) congruence or incongruence of parts of the plans with the theoretical base of the total plan are brought to light; and (3) the best parts of the options can be pooled for developing a plan that meets the needs of the group.

PREDICTIVE PRINCIPLE: Explicit rewards or recognition of individual or group achievement reinforces changing behaviors and promotes continuing efforts toward realization of goals.

The last important strategy for change to be discussed here involves a reward system. There is reward inherent in creating workable changes, which are tangible manifestations of visions. The more emphasis that can be placed on the continuity of the road from the past (what individuals wished to accomplish) to the present (what the total group has accomplished), the greater will be the feeling of success. Beyond the reinforcement of accomplishing goals is the individual group member's contribution to that goal. Often work becomes such a synthesis of so many people's ideas that individual contributions are lost, and an anonymity develops that makes the work itself impersonal and easy to disown as not being a part of each person as an individual. There are some things that change agents can do to keep the personal element in the changes without destroying the group feeling. For instance, when members of a task group, three or four people, collaborate on a special project and generate a piece of the puzzle appropriate for distribution to others or for publication, it is reinforcing to give recognition to the people preparing the product. By-lines, such as "Prepared by Dianne Nicholson and Lucy Miller, in collaboration with other members of the nursing staff of Hillview Health Center," are expressive of the individual work and the contribution of the whole, and thus give special credit to the authors without detracting from the general credit due the group. Following are other reinforcing activities:

1. Encourage and facilitate publication of materials generated.
2. Provide letters, encouragement, and active support for efficiency evaluations and promotions.
3. Speak to "power" people, for example, head nurses, supervisors, and other managers, of specific contributions individuals have made.
4. Promote publicity for innovative endeavors through local newspapers, agency newsletters, and so on.
5. Celebrate milestones of accomplishment with small parties (this activity interrupts flow and marks progress and thus provides a point of reference).
6. Save early work as a starting point marker to make comparisons and provide perspectives on how far the group has come in achieving changes.
7. Distribute general congratulatory letters periodically when particularly effective results have been achieved.

These activities are useful for role modeling the process of valuing the contributions of individuals. Too often nurses tend to devalue their own work and value that of outsiders. Any activity that provides patterns of behavior establishing the value of "home town prophets" builds self-confidence and helps the group make it legitimate to use each other as consultants.

Application of predictive principles of changing

A representative from the evening shift approaches the head nurse and states: "The afternoon personnel have asked me to represent them. They wish to discontinue charting on evening shift patients. It is a meaningless bit of busy work and a waste of time. We could just check off medications and sign the nursing record page that we've seen the patient."

Problem	Principles	Prescription
How to enable the group to determine what changes in charting and charting policies will best meet the needs of clients and staff.	Failure of a nursing care delivery system to meet the needs of its practitioners, clients, or employers ensures changes in or the death of the system.	Make critique of the system legitimate and elicit consensus that change is needed.
	The breakdown of effectiveness of standard procedures and traditional organization patterns causes an increase in anxiety of the individual nursing caregiver.	Elicit agreement to participate in work toward finding workable solution to problem.

Problem	*Principles*	*Prescription*
	Experiencing high anxiety levels provides a need for change or adaptation accompanied by an increase in individual and collective energy.	Channel energy into task groups, goal setting, and goal attainment.
	Need for change or adaptation stimulates personal fantasies of solutions or anticipation of achieving objectives.	Involve group in brainstorming about problems and possible workable nursing recording forms and procedures.
	Free exchange of ideas about goals and subgoals enables the establishment of specific and legitimate goals and collaboration for their achievement.	Brainstorm about a process for change that would involve all concerned and accomplish goals; brainstorm about goals and steps or tasks necessary to achieve goals.
	Explicit participation in and support of the administration for change ensures that the changing group has the power and authority to implement plans for change.	Invite appropriate power people to take part in the discussions from the first or have regular appointments; be sure power people condone or consent to potential change.
	Creating environmental and operational conditions that nurture the change process supports the potential success of the change effort.	
	Use of an organizational pattern for changing that utilizes a framework for guiding the logistics of human resources in a task-oriented system promotes effective and efficient use of energy toward attaining the goal.	Get consensus for an organization for change that uses everyone's potential without regard to status, rank, or position—transient task groups of some kind.
	An explicit and definitive task analysis supports the ability of the client system to have an overall view of the subgoals and tasks to accomplish these goals.	Assign a task group to do a task analysis on overall goal.
	Formation and assignment of task groups according to the task, time limitations, and capabilities of the change participants enables each member to contribute optimally.	Assign task groups to task identified by the analysis group.
	Feedback from an alter group during the planning phase increases the probability that the group product will meet the staff needs, fulfill the task charge, and be useful to the target system.	When tasks are completed, give to feedback group; rework task, based on feedback.

Problem	*Principles*	*Prescription*
	Generating several solutions to a problem to achieve a goal enables the group to select an option most nearly in keeping with group needs.	Be sure that several task groups work on alternative solutions so group will have a choice.
	Explicit rewards or recognition of individual or group achievement reinforces changing behaviors and promotes continuing efforts toward realization of goals.	Acknowledge groups' and participants' contribution; write notes for change participants; acknowledge ideas; give reinforcement for participation; set up mechanism for continued review, testing, and evaluation of planned program of change.

BIBLIOGRAPHY
Books

Alexander, E.L.: Nursing administration in the hospital health care system, ed. 2, St. Louis, 1978, The C.V. Mosby Co.

Bennis, W.G.: Changing organizations, New York, 1966, McGraw-Hill Book Co.

Bennis, W.G., Benne, K.D., and Chin, R.: The planning of change, ed. 2, New York, 1969, Holt, Rinehart & Winston, Inc.

Bevis, E.O.: Curriculum building in nursing: a process, ed. 3, St. Louis, 1982, The C.V. Mosby Co.

Havelock, R.G.: A guide to innovation in education, Ann Arbor, Mich., 1970, Center for Research on Utilization of Scientific Knowledge, Institute of Social Research, The University of Michigan Press.

McLemore, M.M., and Bevis, E.O.: Planned change. In Marriner, A., ed.: Current perspectives in nursing management, vol. 1, St. Louis, 1979, The C.V. Mosby Co.

Saunders, L.: Permanence and change. In Lewis, E.P.: Changing patterns of nursing practice, New York, 1971, The American Journal of Nursing Co.

Seiler, J.A.: Systems analysis in organizational behavior, Homewood, Ill., 1967, The Dorsey Press, Inc.

Periodicals

New, J.R., and Corriland, N.: Guidelines for introducing change, J. Nurs. Admin. **11**(3):17-21, 1981.

Simms, L.L.: Administrative changes and implications for nursing practice in the hospital, Nurs. Clin. North Am. **8**(2):227-234, June 1973.

chapter nine

Predictive principles of leadership behavior

Fundamentals of leadership

Understanding the meaning of authority, power, and influence provides the nurse with a basis for successful leadership.

Understanding personality, behavior, and situational factors that influence leadership provides the nurse with a basis for determining a suitable style of leadership for the work setting.

Consideration of the work situation, manager's leadership style and expectations, and follower's characteristics and expectations results in harmonious goal accomplishment.

Knowledge of theory levels and ability to formulate valid predictive principles promote the leader's ability to identify the levels on which members are functioning to facilitate growth in problem solving and goal attainment.

Effective use of self in time management results in control of self and of the work situation.

Planning for urgent or crisis situations provides proper nurse coverage and reduces negative leadership behaviors as a result of work overload.

Awareness of self

Knowledge and understanding of factors about human beings permit assessment and acceptance of self and others.

Identification of the leader's own needs aids in the identification of needs of others.

Translation of individual needs into behavioral terms allows an objective approach to leadership with respect to need analysis and fulfillment.

Accomplishing goals through assertive behavior enables a leader to exercise the rights of self without denying the rights and feelings of others.

Consistent use of passive behavior ignores personal rights of the leader and leads to lowered self-esteem and maladaptive behaviors.

Achievement of one's goals through aggressive acts violates another person's rights and results in feelings of domination, humiliation and hostility.

Knowledge of the job

The demands of the situation in which a leader is to function influence the qualities, characteristics, knowledge, and skills necessary for successful leadership.

The degree to which the leader is clinically knowledgeable and competent directly influences feelings of security about the appropriateness of nursing activity.

Mutual respect

Understanding and practicing the basic elements of mutual respect facilitate effective leadership.

The leader's expressions of respect for others precipitate acts of mutual respect among members.

Open channels of communication

Knowledge of appropriate organizational channels of communication facilitates efficient utilization of line organization.

The nurse working in an expanded role provides leadership initiative in establishing channels of communication congruent with the role.

Knowledge of participants' capabilities

An understanding of sociocultural backgrounds of members helps the leader to assess job capabilities.

Reactions to stress influence efficiency of performance in the work situation.

Knowledge of a caregiver's preparation and experience promotes fullest use of skills and provides a basis for continued growth.

Environment

A work environment that is open and amenable to valid change assists in personal and professional growth and development.

The word leadership is an exciting one. If asked to name people who are leaders, certain names immediately come to mind such as Abraham Lincoln, Winston Churchill, John F. Kennedy, Martin Luther King. In the nursing world Florence Nightingale probably stands out in the minds of most who are asked to name a single example of a nursing leader. Defining leadership is more difficult. Stogdill[*] points out that "There are almost as many different definitions of leadership as there are persons who have attempted to define the concept." A philosophical approach to leadership is taken by Levinson[†] who states, "The successful leader is a builder of men and women who are bigger than they know and serve better than they dreamed." In formal organizations, leadership is generally defined as *a set of interpersonal behaviors designed to influence employees to cooperate in the achievement of goals or objectives.*

In nursing publications the definitions of leadership contain the basic commonalities of goal setting, participant involvement, and leader behavior. For

---

[*]Stogdill, R.: Handbook of leadership: a survey of theory and research, New York, 1974, Free Press, p. 7.
[†]Levinson, H.: Executive stress, New York, 1970, Harper and Row, p. 143.

this discussion, nursing leadership is defined as *the ability to use the processes of life to facilitate the movement of a person, a group, a family, or a community toward the establishment and attainment of a goal* (see Chapter 1). Leadership is not automatic. Effective leadership is a learned process. The culmination of all nursing activity is the delivery of client care. Scientifically based, problem-oriented behavior that is in the client's interest will produce quality care and is likely to be administered at less cost to the consumer of health services.

This chapter discusses the fundamentals of leadership, awareness of self, and knowledge of the tasks to be performed. Similarly, it is concerned with the capabilities of the leader, as well as with the environment in which nursing care is rendered. Most of these concepts have been integrated into the content of the preceding chapters.

Fundamentals of leadership

Historically, leadership was awarded to the strong. From primitive times to the present, rule of the powerful has been felt on all levels. Cunning and brain power have replaced brute strength, but the system still exists in some milieus. It is a hallmark of an advanced civilization that leaders receive their authority from the groups they lead and maintain their leadership only as long as they meet the needs of the groups they are guiding.

Even in the most democratic of leadership situations, authority and power struggles exist. In nursing, for example, for too long the capable nurse-leaders have not been delegated authority and power commensurate with responsibility for planning and decision making. Traditional management practices reflect the belief that nurses at the operational level require close supervision and control; therefore someone else must retain the power. The divestment of authority from those nurses on operational levels has led to power struggles. If ignored, these power struggles dissipate energy, divide and demoralize the participants, and result in decreased productivity.

PREDICTIVE PRINCIPLE: Understanding of the meaning of authority, power, and influence provides the nurse with a basis for successful leadership.

The terms "authority," "power," and "influence" will be reviewed briefly. *Authority* means the right to give commands, enforce laws, or exact obedience. The one who has authority generally is considered to have the knowledge and expertise in a given field necessary to make judgments and to direct others. Formally, authority is commonly viewed as originating at the top of an organizational hierarchy and flowing downward via delegation. However, authority must be accepted by its subjects before it becomes a reality.

Power implies the ability or capacity to act or perform effectively. It is the ability to impose the will of one person or group so as to bring about certain behavior of other persons or groups. As shown in Fig. 9-1, authority, power, and

AUTHORITY	POWER	INFLUENCE
The right to: Give commands Enforce laws Exact obedience	The ability or capacity to impose the will of one person or group upon another person or group	The behavior of an individual or group affected by the behavior of another individual or group

Fig. 9-1. Differences and interdependency between authority, power, and influence.

influence have different definitions and mean different things. One cannot use them interchangeably. One can have authority (the right to give commands) but because of timidity, lack of knowledge, hesitancy, or confusion not have the power (ability to impose compliance) or influence (ability to effect changes of behavior) to make another actually bend to commands. On the other hand, a person may have the power to impose his will because of influence with persons in authority but may lack the direct official authority (right).

Leadership is enacted through the exertion of power and influence. Management is enacted through the use of authority, power, and influence. As discussed in previous chapters, there are five bases of a leader's power: (1) *reward* power, or the power to compensate or give rewards for tasks satisfactorily completed, (2) *coercive* power, or the power to punish, (3) *legitimate* power, or the power of lawful or formal authority, (4) *referent* power, or the power to cause others to imitate one's personal style or behavior, and (5) *expert* power, or the power of superior knowledge, ability, or skill.

Power implies a relationship of interdependency. The effective leader will honor this concept, knowing that success in any venture rests in collaborative effort of the participants. The use of aggressive, assertive, or passive behavior becomes vitally important in power relationships.

Influence is a relationship in which the behavior of an individual or group is affected by another individual or group. Influence can come from direct or indirect sources. It can be exerted because of certain role expectations of a position, individual, or group. Nurse-worker, nurse-client, and nurse-physician are examples of direct influence. Indirect influence is far more subtle since the major base of influence is intangible. One does not need to have authority and power to exercise influence over another. Motivation for influencing others is couched in terms of gains and costs to be expected. The influencing process utilized by the leader may be in the form of advice, suggestion, discussion, persuasion, or role modeling. The outcome of influence is uncertain because one cannot predict with assurance the effects of influence. Influence can be said to be operational when response by others to the one who influences occurs voluntarily and without coercion.

In summary, authority, influence, and power are distinguishable but interdependent. Each is vital to the leadership role. A leader must have the authority to make decisions affecting the behavior of others. Leaders must have the power and ability to satisfy or not to satisfy human needs, and they must exercise influence directly and indirectly to effect change. The more sources a leader can draw on, the more successful his or her leadership will be.

PREDICTIVE PRINCIPLE: Understanding personality, behavior, and situational factors that influence leadership provides the nurse with a basis for determining a suitable style of leadership for the work setting.

There are three major approaches to the study of leadership: traits, behaviors, and situational. The *trait* approach attempts to determine the personality characteristics possessed by successful leaders. The second approach attempts to identify the *behaviors* associated with effective leadership. Both these approaches assume that an individual with the appropriate traits or behaviors will emerge as the leader in whatever group situation that individual may be placed. A third approach, the *situational* perspective on leadership, assumes that the qualities that determine leader effectiveness will vary with the situation, the tasks to be accomplished, the skills and expectations of the workers, the organizational environment, and the past experiences of the leader and workers. The premise is made that an individual who is an effective leader in one situation might do very poorly in another. These three major approaches will be examined further with implications for nursing leadership.

Traits or characteristics. Since the 1930s, when psychologic testing became popular, the research on leadership focused on personality traits or distinguishing features about a person such as intelligence, shyness or aggressiveness, ambition, or laziness. The intent of these leadership theorists was to isolate a set of characteristics that would describe all effective leaders. Then all an employer need do was to compare the applicant with the list of characteristics and determine the worker's acceptability for the job. Examination of the literature reveals that the list has grown until there are over a hundred characteristics identified as being essential to successful leadership.

A more constructive approach is to look closely at personal characteristics that influence a leader's ability to perform the role of manager effectively. To do this the factors of group and work situation need to be considered. Taken together, there is good evidence that certain personal qualities favor success in the leadership role.* Researchers who have studied men and women in high positions have discovered a disturbing fact: Intelligence and imagination are common among leaders, but there seems to be little correlation between a person's intelligence and effectiveness or ability to get the job done. Many highly

---

*Campbell, L.: Managerial behavior, performance and effectiveness, New York, 1970, McGraw-Hill Book Co.

intelligent people do not know how to become effective as leaders and managers.

Stogdill,* a noted authority on leadership who studied characteristics of leaders for over twenty years, concludes that a selected group of characteristics indicates differences between leaders and followers, and effective leaders from ineffective ones. Following are characteristics he identifies as being distinctive of effective leaders:

1. Self-confidence, with a sense of personal identity
2. Strong drive for responsibility
3. Completes tasks (is persistent)
4. Energetic
5. Willing to accept consequences of decisions and actions
6. Accepts interpersonal stress
7. Tolerant of frustration and delay
8. Can influence behavior
9. Can structure social interactions to accomplish purposes
10. Venturesome and original
11. Excessive initiative in social situations

In an attempt to help nurses prepare for leadership, Bailey and Claus† identify factors that have been associated with nursing leadership:

1. Capacity (intelligence, alertness, verbal facility, originality, judgment)
2. Achievement (scholarship, knowledge, athletic ability, accomplishments)
3. Responsibility (dependability, initiative, persistence, aggressiveness, self-confidence, desire to excel)
4. Participation (activity, sociability, cooperation, humor, adaptability)
5. Status (socioeconomic position, popularity)

While both these sets of characteristics include admirable qualities, variations exist in the degree to which the characteristics are exhibited in individual leaders. There are wide differences in personalities. Also, not all characteristics are found to be present in each person. Many strong leaders are also known to have strong weaknesses. Experience indicates that only a minority of leaders have great talents. Social science research since the 1930s reveals that only a few outstanding leaders have been identified as unusually gifted people. The reality is that most people have strength in one or two areas and need a lot of help in others. Knowledge of the characteristics that have proved to identify effective leaders can help the nurse in preparing for the role of leader and manager. In the final analysis, *leaders and managers are judged to be successful not on their characteristics but on what they accomplish.*

---

*Stogdill, R.: Handbook of leadership, New York, 1974, The Free Press.
†Bailey, J., and Claus, K.: Preparing nurse leaders for the world tomorrow, Nurse Leaders. 1(6):21, 1978.

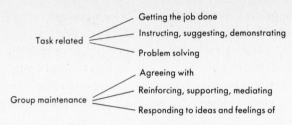

Fig. 9-2. Leadership functions.

Behaviors. When it became evident that effective leaders did not seem to have any distinguishing traits or characteristics that were common to all, researchers tried to isolate the behaviors that made leaders effective. Rather than try to figure out what effective leaders *were,* researchers tried to determine what effective leaders *did*—how they delegated tasks, how they communicated with and tried to motivate workers, and how they carried out their tasks. This approach to study leadership again assumed that there must be one best way to lead. Knowing that, unlike traits, behaviors can be learned, researchers concluded that individuals trained in the appropriate leadership behaviors could lead more effectively.*

Once research results were obtained, it became apparent that leadership behaviors appropriate to one situation were not necessarily appropriate in another. Despite evidence that effective leadership behaviors depended at least partially on the leader's situation, the conclusion was reached by many that certain management behaviors are more effective than others in a wide variety of circumstances, namely leadership functions and leadership styles.

Leadership function. This term suggests that in order for a group to operate effectively, someone has to perform two major functions: (1) task-related/problem-solving functions, and (2) group maintenance or social functions (Fig. 9-2). Group maintenance functions include anything that helps the group function more smoothly. Studies in leadership function have found that most effective groups have some form of shared leadership in this area, depending on the characteristics of the leader and members and on the situation. Individuals who are able to perform task-related and group-maintenance roles successfully will obviously be especially effective leaders.

Leadership styles. Style is an important factor in the leadership process. A style is the way in which something is said or done; it is a particular form of behavior directly associated with an individual. Leadership style is how a leader uses interpersonal influences to accomplish goals. Individual behavior is influenced by experiences in the formative years and by all the input in a person's life thereafter. Thus the style or approach taken by a nurse toward clients, nursing

*Owen, J.: The uses of leadership theory, Mich. Bus. Rev. **25**(1):13-19, 1973.

staff members, and other associates strongly reflects prior experiences. Managers learn that some styles work better for them than others; if a style proves unsatisfactory for the situation, the manager can alter it. However, managers who attempt to adopt a style that is inconsistent with their basic personality are unlikely to use that style effectively.

A single style of leadership is rarely practiced alone. Leadership behaviors that are right for one situation are not necessarily appropriate in another. For example, a nurse may use one style when mobilizing forces to take care of a client who is hemorrhaging or in deciding if a team member may change her day off, another style in encouraging creativity in developing a new procedure, and yet another style in formulating nursing diagnosis and plans for treatment. *One goal of an organization is for its managers to adopt a style of leadership that promotes a high level of work performance in a wide variety of circumstances, as efficiently as possible, and with the least amount of disruption.*

Styles of leadership range from very conservative to very liberal. Effective nurses study (1) their structural environment (hospital organization or other health facility), (2) the task to be accomplished (delivery of quality client care), and (3) the persons they are to lead (nursing staff members), and adopt a style of leadership to complement the situation.

Although theorists label styles differently, offering a variety of ranges of behavior representative of a specific style, all describe the authoritarian, democratic, and permissive styles as basic approaches to management.

Authoritarian style of leadership. Authoritarian styles of leadership range from very rigid to benevolent practices (see Table 2). In the strictest sense, authoritarianism functions with high concern for task accomplishment but low concern for the people who perform those tasks. Likert,* a noted management researcher, characterizes the authoritarian style of leadership as "exploitive," or using the efforts of workers to best possible advantage of the employer without regard to the worker's interests. In the extreme use of authoritarian leadership, communications and activities occur in a closed system. Managers make all work-related decisions and order workers to carry them out. Standards and methods of performance are also rigidly set by managers. The autocratic leader frequently exercises power, sometimes with coercion. Failure to meet the manager's goals may result in threats or punishment. The autocratic personality is firm, insistent, self-assured, and dominating with or without intent, and remains at the center of attention. This kind of manager feels little trust or confidence in workers, and workers in turn fear the manager with whom they feel they have little in common. McGregor† has produced perhaps the most famous description of attitudes assumed by autocratic leaders. He maintains that autocratic leaders view individuals as naturally lazy, lacking in ambition, disliking respon-

*Likert, R.: The human organization, New York, 1967, McGraw-Hill Book Co.
†McGregor, D.: The human side of enterprise, New York, 1960, McGraw-Hill Book Co.

Table 2

Comparative summary of democratic, authoritarian, and permissive styles of leadership*

Democratic	Authoritarian	Permissive
Participative	Conservative	Ultraliberal
Group goals	Organizational goals	Individual goals
Open	Defensive	Open
Facilitating	Restrictive	Permissive
Freeing	Coercive, pressure	Abdicating
Encouraging	Discouraging	Frustration, conflict
Accepting	Rejecting	Accepting and rejecting
Variety	Sameness	Differences
Equality	Inequality	Equality
Trusting	Fearing	Indifferent
Available supervision	Constant surveillance	Supervision as requested
Encouragement, assistance	Force	Self-direction
Freedom of choice	Obedience	Freedom of choice
Cooperation, group loyalty	Competition	Limited group alliance
Opportunity	Exploitation	Uncontrolled
Challenge	Threat	Permissive
Recognition	Praise	Acceptance
Self-discipline	Punishment	Self-gratification
Satisfaction	Reward	Acceptance

*Adapted from Douglass, L.M.: Review of leadership in nursing, St. Louis, 1977, The C.V. Mosby Co.

sibility, preferring to be led, self-centered, indifferent to organizational needs, resistant to change, not very bright, and lacking in creative potential.

Many managerial leaders take issue with those who believe authoritarian leadership to be degrading of persons. Proponents of a more conservative or benevolent approach value workers and their capabilities, but believe there is need for strong structure and order. In the benevolent authoritative approach managers still issue orders, but workers have some freedom to comment on those orders. Workers are given some flexibility to carry out their tasks but within carefully prescribed limits and procedures. A benevolent autocrat may simply give orders, use praise and demand loyalty, or make followers feel they are actually participating in decisions, even though they are doing what the leader wants.

Some form of authoritarian leadership has been used in nursing for many years. It reflects a very directive type of leadership that stresses giving orders by the nurse and taking orders by other members of the nursing team. In this role the leader puts a high degree of emphasis upon basic physiologic and security needs and upon adherence to hospital policy and regulations. If the members do what the leader wants, work will be provided and the paychecks will continue. Individuals are expected to follow orders as given, not to ask questions or to question authority, and the organizational system assumes the predominant role.*

Certain followers are most productive with authoritarian leadership. They derive a sense of security and satisfaction under this style of management. In turn, this type of management provides strong motivation and psychologic rewards to the leader. Authoritarianism allows for the possibility that the manager is likely to think and act faster and more effectively than others. Leaders with authoritarian styles are known for their ability to excel in times of crisis, to be able to get tough jobs done, and to bring order out of chaos when those around them falter.

Permissive style of leadership. The permissive style of leadership is at the opposite end of the continuum from the authoritarian style. Some would say that calling the permissive style "leadership" is a contradiction of terms, for leadership is absent under this system. Under this laissez-faire style of leadership the general climate is one of permissiveness or ultraliberalism in which there is lack of central direction or control (see Table 2). The laissez-faire manager wants everyone to feel good. The free-reign leader avoids responsibility by relinquishing power to followers. Liberal leaders permit followers to engage in managerial activities such as decision making, planning, structuring the organization, setting goals, and controlling the organization.

It has been estimated that fewer than 25% of all employees can operate responsibly with the permissive style and that only 10% of all managers accept and use the laissez-faire, permissive style. According to McGregor,† permissive leaders believe it is the responsibility of the organization to supply money, materials, equipment, and workers, and that managers have the responsibility to direct their own efforts toward achievement of organizational goals. Permissive leaders assume workers are ambitious, responsible, accept organizational goals, are dynamic, flexible, intelligent, and creative. The leader assumes a small role, relinquishing the bulk of the management process to followers. This style can be effective in highly motivated professional groups, such as in research projects where independent thinking is rewarded. The very liberal style of leadership is oriented to higher social, ego fulfillment, and self-actualization needs. But this style is not generally useful in the highly structured health care delivery system where organization and control form the baseline of most operations.

Democratic leadership. In the democratic (participative or consultive approach) the manager is "people oriented," focusing attention on the human

---

*Stevens, W.: Management and leadership in nursing, New York, 1978, McGraw-Hill Book Co.
†McGregor, D.: The human side of enterprise, New York, 1960, McGraw-Hill Book Co.

aspects and building effective work groups. Interaction between manager and personnel is open, friendly, and trusting. A collaborative spirit or joint effort exists, allowing for governance via group participation in decision making (see Table 2). In the open system communication prevails, with the democratic manager consulting with group members and solving problems with them, assuming that others want to be considered in the process. There is a mutual responsiveness to meeting group goals, with work-related decisions made by the group. The democratic manager attempts to develop the group's sense of responsibility for the good of the whole and for individual accomplishments. The goals set by the work group may not always be the ones personally favored by individual members. Democratic managers try to give workers feelings of self-worth and importance. Performance standards exist to provide guidelines and to permit appraisal of workers, rather than to provide managers with a tool to control workers.

There are some decisions that do not permit the nurse-manager to exercise total democracy, but using the participatory process where possible permits each member to identify with the work setting by establishing challenging goals, providing opportunities to change or improve work methods, pursuing professional and personal growth, recognizing achievement, and helping personnel learn from their mistakes. Likert's* studies found that a democratic or participative style of leadership leads to high productivity and is the most desirable form of management in a wide variety of work situations.

Comparison of styles of leadership. There are many similarities and differences in behavior, attitudes, and conditions present in leadership styles. Table 2 provides a comparison of commonalities found in authoritarian, democratic, and permissive styles. As mentioned previously, not all the behaviors are evident at any one time; however, each of the three styles of leadership is usually consistent within its category. A manager will utilize all the styles separately or together, depending on the manager's flexibility and the circumstances inherent in each situation.

PREDICTIVE PRINCIPLE: Consideration of the work situation, manager's leadership style and expectations, and follower's characteristics and expectations results in harmonious goal accomplishment.

Leadership and management by situation. A comparative study of leadership styles would seem to suggest that a democratic or participative style of leadership would be the mode of choice in most situations. However, there are too many factors to consider to make so broad an application. Recently researchers have turned their attention from behavioral classifications that label managers as autocratic, democratic, or permissive to a classification of management by situation. The premise is that styles of leadership should not be ste-

*Likert, R.: New patterns of management, New York, 1961, McGraw-Hill Book Co.

	Highly structured (authoritative)	Moderately structured (participative)	Minimally structured (permissive)
Manager's style of leadership and expectations	←		→
Follower's characteristics and expectations	←	→	
Work situation	←		→

Fig. 9-3. The continuum or range of possible variables to consider when choosing a leadership style of management. (From Douglass, L.M.: The effective nurse: leader and manager, St. Louis, 1980, The C.V. Mosby Co. Adapted from Tagliere, D.: People, power, and organization, New York, 1973, AMACOM, A Division of American Management Associations, p. 32.)

reotyped as either forceful, participative, or permissive; rather, management should be viewed as a process comprised of a range of possible options in which the manager chooses a leadership style complementary to the need.

Tannenbaum and Schmidt* were among the first theorists (1958) to identify forces they believed should influence a manager's choice of leadership style. Those identified were (1) forces in the manager, (2) forces in the subordinates, and (3) forces in the situation. While Tannenbaum and Schmidt personally favored the democratic style, they found that managers need to take certain practical considerations into account before deciding which style of leadership to use. Fiedler and Chemers† are more explicit in their description of factors to consider when determining a style of leadership. The manager is asked to review (1) the work situation, (2) the manager's leadership style and expectations, and (3) the follower's characteristics and expectations. Fiedler and Chemers believe that when the three forces are considered and adaptations made, the situation is likely to be harmonious with a willingness on the part of all those involved to cooperate in accomplishing goals. The continuum or range of possible variables to consider when choosing a leadership style of management is illustrated in Fig. 9-3.

Manager's style of leadership and expectations. How a manager leads is influenced by that person's background, knowledge, values, and experiences (forces in the manager), and the relationships or interdependency between the manager and the other personnel. Managers are likely to choose a style that complements their personalities. The greater the manager's need to control the situation, the more likely it is that an authoritarian or conservative leadership style will be selected. The greater the belief in the followers' competence and in

---

*Tannenbaum, R., and Schmidt, W.: How to choose a leadership pattern, Harv. Bus. Rev., pp. 162-164, May-June 1973.
†Fiedler, F., and Chemers, M.: Leadership and effective management, Glenview, Ill., 1974, Scott, Foresman & Co.

the ability of members to work responsibly, the more likely a democratic or participative approach to leadership will be taken. The greater the belief that workers have the ability to achieve with minimal structure and direction, the more likely a permissive or ultraliberal style of leadership will be taken.

Followers' characteristics and expectations. Characteristics of followers and their expectations also must be considered before managers can choose an appropriate leadership style. Like managers, followers are different from one another in their response to leadership. Ultimately the response of followers to the manager's leadership determines how effective the manager will be.

Knowledge, competency, and level of the workers are important characteristics to consider. For example, capable persons usually require much less supervision than new or inexperienced workers. And less prepared personnel require carefully planned, detailed guidance. The manager's task is to know the qualifications of each member assigned to the nursing team in order to provide each with the right amount of supervision and guidance.

Attitudes and needs of followers are also influential factors in selecting a leadership style. There are those workers who are extremely dependent, preferring a highly structured environment in which the worker makes very few decisions about work activities. This kind of worker is most comfortable with an authoritarian manager. Persons fitting into this category may be a great asset to the organization. They may be very reliable and willing workers who gladly perform the most difficult and distasteful assignments. Also, this structured situation may be a temporary state as for a new worker who needs a period of close supervision during the time of orientation.

At the opposite end of the continuum are the workers who have a strong need for minimal structure, preferring to chart their own activities and to decide what will be done. Such persons are less likely to relate closely with a group or team endeavor. This independent kind of personality is usually driven to achieve and to master every situation, desiring a manager who respects individual ambitions and allows free rein. If the job situation is wrong for such a follower, this person can be harmful to the organization.

Followers who perform best in a moderately structured environment are those who have a part in the decision-making process within limits, but who have others making major decisions. They are usually competent workers who do not require constant supervision, but who prefer democratic or participative leadership that provides reassurance that they are performing correctly and well. In contrast to the worker who wants everything clearly spelled out, the person who enjoys a participative relationship wants to know the goals but also wants to have a voice in how they will be achieved.

The work situation. Fiedler,* using fifteen years of research on leader-

---

*Fiedler, F.: Validation and extension of the contingency model of leadership effectiveness, Psychol. Bull. **76**(2):128-148, 1971.

ship in hundreds of work groups, identifies three elements in the work situation that help determine which style of leadership will be most effective: (1) interrelationships between leader and followers, (2) the task to be accomplished, and (3) the extent of the leader's power.

1. *Leader-follower relationships.* According to Fiedler, interrelationships between leader and followers are the most important influence on the manager's power and effectiveness. If relationships are good, the manager may not have to rely on formal rank or authority. On the other hand, a manager who is disliked or not trusted may have to rely heavily on authoritarian methods to accomplish group tasks.

2. *Task accomplishment.* Task accomplishment is the second most important variable in the work situation. The nurse's responsibility as a leader, for example, includes both providing care for clients and managing people where such services are performed. A manager's task includes not only planning, organizing, directing, and evaluating the work of others but also enforcing the agency's policies and procedures that apply to the manager, workers, and clients. Again, there is a gradation in structure in a work setting, ranging from those activities that are strictly defined in terms of what, who, where, how, and when they must be accomplished to those tasks that are highly unstructured in those respects. High structure is usually desirable in some work environments, such as with specialty care areas where the job must be done in a certain way, or with workers who have limited preparation for their roles.

3. *Power position.* The third factor to consider in a work situation is the power position. Some positions, such as hospital administrator and director of nursing services, carry a great deal of power and authority (Fig. 9-4). Like most upper level management positions, they have great power over the workers employed by the organization. Generally, the larger the work group, the

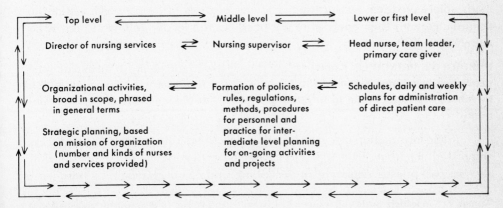

Fig. 9-4. Levels of power and authority in a hospital setting. (From Douglass, L.M.: The effective nurse: leader and manager, St. Louis, 1980, The C.V. Mosby Co.)

greater the geographic spread; the greater the time pressures to make a decision, the more likely the use of an autocratic or conservative style of leadership.

Because of their large and complex nature, it is not uncommon for most health care delivery systems to be structured under a high degree of governance, with limited opportunity for nurses to proceed under their own direction. As work allotment becomes more decentralized, nurses have opportunity to adopt a democratic or participative style of leadership. Nursing leaders are attempting to move away from the confines of rigid control into a structure that allows for utilization of professional knowledge and competency. Progress is slow, but inroads are being made to allow managers more freedom and control in nursing decisions. Any work situation, however, may be designed to provide some flexibility. It is the leader's task to discover where this flexibility exists and to function accordingly.

Flexibility of managers to use various leadership styles. The ideal situation is for a nurse to be able to (1) adequately assess the followers' characteristics and expectations, (2) identify the interrelationships between the leader and followers, the tasks to be accomplished, and the degree of power to do the job, and (3) choose a leadership style that best fits the situation. If managers are relatively inflexible in their leadership style, they will function well only in certain situations. Such a limitation hampers an individual's career, for to use a manager who has only one leadership style an organization must adapt the job to the manager rather than the manager to the job.

Fiedler believes that leadership styles are inflexible, and he is therefore discouraging when discussing the possibility of reeducating managers to use different styles. There are others,* however, who believe strongly that most managers actually have great potential and flexibility in responding to influences in the work setting. They feel that behavior can be changed and managers can develop ability to select and use different leadership styles, from making decisions solely on their own through various degrees of group participation, in accordance with their analysis of the needs of the leader, followers, and work situation.

PREDICTIVE PRINCIPLE: Knowledge of theory levels and ability to formulate valid predictive principles promote the leader's ability to identify the levels on which members are functioning to facilitate growth in problem solving and goal attainment.

The formulation of a valid theory is described fully in Chapter 1. Level I is comprised of *naming* (labeling) and *classifying* (categorizing) the result. Level II also has two phases: *depicting*, or describing, and *factor relating*. The third level

---

*Vroom, V.: Can leaders lead? In Hackman, R., Lawler, E., and Porter, L.: Perspectives on behavior in organizations, New York, 1977, McGraw-Hill Book Co.

is *situation relating*, concerned with causal relationships. The fourth level in theory building is *situation producing*, comprising the formulation of prescriptive theories. Situation-producing theories consist of three aspects: (1) a definable goal, (2) a prescription, and (3) a survey or diagram of specific activities and directions, which, if followed, produce a predicted result or attain preset goals. The final component in the fourth level is a survey list of resources, techniques, and behavioral patterns that can be structured into goal-producing activities. At this stage the wider the leader's knowledge of experiences of related situations, treatment, and results produced, the more reliable the results. In addition, the nurse's behaviors will reflect more effectively the acquired principles or predictive theories, which predict desired outcomes. This knowledge of theory levels equips the leader with the tools necessary to identify the level at which individuals and groups are operating and to provide guidance that will promote growth up through the levels.

PREDICTIVE PRINCIPLE: Effective use of self in time management results in control of self and of the work situation.

Self-management is the most difficult of all management tasks. Effective time management means getting complete control of oneself and of one's own job responsibilities. Getting control depends on (1) determining how the nurse uses time, (2) what is most important in the job situation, and (3) taking steps to see that the job is done correctly. Many nurses perform a set of familiar activities day after day, week after week, year after year, rather than investigate other sets of behaviors that might improve their performance. It takes initiative to change— a valuable trait in a manager. For the process of change to be effective, the desire to change work habits must come from within.

Determining how the nurse uses time. Finding out how nurses use their time is difficult, for it requires analysis of one's habits, an activity that most people shun. Studies of how managers use their time are not very reliable, as it has been found that they consistently overestimate the time devoted to task-related activities and underestimate the time spent on other matters such as planning and interrelationships. Recording and observation are excellent methods to determine how time is used. One recording device is to keep a *log* much like that prescribed for college freshmen to determine study habits. An hour-by-hour account is given of the student's activities for a week. Activities of daily living, school and homework, social activities, and free time are logged and analyzed to determine if priorities are in order. A similar type of log can be used to determine nurse's work activities. It will vary according to the type of role being studied (supervisor, head nurse, team leader, primary caregiver). An example is given in Fig. 9-5 of such a log kept by a primary nurse for one day. For this system to work well, the following should be kept in mind: carry the log with you at all times. Note comments immediately or details will be forgotten. Make entries short but

6:45- 7:00	Prepared individual worksheet
7:00- 7:20	Walking rounds for change-of-shift report
7:20- 7:35	Checked accessability of medicines, linens, and supplies for care-giving (3 meds missing; requisitioned for I.V. supplies)
7:35- 7:45	Talked with patient B's relative by telephone (had to put him on hold while I obtained information)
7:45- 8:15	Visited each patient — discussed plan of care
8:15- 8:25	Reviewed plan of care for patient C with physician
8:25- 8:45	Break
8:45- 9:15	Assisted physician with paracentesis — stayed with patient following procedure
9:15- 9:45	Administered medications
9:45- 10:10	Helped Mary with chemotherapy (first time for this primary nurse)
10:10- 12:00	Gave care to 4 patients; telephone calls ×4; talked with physicians ×2
12:00- 12:30	Helped patients with their meals; revised dietary orders for 2 patients with patients and dieticians
12:30- 1:00	Lunch
1:00- 1:30	Administered medications
1:30- 2:00	Documented care; chatted with nurse friend about her children
2:00- 2:45	Related with patients, consulting, supporting, teaching; updated nursing care plans
2:45- 3:10	Completed documentation
3:10- 3:30	Change of shift walking rounds

Fig. 9-5. An example of a log kept by a primary nurse for one day.

Preparation	Direct patient care	Telephone calls	Conferences	Assisting others	Documentation	Personal
30 min	4 hr, 50 min	30 min	50 min	25 min	45 min	10 min

Fig. 9-6. Analysis of time spent by a primary nurse on a typical day.

specific, record all uses of times, especially interruptions (telephone calls, helping others with their work, errands).

Determining what is most important in the job situation. After a record of activities during a typical period has been completed, an analysis is done to see how much time is spent in various areas. The time is divided into categories that most represent the activities of the nurse, such as preparation, direct administration of client care, telephone calls, conferences, assisting others, documentation, and personal contacts. Fig. 9-6 offers an approximation of the time spent by the primary nurse in one day. In considering use of time, the nurse reviews activities in terms of priority, which means deciding what is essential to the welfare or purposes of the organization or person at the time. Criteria for priority setting in nursing relate to two major goals: (1) those needs that directly affect the client and (2) those needs that affect the management process. Each activity should be considered separately, recognizing that there is great overlap. For example, telephone conversations with the relative of a client might reveal information that influences care. For the primary nurse in the example, six or possibly seven hours could be categorized as activities that affect the client and one or two that affect the management process. This distribution is well within acceptable limits for time allotment. However, several questions should be addressed concerning the workday:

1. *If the activity needs to be done, should I be doing it?* If another person can do it equally well, then the nurse should not be doing it. For example, checking accessibility of medicines, linens, and supplies could be done by a less-skilled person and should be delegated. Teaching another nurse chemotherapy treatment might better be done by an in-service instructor.
2. *If I should do it myself, can it be done in less time? How?* For example, communication by telephone is an important activity but might be structured to conserve time. Arrangements might be made to make most calls at prescribed times. This approach would allow the nurse to acquire necessary information and to impart it in the least amount of time and at a time most convenient for all.
3. *Do I keep to my time schedule, or do I waste my own and others' time?*

If the nurse arrives late for work, she keeps others waiting and must play "catch-up"; this can have a domino effect upon all activities. Or the nurse may have a gregarious nature and be caught up in frequent, lengthy conversations that have no bearing on organizational purpose or client care. Consider the many minutes that have been wasted by nursing personnel who must wait for conversations concerning such things as marital relationships, children, vacations, dates, and recipes to cease before they can carry on professional matters. Unless priorities are kept in mind, nurses are apt to conclude the day's activities, believing that they have done their best and that there was simply not enough time to accomplish all that was necessary. Extraneous conversation is normal and serves positive purposes, but if engaged in to the extent that it hinders goal accomplishment, then behavior changes in this area need to occur.

PREDICTIVE PRINCIPLE: Planning for urgent or crisis situations provides proper nurse coverage and reduces negative leadership behaviors as a result of work overload.

Urgent situations. There are always many demands competing for a nurse's time and many choices available as to how to use it. The matter is compounded when a crisis or an urgent circumstance arises. The urgent task demands instant action and drives other important things from the mind. A common reaction to a high-pressure situation is to drop everything else and deal with the problem, then hurry up and work harder to complete all regular activities. Another solution is to work longer hours. Results of these alternatives are poor. As management consultant McCarthy* states, "People in a hurry cannot reflect. They cannot evaluate alternatives. They cannot plan. The result is poor performance, plus time then spent correcting mistakes, compounding the original burden. Working long hours has similar effects: fatigue, tension, murky thoughts, and poor judgment." One resolution to this problem is for the head nurse or a float nurse to take over in crisis situations, freeing the overburdened nurse to resume routine responsibilities.

Awareness of self

Awareness of self is the ability to be sensitive to one's own needs, motives, and responses to stimuli. Self-awareness enables the nurse to help followers understand themselves and develop their potential. In turn, the more the nurse helps others to grow, the more self-growth will occur.

Traditionally, nurses are seen as self-sacrificing; their individual needs

---

*McCarthy, M.: Managing your own time: the most important management task, J. of Nursing Administration, **11**(11-12):61-65, 1981.

are viewed as unimportant. Even the struggle for economic security is more difficult because of the image of the nurse as a giving person. The nature of nursing draws people to the field who have a need to be useful to others. Recognition of the individual needs of nurses and finding ways to meet those needs can free the nurse to meet the needs of the patient.

PREDICTIVE PRINCIPLE: Knowledge and understanding of factors about human beings permit assessment and acceptance of self and others.

The nurse enters the leadership role with certain needs, drives, and motives and seeks satisfaction from the total work situation. Individual feelings are based on many variables depending on goals and the nurse's ability to reach these goals. A person who follows a normal developmental pattern progresses from dependence (mother-child relationship) to the independent role and on to interdependence (in which a productive and satisfying working relationship with others is established). The basic urge of a human being is toward a state of physical, mental, and social well-being.

Nurses who accept themselves fully will not need continually to defend their actions, strengths, and weaknesses. Liking and accepting oneself makes a person able to accept others for what they are, with all their strengths and weaknesses. The nurse will want to relate to others on a person-to-person basis, rather than as actor-to-actor according to the roles in a script. An organization benefits when the nurse has knowledge of self and is self-accepting, since a person of this kind can function without great loss of time and energy spent in solving problems that occur where insecurity and lack of trust abound.

PREDICTIVE PRINCIPLE: Identification of the leader's own needs aids in the identification of needs of others.

People express needs from birth to death; the degree of importance of each need depends on conditions and circumstances. People do what they do because they have needs to satisfy; unless satisfied, they suffer feelings of tension and unrest. As discussed in earlier chapters, Maslow* believes that people can best be understood through the study of human needs and their influence upon behavior. His theory has probably received more attention and application to organizational environments than any other, for his classifications have direct implications for managing human behavior in organizations. Fig. 9-7 provides an example of human needs. Note the hierarchy is arranged in the form of a triangle, which visually portrays the needs that are embodied in each person.

Physiologic need. Physiologic needs are the strongest of human needs. Before any other requirements can be even approached, the biologic factors of food, oxygen, water, reasonable shelter from the outside climate, sex, comfort, and so on have to be satisfied.

*Maslow, A.: Motivation and personality, ed. 2, New York, 1970, Harper & Row, Publishers.

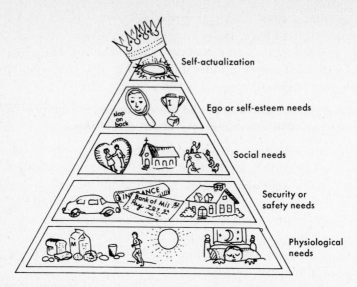

Fig. 9-7. Maslow's hierarchy of needs. (From Douglass, L.M.: The effective nurse: leader and manager, St. Louis, 1980, The C.V. Mosby Co. Adapted from Maslow, A.: Motivation and personality, ed. 2, New York, 1970, Harper & Row, Publishers.)

Security or safety need. With few exceptions, people want to feel protected from danger or threat of physical harm. Regardless of station in life, most persons have a desire for some order in their lives, some stability and predictability. In general, individuals do not want to be surprised about significant happenings, nor do they want to be constantly bombarded by stressful situations.

Social needs. This is the desire to belong, to be accepted by others, and to experience love, affection, and friendship. Social needs are sometimes called "affiliation needs." In Maslow's hierarchical pyramid, the desire for companionship, love, affection, belonging, and approval can be satisfied only after biologic and security needs are satisfied. Managers must not forget that the work environment is a social situation, and the same needs for feelings of belonging and affection apply. Unless employees or staff members feel they are a part of the organization and their fellow workers or team members want them as members, they will be dominated by the need for belonging and will be unlikely to respond to higher order opportunities.

Ego or self-esteem needs. The first is a desire for achievement, competency, and mastery of one's personal and work or professional activities. In organizational terms, persons want to be well trained or well educated or both and be good at their jobs. They also want to feel they are achieving something important when they perform their work role. These are elements that reflect a sense of self-respect and self-confidence. The other type of self-esteem is the desire for prestige, status, importance, and recognition. There are many ways of fulfilling both these types of needs in staff members through such means as providing challenging work assignments, positive feedback about performance, personal encouragement, and recognition for jobs well done or for specific achievements. Maslow offers a word of caution with a further point that the soundest base for self-esteem is earned respect from others, rather than praise that may be superficial and unearned. Another way of meeting ego and self-esteem needs is by involving staff members in goal setting for the delivery of nursing care and in decision making throughout the nursing process.

Self-actualization needs. Employees motivated by self-actualization try to find meaning and personal growth in their work and actively seek out new responsibilities. Maslow maintains that for the self-actualized person, work tends to become the same as play; vocation and avocation become the same thing. Studies* of people employed in work organizations reveal that those with a high need for achievement have several characteristics of interest to managers: (1) they like taking responsibility for solving problems, (2) they tend to set moderately difficult goals for themselves and take calculated risks, (3) they place high importance on concrete feedback concerning how well they are performing, and (4) they are successful in teaching others how to meet their own achievement motivation and, in turn, to improve their work performance.

Maslow stresses that individual differences are greatest at the highest level, and any number of ways may be found to achieve self-actualization on the job. For some nurses, producing nursing care of high quality in the same work area may be a means for self-actualization. For others, self-actualization may come through transfer from one kind of nursing care to another, or from advancement from team leader to head nurse, with the aspiration of one day becoming nursing director of a large hospital or education program.

PREDICTIVE PRINCIPLE: Translation of individual needs into behavioral terms allows an objective approach to leadership with respect to need analysis and fulfillment.

A leader's job is not managing people but managing people's behavior within the parameters of the work environment. When nurses accept employment in a health agency they choose to provide the behaviors required to accomplish the specific job for which they were hired. These behaviors are defined in standards, policies, roles, and procedures appropriate to the role. The professional survival of leaders and all other employees depends upon each person exhibiting those behaviors necessary for goal achievement.

Maslow's hierarchy of needs speaks in general terms but offers insight into motivation. To become useful, behaviors exhibited by self and others can be

---

*Holland, M.: Can managerial performance be predicted? J. Nurs. Admin. **11**(6):17-21, 1981; Lawler, E.: Motivation in work organizations, Monterey, Calif., 1973, Brooks/Cole Publishing Co.

matched with one of the levels on the need hierarchy and be dealt with accordingly. For example, a nurse who often verbalizes the need for an increase in pay is operating at the second level of security need. When a team leader runs to the head nurse frequently with an account of her achievements, she is operating in the fourth level of ego, or self-esteem, needs. The nurse who spends much time organizing birthday celebrations, monthly get-togethers, and recognition activities is manifesting behaviors associated with third level, or social, needs. Approaching needs in self and others through behavioral terms provides the nurse with an objective basis for leadership and management.

PREDICTIVE PRINCIPLE: Accomplishing goals through assertive behavior enables a leader to exercise the rights of self without denying the rights and feelings of others.

PREDICTIVE PRINCIPLE: Consistent use of passive behavior ignores personal rights of the leader and leads to lowered self-esteem and maladaptive behaviors.

PREDICTIVE PRINCIPLE: Achievement of one's goals through aggressive acts violates another person's rights and results in feelings of domination, humiliation, and hostility.

Deciding which style of behavior to exhibit while communicating in the role of leader is often difficult for nurses. Even when the decision is made as to the best approach, the nurse may be hesitant to act. There is no one right way to respond all of the time—the nurse behaves in a specific manner according to circumstance. Imposing one style of behavior on others indicates a desire for the members to respond in kind, with all participants in the communication process becoming victims every time circumstances change and alternate behaviors are warranted. There are three common styles of behavior: passive, aggressive, and assertive. The effective nurse learns the process used in each and their advantages and disadvantages.

Passive behavior. Passive behavior is submissively accepting whatever circumstances are in force without resistance or complaint. The passive individual has low self-esteem and is unable to initiate contact with others and to stand up for individual rights or the rights of clients and staff. Very often, passive nurses see themselves as second class employees, unable to exert influence and power in strategic circumstances, rather than as peers or equals with the right to act on their own convictions. Behaviors familiar to the passive person are apologetic speech ("You're right, I'm wrong, I'm sorry," "I don't really know but . . ."), avoidance or withdrawal, hedging when asked to make a decision, and self-sacrifice. The passive nurse avoids direct confrontation, allowing other people and circumstances to dominate the situation. Unable to speak thoughts or feelings in an assertive manner, this kind of nurse experiences feelings of helplessness and powerlessness, which leads to failure in accomplishing the managerial role.

A usual behavioral pattern of the passive nurse is to engage in self-pity, self-righteousness, and superiority, telling others (usually those outside the work scene) of the oppressive conditions caused by the bureaucracy, the charge nurse, or any other scapegoat. Periodically the typical passive person will reach a breaking point and have an emotional outburst of aggressive behavior (for example, crying, shouting, blaming). Immediately afterward the nurse feels guilty and ashamed and quietly returns to the passive routine. Passive individuals have not learned that each individual is responsible for his or her reactions to circumstances, and they continue to allow their manipulation by others.

Aggressive behavior. With aggression, the individual acts in a bold, attacking, and hostile manner, often accomplishing purposes at the expense of others with injurious and destructive results. Aggression is disagreeing by being unpleasant and cantankerous. Examples of aggressive means of communication are blaming, shaming, refusing to take "no" for an answer, making belittling remarks, humiliating or embarrassing another in the presence of others, stomping feet, banging doors, cursing, slamming the receiver down, and crying.

Assertive behavior. Assertive behavior is maintaining a balance between passive and aggressive behavior. As Table 3 illustrates, assertiveness means expressing one's positive and negative beliefs and reactions openly without infringing on the rights of others. The assertive person makes choices about how, when, where, who, and why actions are taken. This may include choosing whether to be assertive. Assertiveness is being in control of what happens to oneself, of making requests and having needs met, and being able to refuse compliance

Table 3

Comparison of behaviors exhibited by passive, assertive, and aggressive nurses*

Passive	*Assertive*	*Aggressive*
Low self-esteem	High self-esteem	High-low self-esteem
Feels self-pity	Feels self-worth	Mixed feelings of worth
Shy, withdrawn	Forthright	Forward and attacking
Apologetic	Open and honest	Hostile, manipulative
Denies rights and needs of self and patients/clients	Acts in best interest of self, patients/clients	Demands needs be gratified for self and others
Feels victimized	Feels on peer level	Feels must fight for rights
Allows situation to control rather than controlling situation	Controls situation	Attacks situation

*From Douglass, L.M.: The effective nurse: leader and manager, St. Louis, 1980, The C.V. Mosby Co.

with unrealistic demands or requests. Assertiveness helps the individual initiate and terminate conversations with confidence. Assertive behavior allows the manager to act in the best interests of self, clients, and members of the health care team by expressing honest feelings comfortably and without undue anxiety.

Chenevert,* a nurse-educator, offers a list of ten basic rights for women in health professions.

1. The right to be treated with respect. (The nurse takes care of self by speaking feelings and giving self and others credit for such things as knowledge, ability, integrity, tact, skill, dedication, and compassion.)
2. The right to a reasonable work load. (The nurse's guiding question has to be: "Is what I am doing or about to do in the best interest of the client?")
3. The right to an equitable wage. (Nurses need to join together and demand wages that reflect education, experience, and level of responsibility.)
4. The right to determine own priorities. (Nurses have the right to choose the ways in which time and energy are spent.)
5. The right to ask for what is wanted. (Nurses must put desires into words before they can be realized.)
6. The right to refuse without making excuses or feeling guilty. (Nurses are comfortable enough with own ability and worth to decline the request or offer.)
7. The right to make mistakes and be responsible for them. (Some mistakes, such as medication errors, can result in disaster to the client, and specific preventive measures are built into the system to avoid their occurrence. However, the nurse knows that everyone makes mistakes at some time. When this occurs, the assertive nurse admits errors and speaks up or steps up in behalf of the client. This nurse also feels free to question authorities when in doubt about issues or procedures.)
8. The right to give and receive information as a professional. (The nurse has a right to approach any other person in the health professions as one professional to another. The professional nurse uses judgment and discretion as to what, when, where, why, and how information is treated.)
9. The right to act in the best interest of the patient. (The nurse cares about the client, sets fear aside, and holds ground until results are achieved.)
10. The right to be human. (Even though nursing is an important and

---

*Chenevert, M.: Special techniques in assertiveness training for women in the health professions, St. Louis, 1978, The C.V. Mosby Co.

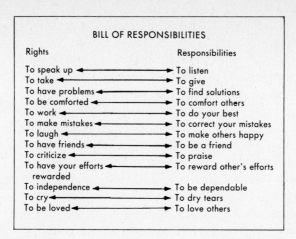

Fig. 9-8. Bill of responsibilities. (Adapted from Chenevert, M.: Special techniques in assertiveness training for women in the health professions, St. Louis, 1978, The C.V. Mosby Co.)

vital career, the nurse should not be expected to shut out all other life experiences. A nurse must be free to learn, cope, play, and make choices concerning lifestyles.)

Chenevert suggests that if nurses feel upset or uncomfortable about any of these rights, they may need to review the meaning of assertiveness. She warns of the danger of becoming lopsided in the approach to individual rights, emphasizing that rights need to be tempered with responsibilities, just as responsibilities need to be rewarded with rights. Chenevert suggests a Bill of Responsibilities for the assertive nurse (Fig. 9-8).

A nurse-leader can learn the art of deciding when to be assertive and how to go about it. The procedure includes learning how to fight internal fears so that one has enough courage to act in behalf of self, clients, and staff, and learning how, through application of the communication process, to insist on rights when they are threatened. In so doing, people will know what is expected of them in terms of responses.

Dyer* suggests the following attitudes and behaviors that can help the manager develop assertive skills.

1. Expect people to accept your leadership and they will respond with respect.
2. Accept responsibility for treatment given by you to others and for treatment given you by others. ("I allowed this to happen to me.")
3. Stop waiting for things to get better; they will not.
4. Do not demand perfection of yourself or others.

---

*Dyer, W.: Pulling your own strings, New York, 1978, Thomas Y. Crowell Co.

5. Practice control when you are being manipulated. (Avoid passive or aggressive behavior.)

6. Practice behaviors and words that tell others your wishes and with the implication that you will not be intimidated. ("I expect you to come to work on time." "Do not call me honey.")

7. When others respond to you with blaming, making excuses, or complaining, describe their behavior calmly with statements such as: "I feel you are spending time complaining when the work must be done." "I feel that is an excuse, not a reason."

8. Accept compliments graciously with a simple "Thank you" or "I'll feel good about that all day."

9. Give criticism in a clear, forthright manner, as near the time of the incident as possible. ("I notice you are going from room to room without washing your hands in between." "Your patients' call lights were going unanswered; please respond promptly or find someone to do it for you.")

10. Do not allow people to elicit feelings of guilt when you are legitimately assertive in your leadership behavior (when angry reactions, hurt looks, pleas, and so on are received).

11. Do not use sentences that invite people to victimize you. ("I did a dumb thing." "I never can do anything right." "I made a terrible assignment.")

12. Eliminate complaining and blaming words and phrases. ("She's the one who did it." "They did it to me.")

13. Learn how to say "no" without hemming and hawing or offering excuses. (Say "No, thank you" or "I will not do that" or "No, I am not interested.")

14. Consistently refuse to do tasks that you dislike and that are not necessarily your responsibility (preparing reports; requisitioning supplies).

15. Refuse to participate in extra assignments (committees, task forces, and so on) in which you have no interest or talent.

16. Find another person to give you candid feedback about your assertive skills.

17. Practice leaving work behind when you go off duty; push out job-related thoughts and concentrate on outside activities.

18. Remember that worth comes from within; then seek promotions and prestige only if you want them.

19. If you dislike or resent your work, consider the consequences of making your feelings known to the proper authority (disapproval, possible denial of an advancement, or loss of job). Then choose either to remain status quo or to confront.

The nurse who chooses assertive behavior as a plan of action will increase in self-worth and self-confidence, maintain individuality, be accountable for quality health care, and will not hesitate to communicate with those who are in control of organizations. Through the assertion process the nurse will also feel freer to listen, teach, direct, and speak out appropriately. In this way rights are recognized and the leader becomes an effective advocate for the rights of others.

Knowledge of the job

The nursing leadership role assumes certain basic knowledge and skills. These attributes are assured and perpetuated through accreditation of schools of nursing and hospitals, through the licensure of nurses, and through the system of rewards and punishments built into the employment situations. Clients depend on the nurse's clinical judgment for giving the best possible service. The nurse is expected to provide direction in all areas of planning, administering, and evaluating nursing care. The extent to which the leader is successful in role adaptation, perception, and response to leadership requirements directly relates to (1) the leader's ability to built theory and utilize it, (2) the range of conscious role learning, (3) role taking, (4) role enactment, and (5) a large role repertoire. An example of behavioral objectives that reflect this knowledge and ability is as follows:

1. Demonstrates a working knowledge of leadership theories and operational definitions that enable the nurse to move toward full maturity and to be optimally useful in nurse leadership practices within the health care delivery system
2. Establishes plans to obtain desired and appropriate care with client and works with people and agencies that may enhance or inhibit care in the promotion of health
   a. Recognizes components of good health practice for each client and identifies rights being threatened
   b. Clarifies with client standard for good health practice, identifies risks involved, and allows client to make an educated choice
3. Implements and evaluates planned change for the purpose of promoting optimal health in client and society
4. Exercises responsibility and accountability for self and others in nursing practice for the provision and promotion of quality health care
5. Collaborates, coordinates, teaches, and consults in diverse nursing settings
6. Demonstrates characteristics and values inherent in the leadership role
7. Assumes leadership in recognizing the need for adaptations as trends emerge and initiates or participates in research that will contribute to the body of knowledge necessary for judicious decision making

PREDICTIVE PRINCIPLE: The demands of the situation in which a leader is to function influence the qualities, characteristics, knowledge, and skills necessary for successful leadership.

It is impossible for a nurse to possess knowledge and skills necessary to function in all aspects of nursing today, for this career is multifaceted and complex. But the practitioner can influence the development of optimal leadership abilities by collaborating with other persons to (1) preassess leadership qualities, characteristics, knowledge, and skills for the job; (2) plan ways and means to acquire additional service tools viewed as necessary for the proposed managerial role; (3) obtain feedback to ascertain increased level of competence; and (4) secure an assignment commensurate with knowledge and ability.

Clinical competence is effectively rewarded by advancement. Hence competent nurses are often assigned to cardinal positions. This clinical expertise contributes to effective guidance but does not ensure that the nurse will possess leadership qualities. The value of technical knowledge or proficiency in facilitating leadership depends on the situation and the tasks to be accomplished. If technical knowledge is not relevant to the goals established, it will be of minimal service either to the leader or to the recipient of services.

Anxiety is generated in situations that make demands for clinical knowledge the nurse has not acquired; this in turn disrupts organizational behavior patterns even in highly skilled nurses. All too often nurses are placed in roles where they are novices, in jobs that depend on knowledge pertaining to policy, procedure, and routine with which they are unfamiliar or that require expertise in unaccustomed clinical areas. This practice generates false incompetence. For example, a nurse fully qualified to function in a pediatric unit may render poor service in an obstetric unit. Clinical knowledge about separation anxiety in the 2-year-old child does not enable the nurse to make good judgments about postpartum bleeding.

Problems beyond the ability of the nurse cause a high anxiety level and an indulgence in activities that in reality only drain off the excess energy generated by such anxiety. An illustration of this is demonstrated by the following:

A group is responsible for the care of an agitated client who needs the constant presence of a caregiver. The nurse's energy and time are spent in trying to get the charge nurse to assign an extra person, attempting to get the nursing service office to send help, trying to get the physician to change his orders or to request a private duty nurse, and trying to get the client transferred to a different unit or put into an isolated or maximum security room.

This nurse spends time in fruitless efforts and activities that do not contribute to the solution of the problem. Admitting ignorance about the care of agitated clients would have damaged the leader's self-esteem; consequently, the nurse avoided this by engaging in activities that were acceptable to the group such as trying to obtain aid. Any consequent difficulties with the agitated client can conveniently be the fault of those who did not respond as requested.

The nurse who is secure and has the ability to care for this type of patient can help the caregivers devise ways of handling this problem. This can be achieved through teaching these skills necessary to care safely and effectively for the client and through planning a cooperative effort. The time and energy spent in teaching and planning for this emergency will profit the whole membership when a similar problem arises. Goal-directed activity generates self-confidence, which is transmitted to others and is reinforced by success. An example of behavioral objectives that reflect an effective teaching-learning process is as follows:

1. Applies teaching-learning strategies and develops plan most useful for each teaching-learning situation in the promotion of health for individuals and groups
2. Identifies own learning needs that are congruent with own strengths, limitations, and potential in the light of own life needs; identifies and evaluates own learning process and makes necessary adaptations; formulates behavioral objectives that are congruent, relevant, and realistic to fulfill self needs and modifies according to outcomes
3. Seeks to establish a learning environment that will permit relationships of trust, security, and feedback and will allow for realistic goal setting, practice, and assessment
4. Serves as a role model in the practice of physical and mental health in nursing practice; is alert to the need and methodology necessary to effect change
   a. Reflects optimal physical and mental health in nursing practice
   b. Establishes goals for self, recognizing own physical and mental capabilities and stamina
   c. Develops adaptive measures for modifying behavior according to individual assessment of physical and mental condition and expectations of the work setting
5. Uses predetermined criteria to evaluate the effectiveness of the teaching-learning process for self and groups

Self-confidence is born of success and reinforced by enough success to allow failures to be perceived not as basic inadequacies but as momentary or transient failures. Self-confidence enables the leader to identify areas of knowledge and ignorance and to instigate activities that will increase knowledge and expand professional expertise.

Continuing education through individual study, in-service programs, or formal programs enable the leader to keep pace with professional technology. Part of the solution to the need for an increase in quality care is in utilization: better use of employees through on-the-job training for specialized skills. Policies that encourage continuing education help to achieve the goals. Because of increased efficiency and fuller utilization of individual productivity potential, the professionally knowledgeable nurse is an economic asset to the public and to the employing agency.

The energy output utilized in attempting to circumvent a nursing situation decreases when the nurse can cope with a situation; energy can be directed toward achievement rather than circumvention.

The recent trend to offer nursing services at the colleague-peer relationship level, as with the primary care nurse who works in contractual agreement with the client, and other special nursing roles—described as extender, expander, assistant, associate, clinical specialist, and practitioner—necessitates preparation beyond that normally provided in nursing curricula.* Whatever the label and however the functions are described, an expanded role requires a corresponding increase in knowledge and skills to meet the challenge. Schools of nursing, particularly baccalaureate and graduate programs, are deluged with requests from federal, state, regional, and local commissions, as well as from individuals, to prepare the nurse with primary skills to provide better health care to increased numbers of people. Major content areas that have been largely absent from nursing curricula in the past are those of physical and developmental assessment and health history. For the practicing nurse, consistent acquisitions of new knowledge requires aptitude and an investment of time and money. The nurse committed to assuming a new role will seek and complete programs of study that will provide the necessary supplementary preparation.

PREDICTIVE PRINCIPLE: The degree to which the leader is clinically knowledgeable and competent directly influences feelings of security about the appropriateness of nursing activity.

Nurses have a responsibility to the client, to their employers, and to those being led to be clinically proficient. Clinical competence gives the nurse self-confidence, which is communicated in both tangible and intangible ways to clients, employers, and co-workers. Nurses who have sound basic knowledge and clinical expertise save time and energy for themselves and others. They understand when procedures are correct, and they are more innovative in devising better ways to accomplish a given task. Clinically knowledgeable nurses use the nursing process to discuss with clients and caregivers the validity of established goals, the appropriateness of planned activities, and the work schedule necessary for achieving those goals. Individuals who turn to the knowledgeable leader for help and advice are rewarded by having their needs met. This reinforces trust in the leader's competence and frees caregivers to rely on themselves and on each other in cooperative efforts. An example of behavioral objectives in the utilization of nursing process through the model of adaptation is as follows:

---

*Management and supervision of patient care, Nurs. Clin. North Am. 8(2):entire issue, June 1973.

1. Extrapolates and applies relevant knowledge from nursing and related fields to the adaptation process with the individual clients and groups
2. Utilizes holistic approach in assessment of needs and implementation of care with each client
3. Assesses the position of clients and groups on the health-illness continuum
4. Assesses the adaptation of individuals in each of the three modes of adaptation—intrapersonal, interpersonal, and environmental—in a complete and logical manner; uses appropriate resources for data gathering; identifies significant relationships between modes and draws justifiable conclusions from data relationships
5. Identifies focal, contextual, and residual stimuli that influence the behavior of client; identifies and utilizes relationships between stimuli in planning care
6. Establishes priorities for provision of nursing care in concert with client
7. Implements nursing interventions designed to promote and support client adaptation
8. Explores opportunities for innovative nursing interventions; encourages clients and nursing staff to exercise initiative and creativity in goal realization

Mutual respect

Maximum productivity results when consideration and respect are given to a health caregiver's total personality; this means that recognition and utilization of the employee's desires, attitudes, interests, and motives are as important as attention to physical efforts.

As consideration for worth and respect of the individual has progressed in health agencies, many current practices have developed. These include recognition of the following: individuals vary in their personal aptitudes and interests; different jobs require different abilities; the emotional makeup of the individual influences job performance; and the prevailing spirit or feeling of the work force affects productivity. The need for mutual respect between employer and employee is gradually being recognized. Both have an interest in the well-being of the other, and the relationship between employer and employee must be harmonious if they are to work together toward common objectives. This same philosophy applies to nurses and co-workers.

PREDICTIVE PRINCIPLE: Understanding and practicing the basic elements of mutual respect facilitate effective leadership.

Maximum utilization of personnel is influenced by mutual respect between group and leader. Determination of basic elements inherent in respect is a difficult task in a society where people from varied backgrounds, free to develop their own philosophies of life, comprise the work force.

In 1951 the National Education Association* published the results of a survey to determine if there was a core of spiritual and moral values for operation in a free society on which all people could agree. The following values were agreed on:

1. There is significance in the individual personality. (This was the basic assumption from which all others were formulated.)
2. The individual has the capacity to assume moral responsibility.
3. Institutions are the servants of people; people are not the servants of institutions.
4. Common consent is a basis for social action.
5. Devotion to truth is necessary for open, trusting human relationships.
6. Excellence in human achievement should be respected.
7. Moral equality is mandatory. No one in a democratic society has the moral right to injure the growth and development of another personality.
8. There should be brotherhood among people. This means the concern of one person for another—the interest of all people in relation to one another.
9. The pursuit of happiness is a legitimate goal.
10. Spiritual enrichment is desirable.

These points were the consensus of representatives from all ethnic groups, creeds, and religions in America as values that could serve as a basis for interrelationships. If the nurse accepts these values and believes there is significance, worth, and dignity in the human personality, behavior, and attitudes, this belief will be indicated to others and respect will be reciprocal.

Members invest authority in their leader with expectation that their worth will be recognized and that the leader will attempt to meet their needs in the work situation and will support their values.

PREDICTIVE PRINCIPLE: The leader's expressions of respect for others precipitate acts of mutual respect among members.

Leaders who care for others enter into relationships with co-workers that have significance and create feelings of mutual satisfaction and respect. When the practitioner's attitude indicates concern for co-workers, a respect model is provided. Knowledge of members' personal problems requires the leader to express feelings of concern and understanding and to construct a work environment that fosters the growth and potentialities of the members.

---

*Educational Policies Commission: Moral and spiritual values in the public schools, Washington, D.C., 1951, National Education Association.

Situations can be structured that will enable members with problems to find ways within the work situation to deemphasize personal problems. However, it must be recognized that the leader's role is confined to prescribed activities within the work situation.

Admiration and respect for others can be expressed in many ways and still be in keeping with commitment. Sometimes the nurse is hesitant to share feelings of esteem for others because of a fear that intentions will be misinterpreted or effectiveness as a leader will be lessened. The mature leader will realize the value of expressing feelings for others on appropriate occasions and will not deprive self and others of the opportunity for successful reinforcement of the positive relationships that come from such expressions. A leader who respects another person will become involved in that person's development, and mutual growth will result.

Attitudes concern feelings and opinions and are revealed in both overt and covert ways. Those who are led expect the leader's attitudes to be constructive. They expect such attitudes as warmth, acceptance, objectivity, empathy, compassion, and respect to be exhibited. When the leader demonstrates to co-workers that others are held in high regard, a pattern of behavior for that group (feelings of trust) will be nurtured and mutual respect will follow. The leader and members will accept and respect one another as peers and work together to minimize weaknesses and maximize strengths.

When the concept of mutual respect is learned by the nurse, constructive attitudes among members will be promoted. The extent to which co-workers adopt the nurse's attitudes toward others is a measure, to some degree, of the effectiveness of the nurse as a leader.

Open channels of communication

Leaders and managers are involved in two kinds of communication: interpersonal and organizational. Interpersonal is the process of exchanging information and meaning from one person to another or in small groups of people. Organizational communication is the process by which leaders and managers use the established system to receive and relay information to people within the organization as well as to relevant individuals and groups outside it. A leader works toward creating an environment that promotes openness and ease in communication among individuals and groups within the formal communication system defined by the authority structure in the agency.

Many nurses feel unaffected by the environment in which they work. They are preoccupied with clients, their friends, relatives, and advocates, other members of the health team, or the administrative staff of the area. Authority figures are frequently equated with punishment and discipline. No previous personal contact with a specific managerial person or position is necessary for the authority figure to cause anxiety in some nurses. Effective utilization of the administrative staff in an agency, of an independent practitioner, or of a primary caregiver presumes knowledge of the position and the function of each job and a broad understanding of the channels of communication. An example of behavioral objectives that reflect open channels of communication is as follows:

1. Selects, applies, and promotes appropriate interpersonal theories that positively affect the communication patterns in health care delivery system (see Chapter 5)
2. Assesses behaviors in self, clients, and community that promote and block communication; develops, actualizes, and promotes alternative behavioral patterns (see Chapter 5)
3. Assesses, plans, implements, evaluates, and revises communication strategies on an ongoing basis

PREDICTIVE PRINCIPLE: Knowledge of appropriate organizational channels of communication facilitates efficient utilization of line organization.

The purpose of health agencies is to provide quality health service to patients. Nurses who know the lines of communication within and without formal health organizational structures can cope with the setting and can devise ways to facilitate and expedite nursing practice.

The line organizational chart from an agency policy manual describes responsibilities of each position to some degree. However, if the organizational structure is to be useful, the nurse needs to acquire knowledge not only of the line organization but also of job descriptions. The line organizational chart and the actual organizational structure may not be the same; some people in the authority structure may be assuming roles and responsibility that have been officially prescribed to others. This can happen by incorrectly established custom or as a result of power struggles. When the nurse finds that such conflicts exist, clarification can be sought from the nurse's immediate superior in written form. Written memos empower the nurse to function more securely by providing a record of clarified channels for future reference.

Confusion, wasted energy, and decreased service to the client as a result of poor use of the organizational structure can result in a situation such as the following:

The staff nurse asks her unit supervisor for permission to hold a class with the ancillary staff about colostomy care. The supervisor gives permission and encouragement. The staff nurse asks the director of central supply to demonstrate use of the equipment. This nurse then posts a notice in the dining room inviting all interested nurses to attend. The in-service education director becomes upset because in-service education is her area of authority and she should have been consulted about the class first.

The nurse could have prevented problems in this situation by using the appropriate chain of command. Casual perusal of the organizational chart and job descriptions would have indicated that the in-service education director was a necessary person to consult before proceeding with plans involving other departments and people from other nursing units.

PREDICTIVE PRINCIPLE: The nurse working in an expanded role provides leadership initiative in establishing channels of communication congruent with the role.

The nurse engaged in collaborative interprofessional relationships, as in the practice of primary nursing care or an expanded role, will establish relevant and expedient channels of communication between employer, client and related individuals, and other members of the health team. The expanded role includes people and functions that contribute to the nurse's caregiving repertoire. The practitioner establishes avenues of communication with these resources so that combined knowledge, skills, and support will be immediately accessible in routine or critical primary care situations. The expanded role requires the independent nurse to be conversant with contributing sources of communication and enables the nurse to function appropriately in a given circumstance.

The nurse-practitioner who functions beyond ordinary discipline boundaries performs without the structure often attendant with regulations of advisory councils, committees, and other direction-giving bodies. An expansion in role does not imply that the nurse is absolved from accountability to organizational framework, whether casual (as with a verbal agreement between client and nurse) or highly structured (as in a complex health agency). Seeking suitable resources, guidance, and other assistance that accrue from established policy and procedure, either within or without the health agency, contributes to the client's welfare and the nurse's professional development.

Knowledge of participants' capabilities

Since World War II, nursing has been deluged with ancillary workers, each with a different background and preparation. These workers enter the nursing field to perform selected tasks under the supervision and direction of professional nurses. They bring to the job a wide variety of sociocultural and educational backgrounds. Leaders who assess the capabilities of each individual with whom they work can delegate tasks and responsibilities appropriately and assist in developing the potential of each worker.

PREDICTIVE PRINCIPLE: An understanding of sociocultural backgrounds of members helps the leader to assess job capabilities.

The advent of educational and training programs aimed at the unemployed and cultural and racial minority groups has brought large numbers of workers from various ethnic backgrounds into nursing. Race, English language skills, economic level, and the cultural experiences of these workers vary from the middle-class, white, third- and fourth-generation Americans who comprise the bulk of professional nurses. It is necessary that the nurse be able to communicate clearly and relate effectively with these workers if their skills and knowledge are to be fairly assessed and their attitudes understood. This assessment helps the nurse to understand the value systems (Chapter 4) of group members, to know how best to motivate them, and thus to know how to communicate with them effectively. A value system is brought to the job as a part of each person's personality. An understanding of value systems enables the nurse to use the entire work force to full advantage and to promote effectively the development of individual and group potential.

Barriers to understanding and rapport, such as race and class, are not insurmountable. Prejudice, caste, and class conflicts exist in nursing, as in society, both openly and subtly. However, because of the changing self-image of subcultural groups and the legal protection of individual rights and dignity, racial and class prejudices are discussed more freely today than ever before. Nurses who ignore the presence of a group member from a subculture or avoid talking about differences in cultural or ethnic background do not prevent conflict; they only drive it underground. The critical problems of today's society will be reflected in each small group and must be faced.

Open discussions about individual differences or similarities will enable a leader to recognize how cultural, class, or ethnic characteristics influence individual value systems and behavior patterns within the nursing group. Talking openly and directly about class, color, and culture is difficult for the average middle-class white nurse; however, success in this area will come with practice. An observant nurse who is sensitive to others can remark on incidents and solicit comments that help promote understanding among members. If a leader does not understand an individual's feelings, openly admitting the lack of understanding invites further exploration and leads to trust. Relationships based on understanding and insight promote the assessment of capabilities and the development of potential in individuals.

English language differences can influence how the leader perceives the caregivers and can influence assessment of capabilities and potential. Dialects, poor grammar, foreign accents, and colloquial expressions along with unusual diction can mislead the unwary nurse. Language differences are environmental, cultural, geographic, and educational; they have little to do with intelligence, ability, and job training. The effective nurse will assess the worker's knowledge, maturity, skill, and experience and avoid assumptions based on language alone.

PREDICTIVE PRINCIPLE: Reactions to stress influence efficiency of performance in the work situation.

Job capabilities are influenced by many factors other than ability, knowledge, and skill. Personal crises absorb energy and drain resources that would normally be utilized in work functions. Thought patterns and observational skills are interrupted or inhibited by preoccupation with personal crises. The skillful leader will observe departure from normal work patterns and try to ascertain the reasons for altered performance. This knowledge enables the leader to change work assignments or supervisory habits to conform to the demands of the new behavior pattern until the personal crisis is past.

Stressful job situations, such as emergencies, unexpectedly heavy work assignments, breakdowns in communications and interrelationships, nursing errors, and conflicts with physicians or supervisors, elicit responses from the leader and other caregivers that are not normally seen in daily routine behavior (see Chapter 10). The leader who knows each worker's behavioral patterns not only can help to prevent disruptions of client care but also can anticipate how best to help the distressed member. Opportunity for members to discuss stressful work factors and their feelings about them as soon after the incident as possible decreases the accompanying anxiety and allows the daily work to progress smoothly. Such discussions while impressions and feelings are fresh give all participants a more accurate picture of what actually happened and furnish insights that contribute to the leader's knowledge of individual capabilities, increase job satisfaction, and save time and energy.

PREDICTIVE PRINCIPLE: Knowledge of a caregiver's preparation and experience promotes fullest use of skills and provides a basis for continued growth.

The leader needs specific information about the education and work experience of each group member in order to delegate the work load appropriately and to determine the amount of supervision and teaching necessary to develop personnel potential. Some of the necessary information may be in employment records, but frequently the personnel files are not open to staff nurses. The nurse often must depend on personal interviews and observations for information necessary to proper utilization of all personnel. The following is an example:

Mrs. Pedersen, a skilled leader, had worked with Mrs. Williams, an aide, for six months. Mrs. Pedersen discovered during a conversation at lunch one day that Mrs. Williams had worked in a home for the aged for 15 years. The aide stated that she had always loved aged people and liked to work with them; she derived satisfaction from getting them to eat and drink and from contriving ways to motivate them. Mrs. Pedersen was able to learn much from working with Mrs. Williams. As leader, Mrs. Pedersen utilized this aide to help other ancillary workers who were assigned to geriatric patients.

A planned assessment interview would have revealed Mrs. Williams' strength much earlier and would have benefited both clients and personnel.

Sources of information

Two basic sources of information are available to the nurse-leader: the assessment interview and observation. The following outline is designed as a guide to activities that will provide needed member assessment data:

I. The assessment interview
   A. Establishment of a time and place that provides privacy and freedom from interruptions
   B. Introduction of purposes of interview and how information will be used
   C. Establishment of rapport conducive to an exchange of information; inquiring about the following to obtain the specific information desired:
      1. Educational background—amount of formal education (grade completed, high school diploma, education after high school, extent of college work)
      2. Formal job training
         a. Length of program and when completed
         b. Formal classroom content (anatomy and physiology; bacteriology and aseptic technique; talking with clients; procedures—list common ones encountered on present job; organizations of work; observations—recording and reporting)
      3. Clinical practice
         a. Real or simulated situation (client care or practice on dolls or fellow students)
         b. Experience in systems of care (primary, case, functional, team)
         c. Type of clients included in experiences (medical, surgical, obstetric, psychiatric)
         d. Nursing setting (home, convalescent hospital, acute hospital, outpatient clinics)
         e. Opportunity for practice of nursing procedures
         f. Amount of supervision
         g. Who supervised (teacher, nurse on unit, others)
         h. Nursing activity preferences and type of clients preferred
   D. Conclusions
      1. Brief summary of notes taken regarding content and tone of interview
      2. Structure for follow-up at later date as necessary
II. Observation
   A. Observation of work in progress during normal workday activities
   B. Survey of work results
      1. Assignments completed as directed
      2. Client appearance
      3. Content of reporting to group and leader or charting
   C. Observation of relationship with other personnel and group
   D. Participation-observation

Assessment interview. Time and place for the assessment interview must be mutually convenient to both parties. A well-planned and structured interview does not take long. A prior explanation of what will occur in the interview should be given so that the caregiver will come prepared and thus reduce the time required for the conference. Fifteen to twenty minutes should be sufficient for such an interview. Keeping appointments punctually and terminating the conference on time are important. Punctuality helps convey the value of both the worker's and the leader's time.

Setting an atmosphere for the interview occurs both during the preliminary discussions about the interview and within the interview itself. Openness and sincerity are behavioral messages that put the interview on an honest, productive basis. Subterfuge, hesitancy, and lack of candidness elicit responses with the same characteristics.

Nurses who ask co-workers instead of the individuals involved about fellow workers' abilities, problems, attitudes, and preparation are engaging in a practice that will create distrust among the members. Often the leader who follows such a practice not only receives fallacious information but also loses the trust and support of the group.

A relaxed atmosphere is helpful to the establishment of rapport. Relaxed informality is not lack of structure; it is naturalness. Any activity, posture, or attitude that helps both parties behave in a normal way helps establish rapport. Both the party interviewed and the leader should feel free to smoke or take refreshment. These are socializing activities that promote naturalness. A room where there is privacy and, if possible, comfort is helpful. Job responsibilities of both persons should be assigned to other caregivers for the duration of the interview; this enables the devotion of attention to the subject and prevents interruptions.

Beginning an interview with a well-defined plan for achieving objectives is likely to reach those objectives. Having a specific and topical list for discussion produces the best results. Keeping the list in view and making notes as the interview progresses are helpful to the interviewer by keeping attention focused on the subject and giving a brief record for future reference.

Evaluation of interview data requires sensitivity to nonverbal responses and interpretation of verbal responses. The nurse who fidgets, fusses, or verbally hedges may be attempting to say what she thinks the interviewer wishes to hear, to mask true feelings, or to cope with anxiety. The interviewer must weigh all the responses (verbal and nonverbal) of the worker and attempt to evaluate them. Clarifying remarks can take the form of statements, observations, or questions, such as "Will you describe what you learned in your classes on aseptic technique so that I understand a little better?" Statements calling for further descriptions, elucidation, and information help the leader to clarify and evaluate responses.

Observation. The leader needs practical and real knowledge of a group member's ability gathered from firsthand observations of the person at work. Assessment of the worker's ability can be made through several observational methods. Observing work in progress gives the leader insight into the worker's effectiveness, safety, and efficiency. Clients who appear clean and comfortable when care is completed and nursing care plans that have been carried through are indicators of worker ability. The content of written or oral reports can also be used as assessment data.

Participation-observation is probably the most effective method of observing for leaders. It will prove useful in assessments, which are done for the purpose of providing a basis for optimal utilization of personnel and encouraging professional growth. Participation-observation is observing another's conduct while participating with that person in job performance, for example, observing how sheets are handled and how a bed is made while helping to make the bed. Participation-observation must be explained to ancillary workers to enable the leader to observe without usurping the worker's role. Participation-observation experiences provide the following opportunities:

1. An opportunity for the nurse-leader to assess the member
2. An opportunity for the nurse-leader to teach and learn
3. An opportunity for the worker to observe the leader in the care of clients (role modeling)

Plans for participation-observation can be arranged in a group meeting with the client or family in which the purposes for the observations are discussed. Arrangements can be made for the leader to work closely with each member at a convenient time. It is essential that the members have a clear understanding of the purposes of the participation-observation experiences.

Observational assessments help the leader to make assignments that fully utilize each person's capabilities. Working together fosters mutual respect and mutual assessment. Since the nurse has prescribed activities, plans must be made for short participation-observations on a daily basis so that observations can be made of routine work as well as of special assignments or new procedures.

The ability to function is dynamic and changes with the variables of conditions, environments, and associations with people. The leader can only try to assess and reassess each worker. This continuous assessment process enables the nurse-leader to delegate responsibility and supervise work appropriately while promoting the greatest development of personnel potential. The outcome of this approach will improve the quality and safety of nursing care.

Environment

In addition to concentration on human motivation and group behavior, the nurse takes into consideration the work environment, which in part determines the scope and limitations of activity.

Technical environment includes the physical geography, organizational layout, equipment, system of supply, scheduling, and methods of administering services. The leader's work environment includes all technical aspects and the conditions, circumstances, and pressures that influence administrative processes.

The findings of much of the research in executive behavior support the conclusion that effective performance of leaders is directly related to the organizational environment.

An alert and interested nurse-leader will find ways to meet personal needs in the work environment, protecting client, employees, and self from harmful environmental factors, taking advantage of desirable aspects, and changing the environment in ways that make it a better source of need satisfaction. To accomplish this, the nurse-leader understands and is able to apply those principles that contribute to a satisfactory environment.

PREDICTIVE PRINCIPLE: A work environment that is open and amenable to valid change assists in personal and professional growth and development.

Work experiences that allow the nurse to satisfy intellectual curiosity enable an acquisition of skills and knowledge necessary for intelligent, efficient work and informed living. Each leader and participant needs opportunities to engage in experiences that promote ongoing motivation to grow professionally. Work environments can make provision for the expression of personality through creative activities. Professional productivity is promoted by identification with the results of one's own activity and taking pride in personal achievements. Creativity is seen at all levels and can be applied to the most ordinary tasks. Creativity that is utilized can increase efficiency. With imaginative design and innovation, job activities may be completed in less time, with less energy expended, and with less equipment used.

Originality of thought can result in increased service to clients and greater job satisfaction. Creativity flourishes in an environment where workers believe that their ideas and opinions are received by leaders and peers and are given the same consideration as those of every other group member. Henry Ford believed that a lazy man who is given a job to do will find the quickest and easiest way to perform the task. In the same vein, a well-prepared nurse will devise the best possible way to perform the assignment.

It is possible to pursue the goals of individuals, organizations, and agencies without destroying human values in the process. The organization has a great stake in developing its people and thus in serving human values and organizational ends. Management that takes specific steps to ensure that the work environment gives employees an opportunity to grow and develop will have more stable and productive personnel. The achievement of emotional maturity in the leader depends on an environment that provides opportunities to express independence and autonomy, to have a part in determining the outcome of efforts, and to participate in significant relationships with others. Innovations that promote desired changes in environment can support optimism and the freedom to be productive.

Application of predictive principles of leadership behavior

You are the leader of a four-member nursing team. One of the members exhibits maladaptive behaviors that are disruptive to the team. She complains to clients and peers about such things as her work assignment, time for breaks and lunch, poor organization, and the team leader's personality. To date, the team leader has ignored the problem, hoping the situation would improve.

Problem	*Predictive principle*	*Prescription*
Disruptive behavior by team member.	Knowledge and understanding of factors about human beings permit assessment and acceptance of self and others.	Team leader assesses that complaining member is acting in passive and aggressive manners, and recognizes that she has been passive in not confronting the member with her behavior.
	Consistent use of passive behavior ignores personal rights of the leader and leads to lowered self-esteem and maladaptive behaviors.	
	Achievement of one's goals through aggressive acts violates another person's rights and results in feelings of domination, humiliation, and hostility.	Team leader arrangers for a meeting with team member in a secluded place. She is open and forthright in her approach: "Laura, for some time now I have observed you complaining to others about [lists complaints]. When you act in this way you not only harm yourself but you cause the other team members to become discontented. I want you to go over your complaints with me one by one so we can resolve the problems."
	Accomplishing goals through assertive behavior enables a leader to exercise the rights of self without denying the rights and feelings of others.	
	A work environment that is open and amenable to valid change assists in personal and professional growth and development.	

BIBLIOGRAPHY
Books

Alberti, R., and Emmons, M.: Your perfect right: a guide to assertive behavior, San Luis Obispo, Calif., 1974, Impact Publishers.

Argyris, C.: Management and organizational development, New York, 1971, McGraw-Hill Book Co.

Auld, M.E., and Birum, L.H.: The challenge of nursing: a book of readings, St. Louis, 1973, The C.V. Mosby Co.

Bower, F.L.: The process of planning nursing care: a model for practice, ed. 3, St. Louis, 1982, The C.V. Mosby Co.

Carlson, C.E.: Behavioral concepts and nursing intervention, Philadelphia, 1970, J.B. Lippincott Co.

Chenevert, M.: Special techniques in assertiveness training for women in the health professions, St. Louis, 1978, The C.V. Mosby Co.

Drucker, P.: Management: tasks, responsibilities, practices, New York, 1973, Harper & Row, Publishers.

Dyer, W.: Pulling your own strings, New York, 1978, Thomas Y. Crowell Co.

Dyer, W.: Your erroneous zones, New York, 1976, Funk & Wagnalls, Inc.

Fiedler, F., and Chemers, M.: Leadership and effective management, Glenview, Ill., 1974, Scott, Foresman & Co.

Gallasi, M., and Gallasi, J.: Assert yourself: how to be your own person, New York, 1977, Human Sciences Press.

Ganong, J., and Ganong, W.: Nursing management, Germantown, Md., 1976, Aspen Systems Corporation.

Herman, S.: Becoming assertive: a guide for nurses, New York, 1978, D. Van Nostrand Co.

Jourard, S.M.: Disclosing man to himself, New York, 1964, D. Van Nostrand Co.

Jourard, S.M.: The transparent self, New York, 1964, D. Van Nostrand Co.

Kramer, M., and Schmalenberg, C.: Path to biculturalism, Wakefield, Mass., 1977, Contemporary Publishing, Inc.

Levinson, H.: Executive stress, New York, 1970, Harper & Row, Publishers.

Likert, R.: New patterns of management, New York, 1961, McGraw-Hill Book Co.

Loye, D.: The leadership passion: a psychology of ideology, San Francisco, 1977, Jossey-Bass, Inc. Publishers.

Maslow, A.H.: Motivation and personality, New York, 1954, Harper & Row, Publishers.

McGregor, D.: The human side of enterprise, New York, 1960, McGraw-Hill Book Co.

Stevens, B.: First-line patient care management, Wakefield, Mass., 1976, Contemporary Publishing, Inc.

Stevens, W.: Management and leadership in nursing, San Francisco, 1978, McGraw-Hill Book Co.

Stogdill, R.: Handbook of leadership: a survey of theory and research, New York, 1974, Free Press.

Periodicals

Bailey, J., and Claus, K.: Preparing nurse leaders for the world tomorrow, Nurse Leaders. **1**(6): 21, 1978.

Chism, S.: The nurse administrator: a long distance runner, Superv. Nurse **12**(1):36-37, 1981.

Fagin, C.: Accountability, Nurs. Outlook **19**(4): 249-251, 1971.

Hall, D.T., and Nougaim, K.E.: An examination of Maslow's need hierarchy in an organizational setting, organizational behavior and human performance, Nurs. Outlook **16**(3):12-16, 1968.

Helmann, C.: Four theories of leadership, J. Nurs. Admin., pp. 18-24, June 1976.

Huckabay, L., and Arndt, C.: Effect of acquisition of knowledge on self-evaluation and the relationship of self-evaluation to perception of real and ideal self-concept, Nurs. Res. **25**(4): 244-251, July-Aug. 1976.

Krueger, J.: Utilization of nursing research: the planning process, J. Nurs. Admin., pp. 6-11, Jan. 1978.

Lindeman, C.: Nursing research priorities, J. Nurs. Admin., pp. 20-21, July-Aug. 1975.

McClure, M.: The long road to accountability, Nurs. Outlook **26**(1):47-50, 1978.

Migut, P.: Self-care for nurses: assertiveness, Nurs. Mgmt. **13**(2):13-17, 1982.

O'Donovan, T.: Leadership dynamics, J. Nurs. Admin., pp. 32-35, Sept. 1975.

Owen, J.: The use of leadership theory, Mich. Bus. Rev. **25**(1):13-19, 1973.

Pierce, S., and Thompson: Changing practice: by choice rather than chance, J. Nurs. Admin., pp. 33-39, Feb. 1976.

Pinkleton, N.: Commitment to nursing and to self, Nurs. Mgmt. **13**(2):39-41, 1982.

Reres, M.: Tapping human resources, J. Nurs. Admin., pp. 18-19, July-Aug. 1975.

Styles, M.: Dialogue across the decades, Nurs. Outlook **26**(1):28-32, 1978.

Tannenbaum, R., and Schmidt, W.: How to choose a leadership pattern, Harv. Bus. Rev., pp. 162-164, May-June 1973.

chapter ten

Predictive principles of preventing attrition

Identifying the issues

Acceptance of myths instead of data results in faulty conclusions that lead to minimally productive solutions.

Types of attrition

Discounting either the complexity or the solvability of the problem of nurse attrition reduces the probability that the problem will be solved.

Multiple and complex problems produce multiple alternative responses.

Manifestations of the frustrated burnout, dropout, or runaway

Inability of the nurse inclined to burnout, dropout, or runaway to change jobs or leave nursing is likely to result in behaviors that are counterproductive.

Causes of attrition—epidemiologic analysis

Use of a scientific method for investigating attrition increases the probability that a clear and accurate picture of etiology and treatment will emerge.

Increasing the resistance of the nurse to factors causing attrition will help provide a stable cadre of nurses willing to work for environmental improvement and control of noxious factors.

Identification of prime candidates for burnout enables preventive measures to be initiated.

Smooth transition to the real work world and good education in how to effect change can increase resistance to dropout and runaway.

Increased recognition of the importance of a career and a realistic view of prospective life work pattern motivates commitment to help create positive working conditions.

Unmet expectations increase nurse dissatisfaction and result in increased number of nurses who drop out or run away.

A sense of powerlessness increases the incidence of burnout, dropout, and runaway.

Prevention of host attrition reduces cost and is easier than curing attrition.

Self-respect and assertiveness increase attrition resistance.

Strong support systems provide a base for growth and security and decrease susceptibility to burnout, dropout, and runaway.

Stability promotes job effectiveness and increases the ability to facilitate positive changes.

The virulence, dosage, frequency, and duration of noxious events in a nurse's work life directly affect burnout, dropout, and runaway.

Limiting the exposure of the nurse to virulent, high dosage, frequently occurring, noxious events of long duration will decrease the possibility of the nurse leaving the job.

A positive unit environment created by middle and lower management increases unit retention rates.

Positive reinforcement increases job satisfaction.

Improving the unit climate creates an atmosphere of caring about the employee, improves the quality of patient care, and decreases unit attrition rates.

Top nurse management committed to creating a positive environment and improving salaries increases job satisfaction and decreases attrition.

Attrition is a universal problem of nursing employees, both in times of plenty and times of scarcity in the supply of nurses. Whether or not there are few or many nurses in the supply pool, nurses historically work no more than two or three years at a job before they leave it. Where they go and what they do is of concern both to nursing organizations and to a public that suffers from the problems in nursing care delivery brought about by this phenomenon. However, to employers of nurses, the greatest concern is that those nurses who were so difficult and expensive to recruit and train will move on and leave a vacancy that must be filled again and again and again.

Most employers tie attrition directly to the shortage of nurses—and there is a connection. However, whether or not there is a real shortage of nurses or only seems to be one is the subject of much speculation. Estimates are that from 25% to 40% of nurses are not currently working. It is known that whenever salaries rise to levels equal to other female professionals of comparable education and responsibility, the number of vacancies in hospitals falls.

According to Aiken, Blendon, and Rogers,* salaries have the most significant influence on the number of nurses in the work force. To support this, they offer the following facts:

1. The twenty-year period from 1946 to 1966 saw an increase in nurses' salaries of 53%. During that same period teachers' salaries increased by 100%, and those of other female professionals and technical workers increased by 73%. Nurses remained scarce while there was an oversupply of teachers.

2. Beginning in 1966, nurses' salaries increased at twice the rates of teachers and technical workers, primarily because of the introduction

---

*Aiken, L., Blendon, R., and Rogers, D.: The shortage of hospital nurses: a new perspective, Am. J. Nurs. **81**(9):1612-1618, 1981.

of Medicare, which enabled hospitals to have enough income to raise sagging salaries. By 1969, income for nurses was 87% that of teachers and had passed average incomes of other like groups.

3. Vacancy rates declined from 23% in 1961 to 9% in 1971. This rapid decrease in the shortage of nurses directly corresponded with the rise in wages brought about by Medicare.

4. In late 1971 nurses' salaries declined relative to other like groups, and hospital nursing vacancy rates climbed to near pre-Medicare figures.

5. Comparing the current income of nurses to like groups finds teachers making 120% to 130% more than nurses, hospital social workers making about 115% of what nurses make, and physical therapists making from 105% to 110% of what nurses make. Nurses' salaries are about equal to the national average for secretaries, which accounts for the increased numbers of position vacancies.

Attrition rates increase during times of high vacancies and low salaries since competition for nurses is great and nurses leave one job seeking better conditions and better pay. But when there are few vacancies and the pay is good, nurses do not tend to move as frequently.

The literature about the phenomenon of nurse turnover or attrition rates is growing rapidly since employers view turnover as important a factor in their staffing problems as a real manpower shortage. However, research often leaves so many unanswered questions concerning attrition that myths grow freely and unchallenged. This chapter examines some of the current problems about nurse attrition and attempts to provide some principles for helping middle and lower management keep those hard-to-acquire nurses working where they are, rather than dropping out, running to another job, or burning out. Creating a stable work group is essential in elevating the quality of care. It may be equally true that elevating the quality of care helps to stabilize the work force. What is clear is that nurse attrition is no simple problem; therefore simplistic answers are not likely to become lasting solutions. This chapter offers no specific diagnoses and no clear-cut prescriptions that pretend to solve the problems. It provides only some guidelines that may prove helpful to nurses in middle and lower levels of management in their attempts to use whatever power and influence they have to reduce attrition on their units.

Identifying the issues

PREDICTIVE PRINCIPLE: Acceptance of myths instead of data results in faulty conclusions that lead to minimally productive solutions.

There are so many myths about nurse attrition that separating fact and fiction is not easy. However, enough facts have been uncovered by shrewd observers to disprove a few of the more obviously misleading conclusions about nurse attrition.

The most popular myth is that *there must be something wrong with nurses*. People who believe this usually back up their argument with unsubstantiated statements such as "Nurses leave nursing at greater rates than other female workers," "Nurses do not want to work the evening and night shifts because educators don't make them do it anymore," and "Reality shock and burnout decimate nursing ranks and cause nurses to leave nursing."

The facts paint a very different picture. According to Aiken and coworkers,* nurses participate in the labor market at one of the highest rates of any predominantly female group. In 1960, only 55% of nurses were active in nursing compared to 75% in 1980. Nurses do leave nursing, but only 25% are absent at any one time. Were this 25% working, it would reduce the shortage, but it would not solve the attrition problem. Much of the attrition is among nurses who change jobs; relatively few leave the work force. It is reported that only about 3% of nurses are working at nonnursing jobs; however, this estimate may be low, since nurses who leave nursing for another field often allow their licenses to lapse and no longer identify as nurses. These would be difficult to count.

Most nurses do not want to work evening and night shifts, which in itself is not surprising. Staffing the night shift has always been a problem. It is difficult to find people who are willing to sleep while everyone else is awake and work while their friends and families sleep, especially when differential in pay for these difficult hours is not very tempting. In the past when training occurred in hospitals that used students as the mainstay of their labor forces, students were required to work nights and evenings. Upon graduation they moved as quickly as possible to jobs where days and free weekends were the routine. The fact that students were required to work nights did not decrease the difficulty in finding staffing for those unwanted hours. However, agencies that offer significantly increased pay for nights and weekends have had no difficulty finding nurses for those times.

The other myth that promotes the belief that there must be something wrong with nurses is that they experience reality shock and burnout to the extent that it decimates the work force. Reality shock does occur. Nurses leave their first job after six to nine months, but they usually seek a job in nursing somewhere else. Burnout results in a decrease in enthusiasm, but seldom is it the single cause for nurses to leave their profession.

Types of attrition

PREDICTIVE PRINCIPLE: Discounting either the complexity or the solvability of the problem of nurse attrition reduces the probability that the problem will be solved.

---

*Aiken, L., Blendon, R., and Rogers, D.: The shortage of hospital nurses: a new perspective, Am. J. Nurs. **81**(9):1612-1618, 1981.

Recruitment costs approximately $4,000 per nurse, although cost varies from institution to institution depending on the size of the agency and the range of its recruitment activities. This estimated cost does not include the lost productivity while new nurses are being oriented to the new work situation. Hospital attrition rates vary but range from 25% to 75% each year. This adds up to a major expense.

The attrition rate has been a chronic problem for so many years that employers now view it as normal. Nurses are seen as transient, always looking for greener pastures, and ever on the move. Because most nurses are women, employers expect a high turnover rate. Raising a family, a spouse's job transfer, and changes in the spouse's income are reasons given for the high attrition rate. However, these rationales discount both the complexity of the problem and possibility of solving it. Few agencies actually ask the right questions of nurses to diagnose the cause of leaving. All agencies want to keep nurses because of the difficulties in finding replacements, but few administrators look at the multicausal aspects of the attrition problem or analyze its effects.

PREDICTIVE PRINCIPLE: Multiple and complex problems produce multiple alternative responses.

There are three basic categories of attrition (see Fig. 10-1): burnout, dropout, and runaway.

Burnout. Literature on burnout is plentiful, and most authors treat the subject as a problem related strictly to the individual. Only a few relate nurse

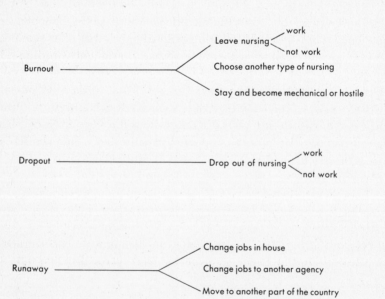

Fig. 10-1. Three forms of attrition and their usual manifestations.

burnout to environmental factors, and most of these hold both the nurse and the environment responsible.

Burnout, according to Pines and Maslach,* is a "syndrome of physical and emotional exhaustion, involving the development of negative self-concept, negative job attitude and loss of concern and feelings for clients." Nurses in burnout feel worked out, used up. They lose enthusiasm and their sense of humor. They feel that the situation in which they work will never improve. In its advanced stages the nurse is depressed, lacks initiative, and does not seem to care about work or clients. She feels both hopeless and helpless.

Burnout will affect all aspects of the nurse's life. The nurse may procrastinate when that has never been the pattern before. Additional symptoms are sleep disturbances, irritability, being distracted and forgetful, and feeling abnormally tired. The individual may manifest a lowered resistance and begin to have repeated infections, headaches, backaches, and other infirmities. The nurse may begin to drink more and enjoy it less or increase tranquilizer intake. Burnout is not a new phenomenon; it is simply the new catchword for the old syndrome of stress. It is a stress response to a specific set of work-related stressors.

The consequences of burnout fall into one or more of three categories as illustrated in Fig. 10-1. The nurse may change jobs in nursing, leave nursing altogether, or occasionally stay on at the same job. For each option there are several choices. For instance, the person who changes jobs in nursing may do so within the institution, as from general duty to orientation coordinator, or from IV therapist to rehabilitation nurse. Within most agencies there will be a group of nurses who have held several different jobs, each position quite dissimilar from the others. By changing, the nurse seeks renewal and rekindling of enthusiasm, dissolution of depression, and regaining a sense of purpose and caring.

When information on burnout first became available, employers jumped at the opportunity to help nurses fight burnout. They reasoned that burnout must account for a great portion of nurse attrition; therefore if nurses could be helped to be stronger and more resistant to burnout they would stay in their present jobs, able to cope with work problems, disgruntled physicians, difficult clients, and their own powerlessness. It did not seem to occur to anyone that burnout must be a result of other factors beyond an individual's weakness or susceptibility.

Burnout is the current name for a very old phenomenon. Where one used to hear "I'm sick and tired of it all," now one hears "I'm burned out." Burnout has been treated primarily as a problem of the individual nurse, and the literature prescribes preventive and curative measures as if some home remedy or over-the-counter patent medicine could take care of the problem. There are

---

*Pines, A., and Maslach, C.: Characteristics of staff burnout in mental health settings, Hosp. Comm. Psych. **29**:233-237, 1978.

things the individual can do—but as in most jobs nursing is like a marriage in that it takes two to make or break it. The "sick and tireds" are a result of two factors: (1) poor work environments brought about by poor nursing care and poor hospital management (all levels) and (2) nurses who do not know how to take care of themselves.

Workshops on burnout, offered as a way to reduce attrition and to provide stability to agencies whose turnover rate ranges between 25% and 75% a year, fail because burnout is only one problem of three attrition pathways and is part of attrition, not a cause of it. The cause is much deeper.

Dropout. Nurses who experience dropout feel they have made a mistake in career choice. They feel their talents and abilities are going unused and unwanted. They feel unappreciated for what they can contribute to client care. They feel remorseful that they have spent so much time and money preparing for a career they do not wish to pursue further. They often are in a dilemma: should they drop out now and cut their losses, or should they stay and perhaps regret that decision for the rest of their lives? These people do not burn out, but sometimes the symptoms are similar.

Some burnouts and dropouts simply leave nursing. Of these some go on to real estate, teaching, or into industry and business. Others remain technically unemployed, not working outside the home.

Nurses drop out for a number of reasons. One survey* states that nursing has a 40% dropout rate. Of these, 75% leave to get married, have children, and bring up a family. The remaining 25% leave for a variety of reasons: 9% leave nursing permanently; 4.4% leave because of job frustrations; 3.9% because of other job-related problems; and more than 6% to continue their education.

Citing the number of nurses (75%) who drop out to raise a family, many experts say there is a limited amount that can be done to stem the attrition. That conclusion ignores the contribution that poor wages and unsatisfying working conditions make to a woman's decision to resign rather than take maternity leave with the intention of returning to work. For many women having a baby is a pause, not a reason to quit, but unless her career is rewarding, there is little incentive to return.

Nurses drop out for varying lengths of time. Donovan* found that 10.6% drop out from one to two years and over 15% for six years or more. In today's fast-moving world, those who drop out for more than five years have problems on returning; their knowledge and skills have become obsolete. They must take refresher courses to refurbish their skills before reentering the work force. This group consists of the prospects most sought after by employers, who use television, newspapers, and letters to plead with these nurses to return to a profession that is critically short of manpower. Every attempt is made to invoke their

---

*Donovan, L.: What nurses want (and what they're getting), RN **43**(4):24, 1980.

feelings of guilt and social responsibility so that they will return to the active work force. Often tremendous and unfair pressure is brought to bear as if these nurses did not have the right to make personal choices about their own careers and life goals.

Refresher courses are offered as a way to attract nurses back into the work force but the number of those who do return to nursing using this route is relatively small. Therefore, as in disease, the emphasis must be placed on prevention rather than remediation.

Runaway. The runaway has not burned out; she neither despairs nor feels hopeless. Quite the contrary, the most outstanding characteristic of a runaway is hope: hope for better conditions, a better job, better pay, better something. So the runaway changes jobs. She may change jobs in-house, go to another agency, or she may go to another part of the country. Sometimes she finds what she is looking for; most often she keeps moving every year or two.

Runaways are perennial optimists. They tend to be romanticists who believe that life is going to be better just over the hill. They feel a commitment to nursing. They feel that their dissatisfaction is the fault of the job or the administration. Often they are assertive and have ability and enthusiasm. However, they do not see the value to themselves in staying in one place long enough to gain credibility and exert influence to make their agency a better place in which to work. They crave changes in their social life and wish a change in environment as much as a change in job. One suspects that were the chronic runaway tied down and immobilized without being helped to see how she can effect changes in the work environment, she would quickly burn out or drop out.

Runaways almost all have the same pattern. They choose to look for greener pastures. They opt for category 1 (see Fig. 10-1) every time. They change jobs in nursing, occasionally at the same institution but most often at different institutions. If the nurse is unincumbered, she moves to a different state. These nurses often wind up in the "romance" spots: Hawaii, California, Colorado, Florida, New York. Runaways are found in coastal towns and resort villages. Increasingly, runaways are attracted to small towns in the Sunbelt. Their work history shows a job change every eight months to two years. During the time they are employed they tend to become oriented quickly, produce well, and show enthusiasm and initiative. These nurses are definitely neither burnouts nor dropouts. They manifest no depression until they stay in one place too long and begin to tire of it.

Data on runaways present a discouraging picture. Statistics show that nurses between 25 and 30 year of age have held their present jobs for little more than 2½ years. Nurses in the profession as a whole average three years, ten months between job changes. Nurses under age 25 change jobs on the average of once every 1.4 years. Of these, from 75% to 85% change not only jobs but also employers. The sad part is that these workers shift laterally without improving their career status. Five jobs ago 75% of these nurses were in staff nurse slots; almost 67% of them are still in staff nurse slots. Fewer than 12% of these runaways improved their job status. For staff nurses moving does not facilitate promotions.

Studies indicate that a large percentage of nurses who change jobs do so with the hope of improving their incomes. What these runaways seek varies. Although job-related intangibles such as self-realization, achievement, helping clients, stimulation, education, and fellowship rate highest on most surveys, about 60% of all survey respondents rate income as a *very* important consideration. And although income is listed as one of the most popular reasons for changing jobs, studies indicate that job-hopping does not substantially improve income.

Manifestations of the frustrated burnout, dropout, or runaway

PREDICTIVE PRINCIPLE: Inability of the nurse inclined to burnout, dropout, or runaway to change jobs or leave nursing is likely to result in behaviors that are counterproductive.

Would-be burnouts, dropouts, or runaways who by circumstances are forced to remain in their jobs have some difficult choices. Immobility is often a result of management or family responsibilities, such as being a single parent or responsible for aging or dependent parents. However, unwillingness to move can simply be unwillingness to take a risk, to give up a known no matter how dissatisfying and move to an unknown. In health care agencies with excellent retirement plans, good salary, good retention and promotion policies, excellent vacation and sick leave options, and educational support plans, the nurse may be immobilized by "golden chains," feeling unable to leave an investment of years in the agency and lose the benefits accrued. For whatever reason, the nurse who remains when she really wants to quit or change jobs can become either an asset or a liability to the agency, depending on what she does with the feelings that are inevitable consequences of frustration. This nurse can become passive and mechanical, no longer caring about clients or the work environment. She can do her job, take her pay, and protect herself from hurt, involvement, activity, and pain. She often builds a wall around herself to keep others out, which cannot help but also imprison her within. She can be, and often is, efficient, meeting her responsibilities, doing whatever is assigned to her, and saying very little. She has little that is positive to add to working committees; when suggestions are made for changes, she often will make statements such as "It won't work" or "We tried that before" or "You'll see, you just haven't been here long enough; when you have, you'll understand why things are like they are." She seldom actually tries to block progress or acts with hostility. She offers no suggestions and no support and does not seem to be committed to nursing or to believe in anything. More often than not, this behavior is the result of true burnout, but it can also result when the nurse who wants to drop out or run away cannot do so.

A second behavior open to the nonmobile person is to become passive-aggressive or overtly hostile. The passive-aggressive person differs from the passive one in that she resists change or cooperation by not responding at all. She will often agree to do something and simply not produce. If asked, she will have several excuses that are always someone else's fault. She rejoices when others get into trouble and often sets up fights between them that she is unwilling to have herself. This nurse is a real energy drain on co-workers. She can be disruptive without appearing to be. She can appear to agree to do things without ever complying. She avoids confrontation. If confronted with her behavior, she denies that anything is wrong. The passive-aggressive person is aggressive through that very passivity. Persons whose burnout manifests itself in this behavior are very difficult to work with because of denial of their problem; if one will not confront a problem, one cannot solve it.

Overt hostility is much easier to work with than passive-aggressive behavior. When burnout cannot be expressed by leaving the work situation but converts into anger expressed as hostility, it is so near the surface that the aggressive person's feelings are available in ways the passive-aggressive person's feelings are not. Such people are often short-tempered, cross, confrontive, and negative. They say negative things in front of anyone who will listen. They do not care whom they hurt, nor do they try to look good to others. They are often proud of their harshness and brag to co-workers about how they aren't afraid of anyone. They lack the insight to know that change is made through positive action, constructive and supportive suggestions, and the building of support systems based on mutual trust and good will. They constantly put themselves in a no-win situation by turning others against them and getting such a negative response to their behavior that their suggestions are not valued.

Another possibility for those who must stay at their jobs when they really want out is to *participate in change*. This channels energy into positive routes that yield new and better work environments and relationships, and it puts new meaning into their jobs. These nurses build networks and relationships. Because of their efforts and participation, they create a workplace so different from the one to which they were averse that the net result is the same as if they had moved. The advantage is that the person that helped to create a new and better work place is therefore committed to keeping it positive and determined to keep it improving.

These three major reactions—burnout, dropout, and runaway—are just that: reactions. Reaction is an effect. The effect is easy to describe, while the cause is harder to diagnose and more complex and difficult to cure.

Causes of attrition—epidemiologic analysis

Burnout literature describes the symptoms and prescribes ways the individual can prevent or treat the syndrome. Indeed, individuals can be taught to be burnout resistant, but they cannot be "burnout proofed." Assertiveness, setting limits, support systems, and having a variety of nonnursing interests are all good preventives for burnout, but they cannot cure the problem or significantly decrease the incidence of staff attrition. Nurses who drop out and run away can also be helped to develop resistance. But to be really effective in keeping the nurses that are currently employed, efforts must focus both on the individual's resistance and on altering the work place. Nor can nurse education be left isolated from the problem. The attrition phenomenon is based upon three keystones—susceptibility, deficiencies in the work place, and deficiencies in the educational setting. Since the employing agency has little control over individual employee resistance and usually no control over the educational deficits, this discussion will center primarily on the work place.

Finding solutions to problems begins with awareness, for awareness leads to assessments and problem identification. A time of expanding assessment is currently occurring in nursing. A number of studies on the causes of attrition are now available. These studies will affect the nursing work place by improving it. Only the early impact of these studies is currently being felt. However, health care is an industry and industry has learned to be attentive to studies that can be cost saving. Slowing attrition rates will save the agency money, and therefore change will occur.

In order for change to occur a clear picture of the causes and a methodology for examining data must emerge. An epidemiologic approach to nurse attrition provides such a method.

PREDICTIVE PRINCIPLE: Use of a scientific method for investigating attrition increases the probability that a clear and accurate picture of etiology and treatment will emerge.

The most effective means for examining attrition is from an epidemiologic point of view. Epidemiologists are aware of the complexity of any problem and how misleading the single-cause/single-effect perception of problems can be. Epidemiology by its very nature requires investigation of multiple factors. In an epidemiologic problem one examines: (1) the host (nurse); (2) the environment (the work place); and (3) the organism (noxious experiences or stimuli) (see Table 4). This is an appropriate methodology, because nurse attrition—a chronic endemic problem—is reaching epidemic proportions.

The host for attrition (the nurse manifesting an attrition problem, whether it be burnout, dropout, or runaway) cannot be cured simply by helping her cope with the problems of nursing. The fallacy of that single-focused attempt has been that the resistance of the organism alone cannot stem the tide of the epidemic. This concentration on the nurse-victim is based on the assumption that *if the host (the nurse) were made differently—were stronger, better, and more nearly perfect—there would be no problem; therefore we must reshape the nurse.* Helping the nurse become more attrition-resistant is possible, but there is no way for the nurse to become attrition proof—thus the need for a broader approach. Unless the noxious stimuli are decreased in virulence, number, duration, and frequency and the environment (work place) is altered so that it is inhospitable to the organism and hospitable to the nurse, attrition will continue unabated (Fig. 10-2).

The following discussion is designed to take each epidemiologic factor—host, organism, and environment—and provide suggestions for dealing with each in order to reduce attrition.

Table 4

Variables in attrition

Host (nurse)	Organism (noxious experience)	Environment (work place)
Resistance	Frequency	Climate
Coping patterns	Virulence	Economic and general welfare
Diversions	Dosage	Distribution of power
Caring relationships	Duration	Quality of nursing care
Information		

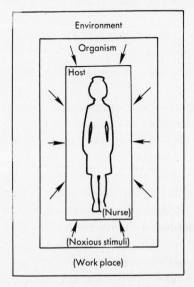

Fig. 10-2. An epidemiologic examination of attrition.

Host: The nurse

PREDICTIVE PRINCIPLE: Increasing the resistance of the nurse to factors causing attrition will help provide a stable cadre of nurses willing to work for environmental improvement and control of noxious factors.

Burnout, runaway, and dropout are the three ways attrition manifests itself, and activities that strengthen the host will help decrease the incidence of all three. Individual nurses can be strengthened, but the ideal is to strengthen a group; for a group of people who have developed insight into the problem and learned to deal with it in healthy ways can provide the stability and energy necessary to help make changes that will reduce noxious stimuli and improve the environment, thereby significantly affecting attrition rates. Nurses, who make up 55% of all health care providers and 45% of hospital workers, can collectively accomplish anything they wish to do.

PREDICTIVE PRINCIPLE: Identification of prime candidates for burnout enables preventive measures to be initiated.

Nurses who are prime candidates for burnout have certain characteristics. This does not mean that others are immune, but only that certain characteristics increase the nurse's chances of becoming burned out. Characteristics common to burnout victims include:

1. Such great enthusiasm for nursing that the nurse volunteers for extra committees, spends off-time going to nursing meetings, discusses and reads nursing literature, and takes extra courses in the subject.
2. Has few interests outside of nursing.
3. Associates almost exclusively with nursing or health-related personnel.
4. Has difficulty in viewing nursing realistically.
5. Has no intimate friends.
6. Experiences trouble at home with husband, children, parents, or siblings.
7. Has a large amount of responsibility at home.
8. Cares about nursing and clients so much that she allows herself to be exploited (works overtime, doubles back, stays on unwanted shifts, accepts transfer to floors in which she has no interest).
9. Feels guilty when there is no cause. Goes to work ill, takes on extra work, sets unrealistic expectations for self and feels badly when they are not met; feels responsible for everything that goes wrong, and often feels that since others seem to be doing okay, there must be something wrong with her.
10. Has no training in burnout prevention.

Nurses with these characteristics seem to burn out quickly. The fewer of the above characteristics one has, the less chance for burnout to occur and the longer it takes. The message here is not to avoid being enthusiastic or caring or feeling responsible, but to do so realistically, to build support systems, to develop interests and friends outside nursing, and to spend some energy changing the system.

PREDICTIVE PRINCIPLE: Smooth transition to the real work world and good education in how to effect change can increase resistance to dropout and runaway.

Some nurses do not realize until they become employed that they do not really like to nurse. Reality shock can be overwhelming and result in temporary or permanent disenchantment with nursing. Because of disenchantment, many nurses drop out for a short time or permanently or change jobs trying to find a more comfortable environment. More frequently than not, schools of nursing and employers do not work together to provide courses geared to enabling transition to the real work world. Faculty, in all good faith and for all the right and educationally sound reasons, protect students from the realities of the everyday work world. In order to learn nursing, the multiplicity of variables in the normal work setting must be decreased so that the learner can concentrate on the factors being taught. However, educators fail to find compromises in the system that would enable a smooth and realistic transition for the new graduate. Caught between the two, new graduates suffer transition problems and as a result drop out or run away. One notable exception is Ohlone College in Fremont, California. Under a Kellogg grant, Ohlone nursing faculty have worked with clinical agencies to establish a carefully structured preceptorship program that has proved effective in enabling a smooth student-to-graduate transition.[*]

It is difficult to work toward controlling the work place environment or reducing noxious factors without a work force that has some awareness of the problems, some sense of power over their problems, and some motivation to alter those problems. There are some direct action methods useful to the unit manager. These can be instituted by middle or lower management personnel. However, to have any long-term effectiveness the management group must support and participate in efforts geared to work satisfaction by staff nurses.

PREDICTIVE PRINCIPLE: Increased recognition of the importance of a career and a realistic view of prospective life work pattern motivates commitment to help create positive working conditions.

Ninety-eight percent of nurses are women, and women have been socially conditioned to be passive and to view their careers as unimportant. Through workshops and work environment changes, nurses can be helped to alter this attitude. Traditionally, women's life expectations have been socially set

---

[*]Limon, S., Spencer, J.D., and Waters, V.: A clinical preceptorship to prepare reality-based ADN graduates, Nurs. Health Care, pp. 267-269, May 1981.

to be active in a career only temporarily. Women are programmed to expect to marry a man capable of supporting them or else to drop out of work while they rear their children. They expect to reenter active nursing when forced to do so by events such as divorce, a husband's illness or death, or when boredom erodes their lives such as when their children are in school. Some women move in and out of the job market as they need more furniture or carpets. These women feel they work only to provide the family with the "extras" they desire.

The fact of the matter is that today more than 70% of the female work force in the United States *must* work. The average length of time a woman works is 25 years, and many work from 30 to 40 years. One in three working women is the sole or major support of herself and her family, and more than two-thirds of working women earn income that is essential to the family's standard of living. Yet the myth persists that a woman's income supplements the family's main income and that her career is temporary. Nursing is seen as some sort of fail-safe insurance policy nurses can turn to in time of need. This belief causes nurses to discount the importance of such things as good working conditions, good salaries, and good retirement plans. As long as the discounting myth is accepted and allowed to persist, nurses will also discount their jobs and will put little effort into improving working conditions and fringe benefits.

More and more working women find themselves divorced after twenty to twenty-five years of married life and living on retirement incomes that are substandard because they failed to face the possibility of having to survive on their own retirement income. If one's job was seen as temporary and as secondary in importance to the spouse's, little energy would have been expended in improvement of working conditions.

Many nurses enter the work place with excellent ideas about how to improve their environment but with little notion of how to bring those changes about. They often start trying to make changes before establishing credibility with those who have been in the setting longer. They suggest solutions before data have been gathered; and the gravest error is to attempt changes without getting colleague consensus and support. The work place needs changes—there is no doubt of that—but what changes, at what rate, and in what sequence are issues that must be addressed using an orderly, planned approach (see Chapter 8). Nurses need more information about change processes in both basic education and in-service programs.

More knowledge of the orderly change process would prevent the new graduate from making errors in judgment when attempting change and would enable the established nurses to channel their energy into orderly changes that promote positive outcomes. The planned change process could enable nurses to alter conditions in the work place and decrease noxious stimuli.

PREDICTIVE PRINCIPLE: Unmet expectations increase nurse dissatisfaction and result in increased number of nurses who drop out or run away.

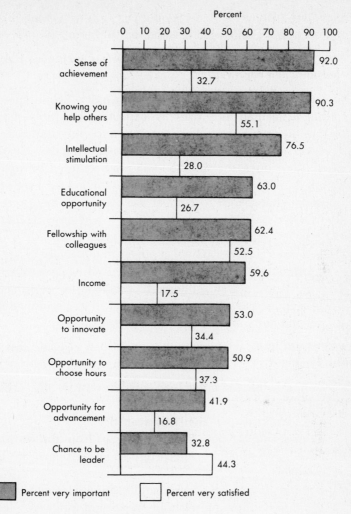

Fig. 10-3. Factors considered by nurses to be very important to their professional lives and their degree of satisfaction with those factors.

One primary reason for dropout is the vast difference between what nurses consider important, and therefore expect from their professional lives, and what they get. One study* compared the factors nurses considered very important to their professional lives with their degree of satisfaction with those factors. The findings are given in graphic form in Fig. 10-3. In only one factor were expectations less than the reality: Of those surveyed 32.8% felt the chance to be a leader was very important and 44.3% were very satisfied that they had realized that expectation. But in most cases, as Fig. 10-3 demonstrates, the dis-

---

*Donovan, L.: What nurses want (and what they're getting), RN **43**(4):22-30, 1980.

appointments are truly great ones. People will simply not stay in a profession where their concerns about what is important to them are so poorly met.

PREDICTIVE PRINCIPLE: A sense of powerlessness increases the incidence of burnout, dropout, and runaway.

Prior to burnout, nurses develop a sense of powerlessness. Powerlessness, according to Seeman and Evans,* is "expecting, or a probability held by the individual, that his own behavior cannot determine the occurrence of the outcomes or reinforcements he seeks." Powerlessness is the deep-seated belief that no matter what one does, the situation will not be altered through effort.

Nurses develop a sense of powerlessness when they are isolated, when they try to make changes, or to combat the system alone. There is power in organization, power in support systems, and power in knowing that others share one's concerns.

Assertiveness is power. There is power in the ability to say "no" courteously, firmly, softly, and without feeling guilty. Power is never taken from nurses; it is surrendered. And once surrendered it is difficult to reassume, because the passivity of surrender has reinforced the belief that the individual nurse can neither change the outcome nor gain desired ends.

PREDICTIVE PRINCIPLE: Prevention of host attrition reduces cost and is easier than curing attrition.

Prevention sounds simpler than it is. Preventive measures include the following:

1. Limit work-related, after-hours activity.
2. Build strong intimate friendships apart from the world of nursing.
3. Build good nursing-related support systems that are loyal and dependable.
4. Build good networks, information, and advice systems.
5. Develop nonnursing-related hobbies and interests.
6. Decrease home and family stressors to acceptable levels or get help to deal with them.
7. Talk about feelings, hurts, happiness, anger, disappointments, and successes.
8. Be assertive, set goals; be positive about achieving them in both small and great things.
9. Don't take abuse, misuse, or exploitation.
10. Be natural with clients—laugh, cry, hug.
11. Don't feel guilty for saying no.

---

*Seeman, M., and Evans, J.: Alienation and learning in a hospital setting, Am. Soc. Rev. **27**(6):272-282, 1962.

12. When feeling spent or strung out, take time off to renew self by doing something you want to do.
13. Take a course in burnout prevention.

Employers spend thousands of dollars dealing with the effects of burnout. They spend an average of $4,000 recruiting and orienting each new nurse; they send nurses to burnout workshops and clinics. They deal with lawsuits and ill will generated by nurses who are forgetful, disturbed, or uninterested. They do all of this in the hope of improving nurse resistance to burnout, lowering attrition, and improving patient care.

PREDICTIVE PRINCIPLE: Self-respect and assertiveness increase attrition resistance.

Women are conditioned to be nonassertive. Assertive women are often perceived as castrating, masculine, or at the least unfeminine. Women have therefore put on a facade of passivity that hides resentment and under pressure turns to aggression. Assertive people recognize their own power and use it to have control over their lives and work. Passive-aggressive people let others control them but resent it and feel angry and hostile. They try to hide these feelings, and then something happens and the hostility comes out in inappropriate ways. Note the following example:

Dr. Jones was a swaggering, loud man who entered the nursing unit with a busy bustle. He never addressed the nurses by name but called each of them "Honey." The first nurse encountered was always addressed, "Honey, run get me a cup of coffee." All the nurses hated to comply as they felt demeaned. They, too, were busy.

Mrs. Burroughs was a new employee who had not been warned about Dr. Jones. Their meeting was memorable. Entering in his usual whirlwind, he glanced at her and said, "Honey, get me a cup of coffee." She replied, "I don't believe we've met. My name is Mrs. Burroughs. You are . . . ?" "I'm Dr. Jones," he sliced in. "I'm glad to meet you, Honey." "Dr. Jones, I'm Mrs. Burroughs, not Honey. The coffee is in the conference room. You are welcome to a cup. When you are ready, I have three of your patients and I'm available to make rounds on them and discuss them with you."

The other nurses watched in amazement. One nurse confessed that she always supplied him with coffee. The doctor likes it black and unsweetened so she put in three tablespoons of sugar when she prepared it. Another said, "When I hear him coming, I disappear." Another stated, "I do it; I just never say a word."

It is easy to compare those nurses who acted in a passive or passive-aggressive way to the one who was assertive. Assertiveness can be taught on the unit using real life situations. Assertiveness conferences can be held once a week and real events replayed and talked through until assertive behaviors are worked out and rehearsed in role play, then tried out at the next opportunity.

Hospitals tend to be microcosms of the larger society, with the physicians playing the traditionally male roles and nurses the traditionally female roles. These roles are usually enacted regardless of the gender of the physician or nurse. The more gender-related the physician/nurse modes of communication, the less collegial the relationship.

For example, a nurse wishing to communicate to an attending physician that the increasing levels of inattentiveness and forgetfulness of a client are probably drug related would, when interacting in the traditional male/female way, approach it somewhat like this: "Doctor, it seems that Mr. Barnes has been getting more and more forgetful lately. *Do you think* it could be related to his Darvon?" The collegial way of handling the same problem would be: "Doctor, since Mr. Barnes has been on Darvon every four hours for his arthritis, he has shown decreasing alertness and increasing forgetfulness. Would you be willing to try him on a drug that may be less disruptive to his mental acuity? He and his family feel he is getting senile but *I think* it's the Darvon."

In the traditional role approach the nurse (female) manipulates to get the doctor (male) to "think of it" himself, to be the big decision-maker filling in the gaps for the "poor nurse." The nurse tries to avoid any reference to her own expertise, the information gleaned by her bedside observations, and the obvious connections that a nurse is in a unique position to make because of the eight hours per day spent with the client.

On the other hand, the nurse who approaches relationships with physicians in a collegial fashion takes for granted that nursing information and conclusions are valuable and valid because of her knowledge, skill, and time spent with the client. This nurse approaches physician/nurse communications with respect for nursing knowledge and its unique contributions. The collegial nurse is never heard to say, "I'm *only* a nurse." "Only" is a discount. Nursing is not less than nor greater than doctoring, just *different from;* and it has a special and equal contribution to make. The inherent discounts by oneself, physicians, and other employees contribute to nurse attrition.

PREDICTIVE PRINCIPLE: Strong support systems provide a base for growth and security and decrease susceptibility to burnout, dropout, and runaway.

One of the most important aspects of increasing resistance to attrition is building support systems. Nurses are usually taught in their educational programs to do any job alone. Teachers want to observe what a student can do without help; not only do they not encourage working together in clinical settings, they actively discourage it. Additionally, grading methodologies are normative. Normative grading, by its very nature, promotes competition. Students are pitted against each other because they are ranked or compared. If one student helps another, that help may be used to achieve a better score or ranking and therefore hurt the helper. As long as normative, ranking, or comparative grading systems are used in schools of nursing, nurses are going to find it difficult to unlock themselves from the competitive mode and be supportive of one another.

Competitiveness is built into society's conditioning of females. Again, this is one more way nursing has suffered by incorporating some of the most harmful aspects of the socialization of women in American society. Females are taught from birth not to trust one another, not to help one another. They compete for boys' attention, for being the prettiest and the sweetest, for having the best clothes, the nicest hair. They do not trust even their best friends with their boy-friends or husbands. Nurses have a difficult time learning not to be competitive and not to hurt one another deliberately. Colleagueship and support systems can be taught. The simplest and most direct approach is to discuss the usual female social conditioning and to have everyone on the nursing unit participate in compiling a list of things that have happened and how they could have been avoided. From that can be derived a list of ground rules for how to treat the people one works with in order to develop supportive, caring relationships.

JoAnn Barclay and Bridget Baker worked together on a medical unit. JoAnn confided to Bridget that she was angry at Dr. Deriso. When a client with cancer had asked him a reasonable question about treatment, he had laughed and teasingly said, "I think we'll just experiment on you a bit. Then maybe we will find something that will work." Actually the neoplasm had not metastasized and the client was expected to recover and do well. The client was very upset and thought she must be very sick and people had lied to her about her condition not being serious. She was convinced from the doctor's comment that she was going to die. JoAnn had deferred talking to Dr. Deriso about it until she was less angry and upset. She knew Dr. Deriso was young and touchy. She needed to think of a way to handle this so that he would not become defensive and could use the experience to grow.

JoAnn was doing her morning charting when Dr. Deriso rounded the corner with fire in his eyes. "I hear you don't like what I said to Mrs. McLeod! Well, let me tell you a thing or two. What I say to her is none of your business. It's my prerogative; I'm her doctor. The trouble with you nurses is that you've got enough education to get a big head and not enough to know when to stay out of someone else's business. Let me tell you something, you stay out of mine or I'll get you fired!" JoAnn was so shocked she just sat there. When she looked up, Bridget was smiling with a satisfied grin.

This is a classic example of "Let's you and him fight." JoAnn had conferred with Bridget to help get things off her chest and clarify her thinking, hoping to be able to approach the doctor with positive results. Bridget had used the information to set up a fight so that Dr. Deriso would be angry at JoAnn and think more of Bridget. The sad thing is that this ploy so often works.

Incidents like this can be handled in unit conferences to decrease the consequences of nonsupport, lessened trust, and disruptive, energy-consuming incidents. In the above example it is very possible that Dr. Deriso's anger will block growth that might have occurred had the incident been handled in a more constructive way. The clients, current and future, are the losers.

Had Bridget been supportive instead of competitive, she would have listened to JoAnn's anger, let her express it and cool off, helped her to think of constructive ways to approach Dr. Deriso, and then left them alone to give JoAnn a chance to discuss it in private. The outcome would have had a much greater chance of being positive for all concerned, and far less energy would have been required to deal with the issue.

Nurses who learn to support one another, help one another with clients, share difficult responsibilities, respect one another's special areas of expertise, and give warmth and caring to one another in the same understanding way they care for and about clients have the most valuable asset for immunization against attrition: caring, supportive, colleague relationships. With these support systems the nurse is never alone with a difficult decision, never without understanding during and after a rough day or an upsetting experience, never without a hug when things go wrong, and never without someone with whom to share joy and excitement when things go right.

Middle management, head nurses, and supervisors are in a prime position to create the kind of environment that promotes the growth of caring, supportive, colleagueship behavior and relationships.

PREDICTIVE PRINCIPLE: Stability promotes job effectiveness and increases the ability to facilitate positive changes.

It takes one to three years in a setting for a nurse to become maximally productive in that agency. This includes establishing credibility, earning the respect of peers and superiors, and becoming familiar with the agency's political system, policies, procedures, and personalities. These things are necessary to be effective in bringing about improvements. When one moves every year or two, these advantages are forfeited. Disappointments and frustrations mount, making disenchantment and burnout inevitable.

Aside from the usually frustrated hope of substantially increasing income, why is there so much job-hopping? Some of the answers may be in a survey made by Donovan.* She lists nurse dissatisfactions in order of priority as:

1. No input on matters concerning them
2. Low client care standards
3. Excessive job demands
4. Inadequate salary
5. Not enough say in client care
6. Too much paperwork

---

*Donovan, L.: What nurses want (and what they're getting), RN **43**(4):22-30, 1980.

7. No chance for advancement
8. Limited educational opportunities
9. Insufficient challenge
10. Lack of recognition

These are legitimate concerns and can be changed. To do so, nurses, for the most part, must remain in their present jobs, focus their energy, and commit themselves to changing the environment and conditions under which they work.

Organism: Noxious experiences or stimuli that create adverse reactions

The second factor in any epidemiologic study is the organism. In the case of nurse attrition, the organism is likened to a series of events—events that occur in the normal course of duties in nursing. These may be client events such as death, disfigurement, suffering, or grief. These are everyday events to a nurse and inevitably take their toll. Some special places where nurses work inexorably wear away at the spirit because of the amount and degree of human suffering and the threat to and loss of life encountered there. These are such places as oncology units, burn units, pain units, and all of the special care units. Each group of nurses has a different organism, a different series of events comprising the work experience: for the public health nurse it may be the poverty and neglect encountered every day; for the home health nurse and the gerontologic nurse it may be the despair, loneliness, and senility of old age in a neglectful society. For all nurses it is discount, abuse from some physicians, the rigidity of bureaucracy, the lack of support from nursing administration, and the constant demands to give more, work overtime, and spread thinner their diminishing reservoir of energy.

When examining the organism, epidemiologists investigate virulence, dosage, frequency, and duration. *Virulence* means severity; some work settings expose nurses to more tragedy than do others. Some have more pain and despair, or present negative working relationships or poor standards of care. Virulence is the degree of impact of these events.

Dosage is used in the same sense as it is in medicating—how much of something one gets. For example:

Dr. Jones finds his patient Mrs. Ebersole in bed in her own incontinence. Without investigating any of the circumstances, he finds the nurse assigned to Mrs. Ebersole and begins screaming and cursing. Afterward he finds the head nurse and lets her have his opinion of the way she runs the floor. But having unloaded once already, the dosage he gives the head nurse is less than the dosage he gave the staff nurse.

Frequency refers to how often the traumatic episode occurs. On specific units, such as oncology, the frequency of seeing young people die and families grieve is high. In intensive care units there is a high frequency of stressful events where the speed and skill of the nurse are crucial. People can cope more easily with unpleasant or stressful events that are infrequent or widely spaced. Even very virulent events of high dosage can be tolerated if they are relatively infrequent. Frequency seems to be a key event factor in nurse attrition.

The last factor in examining the organism, or event in nursing, is *duration*, the length of time an event lasts. Taking care of a client with a very difficult problem for a long period of time fits into this category. Examples are caring for the chronically ill, being involved in a running battle with a physician or supervisor, or struggling constantly with a machine that does not work properly. Events of long duration are like water dripping on stone. No matter how strong, eventually the nurse will wear down until all resistance is exhausted.

PREDICTIVE PRINCIPLE: The virulence, dosage, frequency, and duration of noxious events in a nurse's work life directly affect burnout, dropout, and runaway.

Nurses burn out, drop out, or run away when the organism is very virulent and they are exposed to a high dosage, frequently, and over a long duration. No amount of "immunization" will prevent the inevitable consequences.

The following disguised but true event took place in a Midwestern hospital where the ancillary personnel had union contracts that were specific about the jobs each category of employee could perform.

Jody Antonio was raised in the rough side of Calumet City. She escaped to a nursing school in Chicago, was graduated, and left to make the world a better place than she had found it. Settling in a large Midwestern city, she took a job which she loved. Her enthusiasm ran high, she learned quickly, clients loved her, and physicians asked that she be assigned to their clients who required special quality care.

The restrictions of union contracts bothered Jody, especially housekeeping. The maids were not allowed to wipe down the sides of the bedside tables because, through neglect, the contracts specified only the cleaning of tabletops; the stairwells were never cleaned and littered air conduits plagued infection control—all because someone had neglected to specify their upkeep in the contract. It seemed that every time Jody wanted something from housekeeping the response was, "That's not my job." The irritations were minor (low virulence, low dosage) but seemed constant (high frequency and duration).

One day Jody passed by a room where the housekeeper was mopping and she looked in to find the client, Mr. Nelson, in the throes of an obvious cardiac arrest. She rushed in and asked the housekeeper, "Why didn't you call me?" "That's not my job, I mop" was the reply. She glared at the man. Mr. Nelson weighed about three hundred pounds and was on the bedpan. Jody struggled to slide it out from under him, while the man kept mopping. Finally she was able to remove the pan. In the meantime she had signaled for help. Hastily, knowing that every second counts in cardiac arrest, she held the full pan out to the mop man. "Take this, please," she cried. "That's not my job," he said as he kept on mopping. Without a pause to catch her breath, Jody stepped to the hall, turned the full bedpan upside down, and then let it clatter to the floor. "Now it's your job." She then returned to Mr. Nelson and began cardiac resuscitation.

The patient lived, Jody survived an inquiry, and the union hierarchy were very upset. Resistance breaks down with events of high frequency and long duration. Jody moved to a hospital where there were no union contracts, but other events (organisms) plagued her and she moved again. Jody may still be looking for that place to work where there are virtually no problems. She will be a chronic runaway.

PREDICTIVE PRINCIPLE: Limiting the exposure of the nurse to virulent, high-dosage, noxious events of long duration will decrease the possibility of the nurse leaving the job.

Management can affect the exposure of the nurse to noxious stimuli. In any situation there will be stressful events. By its very nature nursing interacts with people during life crises. Hospital personnel will always have a certain amount of interpersonal difficulty. But certain aspects of exposure to organisms can be managed to decrease the likelihood of nurses leaving the environment. Many of these are currently in place in health agencies. Many more should be.

The secret to managing the organism is, obviously, to concentrate on the reduction of the virulence, the dosage, the frequency, the duration, and above all the exposure. Examine the following ideas about how management can initiate changes that will effectively reduce attrition due to noxious stimuli.

1. Rotate nurses out of high intensity settings such as special care units and oncology units one month out of every four. Rotation interrupts the duration of stimuli and allows for regeneration.
2. Rotate nurses providing care to clients with difficult nursing problems to lessen the stress to any one nurse.
3. Provide training to management personnel in how to intervene protectively when physicians complain about nurses, and insist that physicians use the correct communication channels. No one has a right to castigate others and treat them disrespectfully. The agency can put a stop to such abuses.
4. Use a nursing agency to fill in when adequate coverage is unavailable from within the agency, so that excessive demands are not placed on the nurse.
5. If nursing coverage is not available, temporarily decrease admissions. This hurts the hospital but may be less expensive in the long run.
6. Do not let a problem continue to exist until it is too late. Intervene early.

Middle and upper nursing management can institute measures that affect the organism (noxious events). Staff level personnel can do very little to alter the pattern of these events. Among the primary activities in head nurse and supervisor meetings should be the identification of noxious events and the planning of controls for them. Positive action is likely; upper management is presented with a realistic, cost-effective plan to reduce the exposure of nurses to organisms causing attrition.

Environment

PREDICTIVE PRINCIPLE: A positive unit environment created by middle and lower management increases unit retention rates.

The factor most available to manipulation by lower (team leaders) and middle management (head nurses and supervisors) is the environment. The immediate environment can be shaped by middle management to be inhospitable to some noxious stimuli and to be welcomed as a place for nursing personnel to work, interact, and grow. Such environments can be created where the host (nurse) develops resistance, where nurses are nourished, where organisms that erode away at nurses fail to thrive. Best of all, many things in the immediate environment can be changed by lower and middle management without cost to agencies and without changes in institutional policy and inclusion of policy-making groups. It is surprising how much can be done and how much more tolerable are the irritants in an institutional environment when the immediate work environment is healthful.

Three environments need attention: the immediate environment, the agency environment, and the health care system environment. The focus of this discussion is on the immediate environment, for it is in this realm that lower and middle management really influence events. Therefore, little mention will be made of the health care system and the agency environment.

PREDICTIVE PRINCIPLE: Positive reinforcement increases job satisfaction.

Positive reinforcement is one of management's most available tools and one of the easiest to use. Inhibitors in the social system teach nurses to be sparing with positive strokes (see Chapter 5). The nurses in leadership and management positions who can find creative ways to reinforce staff personnel will find attitudes improving and people feeling better about themselves.

There are ways to reinforce, and there are also ways that may seem reinforcing but are really negative reinforcers:

Mrs. Lathrop, a nurse's aide, is an experienced, cheerful, rapid worker. She can work circles around most of the other aides on the floor. Flora Hilton, the head nurse, gave her five difficult patients on Monday. Mrs. Lathrop cared for them rapidly and well, and Mrs. Hilton complimented her by saying, "You certainly did a good job on that assignment, Mrs. Lathrop, and you did them so fast, too. Since you are through early, you may take all the admissions and discharges today."

It is no reward for a job well done to be given another difficult job. Compliments and reinforcements must not be coupled with punishments (or what can be perceived as punishment) for being good, fast, and able. Reinforcements must be given unencumbered. Evaluation instructions offer the advice that a negative evaluative comment is easier for the employee to accept if it is accompanied by a positive comment. When the manager tries, it often comes out like this: "Mrs. Lewis, you did a very nice job on your patients this morning, but why haven't you done the supply inventory yet?" Mrs. Lewis is not going to register the positive comment; she is going to register the criticism implied by the question.

PREDICTIVE PRINCIPLE: Improving the unit climate creates an atmosphere of caring about the employee, improves the quality of client care, and decreases unit attrition rates.

The climate of a working unit is an intangible but is influenced by very tangible practices. To improve the climate of an environment and make a unit an island of positiveness, try some of the following ideas:

1. At reports and conferences, describe achievements, ideas, creative solutions, and small successes of the staff.
2. Design a Nurse-of-the-Week award and make all nursing personnel eligible. Ask the group to draw up the criteria, take pictures, and each week post a winner and the reason why the award was won. Do not permit it to become a popularity contest, but give it for nursing excellence, good colleagueship, nursing care provided beyond the call of duty, creative care, patience in a difficult situation, consistency, perseverance and follow-through, nurturing, and caring.
3. Be aware of the short-term goals of the staff. ("Jerry wants to get off early today, as he's on his way to Florida. Let's see that he gets away.")
4. Ask the unit personnel to list individually their professional goals and share them. Then provide support for meeting those goals.
5. Do not confuse being a good leader with being a better person than others.
6. Post an award for the laugh of the week so that funny events (not putdowns, goof-ups, or slipups) are surfaced. A good laugh renews the heart and relaxes the face.
7. Keep good records so that achievements and awards are recorded in evaluation forms, letters, and memos to higher level management. Commendations of this kind are real morale boosters. Carbon copies sent to the employee are very affirming.
8. Always allow unit personnel to participate in decisions that affect

them. Announcements such as "I'm reorganizing teams next week; let me know your preferences" and "We're examining the postoperative care routine for gastrectomy, I want your input" provide a real sense of participation and value.

9. Be fair in distributing work. Unfairly apportioned work loads create dissension and unhappiness more rapidly than does any other problem.

10. Recognize special events, birthdays, births, deaths, and weddings, so that there is acknowledgment of the individual as a person in addition to the individual's function as a worker.

PREDICTIVE PRINCIPLE: Top nurse management committed to creating a positive environment and improving salaries increases job satisfaction and decreases attrition.

The institutional environment is difficult to alter, since much of the climate in an agency emanates from the top and from tradition. Directors of nursing service are often not aware of the power they have to set climate. Strict attention to quality of care, support for nursing services having control over their domain of practice, alternative work schedules, and allowing staff to work part-time on "hot spot" hours are some ways to provide a positive climate (see Chapter 3).

Salary and fringe benefits matter most, but without the intangibles of quality, support, and positive reinforcements, the big things will not suffice. Nurses who have good pay, good fringe benefits, and a positive environment remain in their positions and stay fairly happy. Top nursing management increasingly articulates nursing needs to administration. It conducts cost studies that demonstrate the monetary savings of keeping a stable staff rather than recruiting a new one. Staff nurses increasingly have leaders and managers who represent their needs well. Incentives for staying on rather than bonuses for recruiting other nurses help. An example is the Army that pays a reenlistment bonus, which is quite successful in reducing attrition. Incentives for further education and flexibility of hours keep some of the potential dropouts working. Special arrangements for the care of children and the elderly, with the agency paying a percentage of the cost is a simpler, less expensive approach to the family care problem than agency-owned nurseries and day care centers. Special perquisites help, such as low interest loans, special new car deals, discounts on large purchases, and support for a specified number of continuing education units per year away from the institution.

The ideal place to start in an agency is with top management. However, head nurses and supervisors cannot always wait for top management changes to filter down to the unit level. In fact, some of the most effective changes are in the environment immediately surrounding the nurse's daily work. These changes alone will not significantly affect the total agency attrition rate but will alter attrition rates on individual units. Success on the nursing unit level can demonstrate for a whole agency which environmental conditions are effective in increasing nurse contentment and therefore promote retention.

Two of the three epidemiologic factors—the organization (events) and the environment—are in direct control of management. Yet human managerial energy is still focused on the one factor least in control of management—strengthening the host (nurse). The ultimate victim, the nurse, can develop some resistance; but without changes in the organism or events within the work place and the environment, the consequence is that burnout, dropout, and runaway will continue to sap at the very foundations of good client care.

There is tremendous potential for good results as nurses sense their power and test its limits. Nurses are becoming aware that they comprise 55% of all health care workers—and that's a lot of power. The danger exists that they can be seduced away from the goals of safeguards and better care for clients to a total concentration on economic security for themselves. Historically, nurses have remained concerned about quality care.

To stem the tide of nurse attrition, close attention must be paid to all three epidemiologic factors: the nurse as the host, the environment as work place, and the organism as noxious experience or stimuli that create adverse reactions. Nurses, united in their efforts to provide better working conditions and to decrease attrition, would do well to formulate and adopt a nurses' bill of rights. The sample bill of rights presented here incorporates aspects from all three epidemiologic factors.

NURSES' BILL OF RIGHTS

1. The right to be treated with respect by physicians, supervisors, colleagues, and ancillary personnel.
2. The right to work with others who are safe and competent.
3. The right to work in a clean, aesthetic environment.
4. The right to a wage commensurate with responsibilities, experience, and education.
5. The right to expert advice and supervision.
6. The right to control over nursing's domain of practice.
7. The right to free choice of clinical specialty placement.
8. The right to participate in decisions that affect the nurse.
9. The right to good fringe benefits, including but not limited to Social Security, retirement plans, disability, liability, health and dental insurance, vacation and sick leave, and educational opportunity and support.
10. The right to use knowledge and skill creatively on behalf of clients and colleagues.
11. The right to control nurse/client ratios for safe, comprehensive, quality care.
12. The right to safeguard clients from being cared for inappropriately by persons who are not registered nurses.

13. The right to safeguard high standards of care through quality control mechanisms.
14. The right to positive reinforcement for a job well done.
15. The right to straight, honest evaluation.
16. The right to good staff education programs.
17. The right to join together with other nurses to effect change and improve nursing care quality, job satisfaction, and economic security.
18. The right to intellectual stimulation.

Application of predictive principles of preventing attrition

Linda is a 28-year-old, single nurse. She is competent, has a good personality, and works well with the other RNs, LPNs, and aides. She has had experiences in six different cities in seven years and has worked in several different hospital areas. She has good ideas and is productive on committees. She has been staff nursing on Adult Medicine eight months. Over coffee one day she mentioned to the head nurse that she is thinking about going to work at another hospital. She feels City Medical Center is so big that no one could change anything, and things are not as she had hoped they would be.

Problem	*Predictive principles*	*Course of action*
How to help Linda prevent a continuation of her runaway pattern.	Unmet expectations increase nurse dissatisfaction and result in increased number of nurses who drop out or run away.	Talk with Linda about her expectations for this unit. Work with her to develop a list of what things are not right.
	A sense of powerlessness increases the incidence of burnout, dropout, and runaway.	Facilitate building a plan for altering the work setting that would improve conditions and make it more congruent with her expectations. Include in the plan means for involving colleagues in making changes.
	Strong support systems provide a base for growth and security and decrease susceptibility to burnout, dropout, and runaway.	Encourage Linda to call a meeting of other concerned personnel and involve them in planning and implementing changes in ways that help create a supportive work group.
	Stability promotes job effectiveness and increases the ability to facilitate positive changes.	Help Linda see that through her own efforts she has the power to influence her work environment and this power will increase as she learns how to work with the policies, procedures, and personnel, and political system of the hospital.

BIBLIOGRAPHY
Books

Lindsmith, A., and Strauss, A.: Social psychology, New York, 1968, Holt, Rinehart, & Winston.

Marram, G., Barrett, M., and Bevis, E.O.: Primary nursing: a model for individualized care, ed. 2, St. Louis, 1979, The C.V. Mosby Co.

Patrick, P.: Health care worker burnout, what it is and what to do about it, Glenview, Ill., 1981, Inquiry Books.

Wandelt, M.A., and others: Condition associated with registered nurse employment in Texas, Austin, Texas, 1980, Center for Research, School of Nursing, University of Texas at Austin.

Periodicals

Aiken, L., Blendon, R., and Rogers, D.: The shortage of hospital nurses—a new perspective, Am. J. Nurs. **81**(9):1612-1618, 1981.

Beyer, J., and Marshall, J.: The interpersonal dimensions of collegiality, N.O. **29**(11):662-665, 1981.

Christman, L.: Accountability and autonomy are more than rhetoric, Nurse Educ. **3**(4):3-6, 1978.

Clark, C.: Burnout: assessment and intervention, J. Nurs. Admin. **10**(9):39-43, 1980.

Donnely, G.: The insubordination game, RN **43**(4): 58-69, 1980.

Donovan, L.: What nurses want (and what they're getting), RN **43**(4):22-30, 1980.

Duldt, B.W.: Anger: an alienating communication hazard for nurses, Nurs. Outlook **29**(11):640-644, 1981.

Forsyth, D.M., and Cannady, J.: Preventing and alleviating staff burnout through a group, J. Psychosoc. Nurs. Mental Health Ser. **19**(9):35-38, 1981.

Fredenberger, H.: Staff burnout, J. Social Iss. **30**(1):159-166, 1974.

Getting fed up? Cover story, R.N. **44**(1):18-25, 1981.

Holloran, S., Mishkin, B., and Hanson, B.: Bicultural training for new graduates, Nurs. Educ. **5**(1):8-14, 1980.

Homer, Y.: The dynamics and management of burnout, Nurs. Manag. **12**(11):14-20, 1981.

Lambert, V., and Lambert, C.: Role theory and the concept of powerlessness, J. Psychosoc. Nurs. Mental Health Ser. **19**(1):11-14, 1981.

Limon, S., Spencer, J.D., and Waters, V.: A clinical preceptorship to prepare reality-based A.D.N. graduates, Nurs. Health Care, pp. 267-269, May 1981.

McConnell, A.: How close are you to burnout? R.N. **44**(5):29-32, 1981.

McGenley, R.E.: Back from burn out, R.N. **44**(5): 32-33, 1981.

Pines, A., and Maslach, C.: Characteristics of staff burnout in mental health settings, Hosp. Comm. Psych. **29**(4):233-237, 1978.

Seeman, M., and Evans, D.: Alienation and learning in a hospital setting, Am. Soc. Rev. **27**(6): 772-782, 1962.

Stehle, J.: Critical care nursing stress: the findings revisited, Nurs. Res. **30**(3):182-187, 1981.

Appendix

*

Derivation of predictive principles from several authoritative sources

Principles are derived from events. People observe events and record the logical serial order of the occurrence of the event. A theory is established about the cause and effect of the event, which then must be tested for validation. If a theory or hypothesis can be validated, it becomes a law; if it cannot be validated, but evidence seems to support the theory, it is still a usable tool.

The nurse-leader is seldom the originator of a completely new fact, concept, law, or principle. In most instances the nurse depends on the published work of authorities to provide the sources from which predictive principles may be extracted. Those who would compile predictive principles of any given topic must search the literature for pertinent material, critically evaluate the validity of the material, and convert the concepts gleaned from the literature into predictive principles. This process can be described in nine steps. The following are the operational steps in extracting predictive principles from the literature:

1. Determine the topic or area to be considered.
2. Search the literature for books, articles, or pamphlets germane to the subject.
3. Read extensively in the field; keep a list of frequently recurring concepts (and include the source of each concept for reference).
4. Identify in the literature statements about how concepts influence or are related to each other and make appropriate notations on the cumulative list.
5. Select from the accumulated list material relevant to the concept of the circumstances, conditions, or behaviors (CCB) triad.
6. Determine from the authoritative sources on the accumulated list the predicted outcome of the CCB triad concept selected.
7. Determine the appropriate active verb phrase that will connect the concepts selected.
8. Add the qualifiers that will precisely indicate the specific delineations necessary to make the predictive principle valid and relevant.

9. Repeat steps 5, 6, 7, and 8 for each additional predictive principle for the determined topic until all major concepts on the list have been formulated into predictive principles.

The following is an example of the extraction of one predictive principle from an authoritative source using the first eight steps.

Problem: To make progressive changes in the nursing team routine.

1. *Determine the topic or area to be considered.* The topic is determined by the problem to be solved. In any given problem it will be necessary to use predictive principles from several areas. In this instance, the nurse-leader would draw on a variety of topics or areas for predictive principles to use to accomplish the desired goals. Some of these areas would be leadership, teaching-learning, group dynamics, and interpersonal relationships. From each of these areas the nurse would select or formulate the appropriate predictive principles for the task and designate them as "principles for making changes." This topic then becomes the area of desired predictive principles.

2. *Search the literature for books, articles, or pamphlets germane to the subject.* The objective for the review is to identify and extract those concepts that will form the basis for activities and behaviors that will stimulate and enable group change. The searcher seeks any resources it is postulated will be helpful in the determined subject area. For the objective given the nurse-leader would search the literature of such fields as psychology, sociology, business and industry, education, and nursing.

3. *Read extensively in the field; keep a list of frequently recurring concepts (including sources).* Certain topics or concepts recur frequently in the literature of any given subject. A list of the recurring concepts enables the leader to determine the salient themes in any given subject with minimum effort and maximum speed. A list for the selected topic would contain such concepts as the objective of change, motivation, need, problem identification, group involvement, group commitment, individual security, careful planning, design and sequence for change, and optimum pace.

4. *Identify in the literature statements about how concepts influence or are related to each other and make appropriate notations on the cumulative list.* These notations are for the purpose of clarifying concept relationships and will readily facilitate the formulation of principles. The following is a cumulative list of concepts with notations that clarify concept relationships.

Concepts	Notations about predicted outcome and relationships
1. Clearly establish objectives of change	1. Direction, evaluation, minimum sidetracking
2. Group involvement	2. Related to commitment to outcomes of change
3. Group commitment	3. Grows with increasing participation in planning and decision making

<center>Concepts</center>	<center>*Notations about* *predicted outcome and relationships*</center>
4. Individual security	4. Providing individual with knowledge and skills and right to err with ego support during change
5. Careful planning	5. Logical order, central authority
6. Design and sequence	6. Purpose, focus, pace, progress, individual security, limitations
7. Optimum pace	7. Imposed by time and available materials
8. Motivation	8.
9. Need	9.
10. Problem identification	10.

The list is incomplete, as there are no notations for concepts 8, 9, and 10. The investigator need only follow the prescribed outline. Bibliographic data must be kept during the task so that credit may be given to the sources used.

5. *Select from the accumulated list material relevant to the concept of the CCB triad.* If the concept list and notations are complete, this step requires only that the appropriate concept be selected from the list. For example, "design and sequence" might be selected as the CCB triad concept.

6. *Determine from the authoritative sources or the accumulated list the predicted outcome of the CCB triad concept selected.* As previously, if the concept list and notations are complete, this step requires only that the appropriate predicted outcome be selected from the notations on the list. For example, the principle formulator selects "purpose," "focus," and "progress" from the alternatives on the compiled list.

With the CCB triad and the predicted outcome concepts selected, all that remains is to relate them in some logical, meaningful way.

7. *Determine the appropriate active verb phrase that will connect the concepts selected.* The active verb is important because it determines the extent and degree of the relationship between the CCB triad and the predicted outcome. The writer of the principle could choose words such as *ensure, influence,* or *promote* for the active verb.

The principle formulator has found evidence in the literature that **purpose, focus,** and **progress** are influenced by many factors in addition to **design and sequence.** With this evidence in mind, the formulator selects "promote" rather than "ensure" as a more valid active verb.

At this point in the construction of a predictive principle the components appear as follows:

<center>CCB triad</center>	<center>Active verb</center>	<center>Predicted outcome</center>
Design and sequence	promote	purpose, focus, and progress

Although stated as a principle, qualifiers are needed to give the concepts context and limitations.

8. *Add the qualifiers that will precisely indicate the specific delineations necessary*

to make the predictive principle valid and relevant. This is the final step in constructing a single principle. The choice of articles, adjectives, adverbs, and other parts of speech that set its limits is important because qualifiers affect the predictive principle's validity and clarity and may be necessary to make the predictive principle a complete sentence. A predictive principle using the selected components complete with qualifiers could read as follows:

Carefully predetermined **design and sequence** for change **promote** work that is **purpose focused** and **progress** that proceeds as rapidly as possible.

Derivation of a predictive principle from a single authoritative source

The writer of predictive principles may find a paragraph in an authoritative source clearly stating a predictive principle within the text itself. The formulator will find it expedient to identify the parts of the predictive principle and extract it directly from the literature. Such a paragraph is quoted here, and the components of the predictive principle are identified within the text.

Attaching the label of evolutionary to change might be viewed by some as an opportunity to forestall any real innovation or as an excuse for lack of progress. To the contrary, although the suggested pace is less rapid, *evolutionary change requires a carefully predetermined* **design with definite sequence,** *pace and substance. These considerations are necessary to* **insure** *that* **purpose** *is always centrally* **focused** *and* **progress accomplished** *with all deliberate haste.**

In this quotation the concept of the CCB triad stands out clearly as "**design with definite sequence.**" The predicted outcome appears within the text as "**purpose . . . focused and progress accomplished.**" The critical principle formulator will find "**insure**" unacceptable as a valid active verb and will substitute a more realistic one such as *promote.* The result is a predictive principle derived directly from an authoritative source. It will read as follows:

A carefully predetermined design and sequence for change promotes work that is purpose focused and progress that proceeds with deliberate haste.

Common errors in formation of predictive principles

Blunders or errors in predictive principle formation have some similarity to principles and are often confused with predictive principles. Discriminating between predictive principles and nonprinciples is often difficult. Familiarity with common errors in formation of predictive principles can prevent miscon-

---

*From Beggs, D.W.: Team teaching, Indianapolis, 1964, Unified College Press, Inc. (Italics and boldface added.)

ceptions, reinforce valid examples, and help the beginner avoid errors. Most common errors in principle formation take the form of directions, descriptions, statements of fact, or pseudoprinciples. Examples of common errors in principle construction using the predictive principle stated previously are listed below.

Directions. Directions either state how to do something step by step or contain the words *should* or *ought to*. These are actually level IV situation-producing theories.

The effective leader should do the following:

1. Gather data pertinent to the current situation
2. Decide which data are applicable
3. Use data to make decisions

Descriptions. Descriptions state how a person behaves or what an activity is like. Descriptions often take the form of characteristics; there is no *active* verb.

A good leader will always have knowledge pertinent to the current situation on which to base decisions and judgment.

Facts or valid statements. Facts or valid statements are usually about the circumstances, conditions, or behaviors, or about the predicted outcome; however, they do not show relationship.

Knowledge is of use only if it is pertinent to the current problem.

Weak predictive principles take the form of principles in that they have a CCB triad connected to a predicted outcome; however, the active verb lacks the quality of certainty. Such words as *apparently, might, may,* and *perhaps* make the predictive principle so weak that it is almost useless as an action base.

Leaders who have knowledge pertinent to the current situation might make valid judgments and decisions.

Invalid principles. Invalidity is the most common form of error. Predictions that use erroneous material or fail to use modifiers appropriately are often invalid.

Index